# Manipulation Under Anesthesia
## Concepts in Theory and Application

Edited by
### Robert C. Gordon, D.C., DAAPM
Cornerstone Professional Education, Inc.

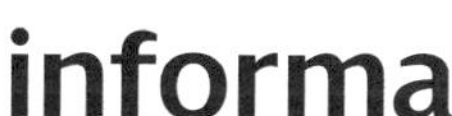

informa
healthcare

New York  London

Informa Healthcare USA, Inc.
52 Vanderbilt Avenue
New York, NY 10017



International Standard Book Number-10: 0-8493-1700-2 (Hardcover)
International Standard Book Number-13: 978-0-8493-1700-2 (Hardcover)



**Library of Congress Cataloging-in-Publication Data**

Manipulation under anesthesia
    edited  by Robert C. Gordon.
       p. ; cm.
    Includes bibliographical references and index.
    ISBN-13: 978-0-8493-1700-2 (hardcover : alk. paper)
    ISBN-10: 0-8493-1700-2 (hardcover : alk. paper)
    1. Manipulation (Therapeutics).
    2. Anesthesia.
I. Gordon, Robert C.

RM724.M345  2004
615.5'3--dc22                                                                                 2004054511

# *Dedication*

---

*I dedicate this textbook to the love of my life, my partner, and my best friend, my wife Yvonne.  Yvonne has been with me since we were high school sweethearts, and today after years of ups and downs, good times and bad times, she still remains the mainstay in my life.  I could not fathom completing a work of this magnitude without having her by my side.  She has been my confidant, my editor, my comrade, and my partner in this effort, and if my name is on the book as the editor, her name will always be the core of my inspiration.*

# Preface

Manipulation in various forms has been performed for hundreds of years. Adjustive procedures specific to chiropractic and osteopathic practitioners have been used and practiced for more than 100 years. From the time these procedures were first used, they carried with them an aura of both allure and mystique. Scientific validation was not a prominent focus by many of the early practitioners, and techniques were passed on from one practitioner to another. The use of these manual techniques provided positive results for patients, and practitioners were not concerned with using controlled studies to prove the results. Some have referred to this as a period of anecdotal results — "Stories of improvement with no actual proof." Sadly this was the way manual practitioners approached their techniques and how they looked at the concerns of the scientific community. Today, as more research is conducted, and as more knowledge of manual therapy becomes available, the scientific community is starting to recognize that those practitioners who were scorned and scoffed at for so many years really did have something to offer.

Even so, we still see educated men and women using pragmatic discourse in their denial of the thousands of cases that have been and are daily being positively affected by the use of manual therapy.

## ADVANCED MANUAL THERAPY

With the advent of more research and more specific types of manual therapy, a technique that has been used for more than 70 years by osteopathic, orthopedic, and chiropractic practitioners is being revisited with regularity. This technique is using manual/manipulative therapy while the patient is under the influence of anesthesia or, to use a more updated vernacular, medication-assisted manipulation. Today this technique is referred to as the fibrosis release procedure using medication-assisted manipulation under IV sedation.

This text is written at a time when manipulation under anesthesia (MUA) is controversial but being practiced with regularity. Third-party payors believed that if they labeled it as experimental, it would go away, even though there are some 70 years of documented proof of its efficacy.

Our greatest challenge today is to prove the efficacy of MUA beyond all reasonable doubt. Our challenges will still be present, but the argument of being experimental will not survive the scrutiny of the scientific community because there will no longer be a platform for unrealistic dialogue.

MUA has indeed been a part of the growth of our health care delivery system. It is part of our heritage now, and it is up to those who wish to study its effectiveness to continue to develop more research into its clinical validity. It is our hope that the material contained in this text will help start your discovery of this wonderful form of therapy. We also hope that it will instill in you a desire to continue your study so that future practitioners will have the benefit of your study to perpetuate the procedure known as manipulation under anesthesia.

This book focuses on all of the aspects of the MUA technique. It presents the scientific basis of the procedure; provides information on patient selection criteria; documents outcomes from patient procedures; and examines policies, protocols, and standards by which the procedure should be incorporated in treatment facilities. It also provides step-by-step guidelines of the generic procedure and policies for documenting results; addresses the "pain management" aspect of MUA; and discusses the overall use of the procedure from pre-MUA through post-MUA rehabilitation. It is my hope that this book will provide the tools needed to investigate this procedure so that it can become an acceptable addition to mainstream health care delivery.

# Acknowledgments

The book that you are about to read has been in the works for the past 4 years and in the mind of the MUA practitioner for the past 70 years. My father used to say that "there is no limit to the good a man can do if he doesn't care who gets the credit."

The men and women who have put their hearts and souls into making MUA the technique that it is today and what it will become in the future is why this book is being written. I have had the privilege of meeting some wonderful people in the field of manipulation under anesthesia. To say the least, they are some of the hardest working people that I can ever remember meeting in my lifetime. To make this book work, I had to have the advice, understanding, caring, concern, and love of many people. This book is a culmination of 15 years of my life dedicated to the MUA field, and it is a tribute to the many folks who have been a part of those years by helping to make MUA what it is today.

Of special acknowledgment are my contributing authors. It is through their hard, tireless, and sometimes frustrating efforts that we have this complete written work that I envisioned so many years ago which would support the doctors who are involved in and who perform MUA every day in the course of their practices. I'd like to thank all of the people who in last minute desperation helped complete sections of this text. Drs. Ed Cremata and Sarb Dhesi from California worked diligently every day for the rights of the practitioner to continue to use this wonderful technique and helped with pictures and comments in the formation of several sections of the book. The National University of Health Sciences stayed with me and has sponsored my course since 1994; I thank them for their support and confidence in this procedure. Drs. Bill Waln, Dana Lawrence, and Jonathan Soltz, the postgraduate deans at National, have played a great part in helping me to grant MUA certification to doctors over the years. I'd like to thank the Forest Surgery Center in Paramus, NJ, for allowing me to take the procedure pictures in their operative suite. A special thank you is in order to the doctors who took the time to help me show the proper techniques for this procedure in picture form, Dr. Don Alosio and Dr. Anthony Riotto. Many people have been responsible for making this book a reality, but three people had an initial vision that my syllabus used in teaching the course could become a book: my wife, who is my partner, and Dan Hovland and Chris Sepulveda from Shark Creative, who through the years have helped me with a great deal of the media production that I have made available in my course for this procedure. Finally I'd like to thank Barbara Norwitz and Erica Dery from CRC Press, who saw potential in a syllabus used in a class setting that would become the book that you are going to read. It takes special people to see the vision of a completed book, and although I have resisted them in many phases of the completion of this text, it is their hard work and dedication to this material that made this come together.

# Editor

**Robert C. Gordon, DC, FRCCM, ABCS, DAAPM**, is a postgraduate faculty member of the National University of Health Sciences. He holds active licenses to practice chiropractic in Florida and New Jersey. Dr. Gordon earned his undergraduate degrees from Florida State University in physical education, recreational science, and sports medicine and was involved in the masters program in exercise physiology.

Since graduating from the National College of Chiropractic in 1975, Dr. Gordon has specialized in the fields of sports medicine and industrial chiropractic, and it is within these fields that he pursued his early interest and training at the Texas College of Chiropractic in the science of manipulation under anesthesia (MUA). Most of the early research for his work in MUA was completed at the Southeastern University of Health Sciences (which is now Nova Southeastern University), an osteopathic college in South Florida.

Dr. Gordon has been actively teaching and researching MUA since 1992 and has been involved in compiling information on the subject since 1985. His interest in the industrial field led him to receive his training as an authorized trainer for the Occupational Safety and Health Administration (OSHA) in 2001, and it is in the sports medicine and industrial fields that Dr. Gordon has used the MUA procedure to bring recovery to many injured employees and athletes over the years. Dr. Gordon holds many awards from his years in the chiropractic field, including Chiropractor of the Year from the Broward Chiropractic Society and the KUDO award from the Florida Chiropractic Association for his work as the state chairman for scoliosis.

Dr. Gordon is the executive director of the National Academy of MUA Physicians and is an active member of the American Academy of Pain Management. He was an active member of the American Chiropractic Association for many years, as well as an active member of the Florida Chiropractic Association, and he held many offices in the Broward County Chiropractic Society, including president. He is currently active with the North Carolina Chiropractic Association as an associate member and lectures on manipulation under anesthesia regularly for many organizations and universities, including the American Academy of Pain Management. He is a consultant for the MUA procedure for many hospitals and ambulatory surgical centers throughout the U.S. and has taught more than 1600 doctors of chiropractic and osteopathy.

Dr. Gordon was recently inducted into the Royal College of Physicians and Surgeons (U.S.) and is vice chairman of the newly formed Royal College of Chiropractic Medicine (FRCCM) of the United States. Dr. Gordon will also assume the position of Professor of Chiropractic Medicine at the American International University. Through the Royal College of Chiropractic Medicine, the American Board of Chiropractic Specialists (ABCS) has been formed, which recognizes board certification in MUA, neurobiomechanics, and hospital emergency room procedures.

# Contributors

**David Basch, MD**
Fellow, American Board of Orthopedic
  Surgeons
Diplomate, American Board of Orthopedics
Sparta, New Jersey

**Ramona Carter, MD**
Department of Family Medicine
University of Texas Medical Branch at
  Galveston
Galveston, Texas

**Robert S. Francis, DC, PhD**
Associate Professor
Course Director Postgraduate Studies
Texas Chiropractic College
Pasadena, Texas

**James Giordano, PhD**
Director of Clinical Research
Professor of Pathology
Texas Chiropractic College
Pasadena, Texas

**Timothy S. Kersch, DC**
Vista, California

**Robert Mathews, MD, PhD, FACS, FICS,
FRCS (US)**
Pain Intervention, American International
  University
Royal College of Physicians and Surgeons (US)
Fellow, American College of Surgeons
Fellow, American International College of
  Surgeons
American Academy of Orthopedic Surgeons
Lancaster, Pennsylvania

**Matt Miller, PA-C**
Lancaster, Pennsylvania

**Anthony B. Morovati, DC**
Glendale, California

**Lawrence Petracco, DC**
Jersey City, New Jersey

**Anthony Rogers, MD**
Fellow, American Board of Anesthesia
Fellow, American Board of Pain Medicine
Lake Worth, Florida

**B. H. Rubin, DC, DABCO**
Hampton, Virginia

**Fred E. Russo, DC**
Tallahassee, Florida

**Thomas Schultea, PhD**
Professor of Pathology
Texas Chiropractic College
Pasadena, Texas

**Dan West, DC**
East Earl, Pennsylvania

# Contents

# *PART II*

# Part I

# 1 An Historical Perspective on Manipulation Under Anesthesia

*Robert S. Francis*

## CONTENTS



## INTRODUCTION

In the past, if patients were not responding to standard conservative manual/manipulative care, whether manually or in combination with physiotherapy, but were candidates for more extensive physical medicine and/or manipulations, they were referred out for orthopedic or neurological followup. Regretting that transfer as a failure, but without much, if any, recourse, we aligned ourselves with practitioners who would recognize the value of manipulative care, but were able to offer pharmacological intervention or other invasive techniques as an adjunct to what we were not able to provide the patient.

The patient who was a candidate for adjustments/manipulation was either constantly in too much pain, or had a difficult time being adjusted due to muscle contracture and/or articular fixations no matter what procedures were used.

With the introduction of manipulation under anesthesia (MUA) into their practices, certified manual therapy professionals are now able to take those same patients, who once had to be referred out for medical intervention and borderline surgery, and perform MUA with remarkable success. This chapter is written by one of the first practitioners in the chiropractic profession to bring this technique back to the forefront. He is a leading authority in the field of MUA and has been a friend and colleague of mine over the years. Robert Francis has been a continuous contributor to the field as we try to bring this procedure into mainstream manual therapy.

## MANIPULATION UNDER ANESTHESIA: HISTORICAL CONSIDERATIONS

Manual medicine, or therapeutic application of the hands in patient care, is as old as medicine itself. It is found in ancient civilizations and in modern times throughout the world. As early as 6000 years ago in ancient India and by 5000 years ago in the eastern Mediterranean, spinal manipulative therapy was utilized in the treatment of various conditions. Appearing simultaneously

---

* Introduction by Robert C. Gordon.

in Mesopotamia and Egypt, the origins of Western medicine were forged by an early class of physician. Ancient Indian and Chinese texts include spinal manipulative therapy for the improvement of posture, locomotion, paralysis, and various disease states. As the art of medicine evolved, so too did the theoretical basis for manipulative interventions. It is in Greece that medicine was first documented to have become committed to scientific objectivity and where we find definite confirmation of the practice of spinal manipulation. Hippocrates, in his book *On Joints*, first described techniques of spinal manipulation to treat curvature of the spine and misalignment of the vertebrae.

The influence of Hippocrates was vast and persisted for more than 2000 years. His teachings spread back to the East, where manipulation had its origins and where during the Middle Ages manipulation was championed by the influential physicians of the time. At the same time, manipulation spread to the West, where the influence was seen with a myriad imminent physicians such as Ambroise Paré, Friar Thomas Moulton (who published *The Compleat Bone-Setter*) and Johannis Scultetus (who describes Hippocratic methods of manipulation in his *The Surgeons Store-House*).

In the mid-19th century, James Paget, one of the most famous surgeons of his time, reported in the *Lancet* that doctors would do well to observe bone-setters and learn from them.

During the late 19th century, Daniel David Palmer founded chiropractic and Andrew Taylor Still founded osteopathy. Both disciplines give emphasis to the treatment of musculoskeletal lesions and organic diseases through spinal manipulative therapy. These two eclectic healers fathered the two disciplines most comprehensive of spinal manipulative therapy, chiropractic and osteopathy, both establishing academic institutions and professions that continue today, with emphasis on spinal manipulative therapy being more prominent in the chiropractic curriculum.

In the past century increasing interest throughout the orthodox health care delivery system has brought about many interprofessional associations and organizations toward an effort to establish scientific principles and clinical applications of manual medicine.

Manual treatment of spinal disorders is perhaps the best-studied remedy for spine-related disorders. Clinical description and controlled studies provide advances in scientific knowledge about manual treatment methods and the disorders to which they are directed. The common factor for all manual methods is that they apply an external load to the spine and its surrounding tissues. Merging of the efforts by basic scientists, engineers, and clinical-scientists has resolved some of the underlying scientific ambiguity surrounding these issues. Specifically decisive efforts in biomechanics have emerged to describe and understand their treatment, the spinal disorder for which it is used, and the physiological effects of treatment.

Manual treatment of spinal disorders is performed under a variety of descriptions and nomenclature, including massage, mobilization, stretching, muscle "energy" techniques, adjustment, and manipulation.

Spinal manipulation is the remedy for spine-related disorders that has received the most scientific attention using controlled and cohort studies.

Alliance, coalition, and association of the chiropractic physician with basic scientists and engineers have provided opportunities to explore fundamental questions, the answers to which have provided further theoretical basis and clinical efforts to study the nature of the manipulative lesion, define and optimize effects of treatment, and set criteria for training.

MUA developed in the early part of the 20th century as a specialized manipulative procedure that was a natural progression of therapeutically credible spinal manipulative therapy. Spinal manipulative therapy gained recognition during the 1980s by mainstream medicine with supporters such as James Cyriax, MD; John M. Mennell, MD; Scott Haldeman, DC, PhD, MD, and, recently, many other physicians who hold academic and clinical appointments at medical and chiropractic colleges and with multidisciplinary research and professional organizations supporting spinal manipulative therapy. The National Institutes of Health has provided educational research grants to medical schools across the United States specifically designed to incorporate complementary and alternative medicine (CAM) into medical school curricula. This author is a member of the Core Curriculum Committee at the University of Texas Medical Branch Department of Family

Medicine, charged with the design and development of medical school curricula that meet the objectives of NIH educational grants regarding CAM curricula.

While Dean of Clinical Sciences and serving as Director of Hospital Rotations at Texas Chiropractic College, the author developed the first program designed to integrate chiropractic students into the medical community through hospital and private medical service rotations in the disciplines of orthopedic surgery, neurosurgery, internal medicine, family medicine, pain management, anesthesiology, and radiology. This interaction of chiropractic interns, chiropractors, and medical physicians effectively bridged the historical chasm of communication that has existed between the different health care communities.

As a result of this increased communication between the medical and chiropractic communities, chiropractors were offered hospital privileges and began to co-manage patients with medical physicians. This author was initially proctored by board-certified orthopedic surgeons in MUA and subsequently developed the first certification course in MUA for chiropractors in the mid-1980s while Dean of Clinical Sciences at Texas Chiropractic College. Subsequent to the first academic program at Texas Chiropractic College, other colleges followed suit, making MUA training programs available to chiropractors across the country.

The ensuing years saw a variety of educational programs and standards for MUA taught by proprietary organizations not affiliated with Council on Chiropractic Education (CCE)—-accredited institutions.

Specific standards and protocol for the MUA procedures have been developed by academic institutions and national and international organizations. This development is an effort to recognize training programs and clinical outcomes that establish a safe and effective means of implementing this procedure across the country in appropriate hospital and ambulatory surgical settings. The first national organization, the National Academy of MUA Physicians, was developed in 1995 in an effort to solidify national standards and protocol for MUA. Most recently, the multidisciplinary European MUA community organized the International MUA Academy of Physicians to provide an avenue for the dissemination of a valid and authoritative database of current research and new scientific developments in the field of MUA for physicians dealing with chronic difficult cases. It is through efforts to develop evidence-based principles for MUA clinical application and practice that these organizations have promulgated effective and consistent standards and protocols for MUA.

These organizations make available to the practicing MUA community of physicians continuing education, national, and international conferences designed to accomplish, implement, fulfill, and discharge the purpose and intent of this mission. The objectives of these continuing education conferences are to present by an authoritative and interdisciplinary faculty a state-of-the-art review of the present knowledge in the field of nonoperative care; interventional, diagnostic, and therapeutic procedures; and other relevant treatment modalities affecting the spine.

MUA has been utilized in manual medicine for over 70 years. Increased participation of chiropractors on hospital medical staffs and with medical physicians has made both the facilities and the training more available for performing and credentialing this procedure.

Multiple prospective and retrospective clinical studies have been performed evaluating MUA in chronic unresolved back pain, acute and chronic disc herniations, cervicogenic cephalgia, and many other neuromusculoskeletal conditions with attendant articular dyskinesia. Robert Mensor,[6] orthopedic surgeon, compared the outcomes of MUA and laminectomy in patients with lumbar intervertbral disc lesions and found that 83% of MUA patients had good to excellent results while only 51% of the surgical patients reported the same outcome.

Donald Chrisman,[1] orthopedic surgeon, reported that 51% of patients with unequivocal disc lesions and unrelieved symptoms after conservative care had been rendered reported good to excellent results post-MUA at 3 years' followup.

Siehl[2] reported on 723 MUA patients, the largest clinical trial conducted on MUA procedures. They found that 71% had good results, 25% had fair results, and 4% ultimately required surgical intervention.

Krumhansl and Nowacek[5] reported on 171 patients who experienced constant intractable pain, from several months to 18 years' duration, and who underwent MUA. All of the patients had failed at previous conservative interventions. Results reported that, post-MUA, 25% had no pain at all and were "cured"; 50% were "much improved," with pain markedly reduced and activities of daily living (ADLs) essentially unaffected; 20% were "better" but pain continued to interfere with activities; and, finally, 5% had minimal or no relief.

West et al.[10] reported on a study of 177 patients, in which 68.6% of the patients who were out of work were able to return to unrestricted work activities after a series of three consecutive MUA procedures at 6 months post-MUA; 58.4% of the MUA patients receiving medication prior to the procedure required no prescription medication post-procedure; and 60.1% of patients with lumbar pain had the pain resolved after a series of MUA procedures.

Palmieri et al.[7] demonstrated the clinical efficacy of MUA performed in a series of three consecutive procedures. The average Numeric Pain Scale scores in the MUA group decreased by 50%, and the average Roland-Morris Questionnaire scores decreased by 51% compared to the control group.

Samuel Turek (1984), orthopedic surgeon, reported in his textbook, *Orthopedics: Principles and Their Application*, that "good to excellent results" can be expected with lumbar herniated nucleus pulposus with manipulation under anesthesia.

Kohlbeck and Haldeman[3] reported that, although much of the literature in the 70 years that MUA has been in use relates to clinical observation and is considered somewhat anecdotal, there is sufficient evidence to warrant further controlled trials.

Kohlbeck et al.[4] reported that medication-assisted manipulation appears to offer some patients increased improvement in low back pain and disability when compared to usual chiropractic care. Further investigation of these apparent benefits in randomized clinical trial is warranted.

In addition to the extant literature, there are currently ongoing prospective clinical trials with appropriate outcome instruments assessing the clinical and fiscal efficacies of MUA in a selected patient population.

The medical literature is replete with case studies and literature reviews on MUA, in addition to clinical trials, all of which report positive clinical outcomes. Further research is ongoing. It is important to note that to date there has been no clinical trial that demonstrates MUA to be ineffective in an appropriately selected patient population.

Toward an effort to satisfy all disciplines, I offer here a definition for manipulation that may be universally accepted by all disciplines. Manipulation consists of accurately determined and specifically directed manual forces to areas of restriction, whether the restriction is in ligaments, muscles, or joints, the result of which may be improvement in posture and locomotion, improvement in function elsewhere in the body, and the enhancement of the sense of well-being.

Chiropractors constitute the group of physicians who most actively practice MUA. This author has trained and certified MDs, DOs, and DCs in the United States and in Europe. Although, in Europe, MDs and DCs actively practice spinal manipulative therapy, it nevertheless remains largely the clinical domain of the chiropractor.

Currently MUA certification courses offered through accredited chiropractic college postgraduate departments are recognized by malpractice carriers for inclusive coverage. It has been important to regulatory agencies, academic institutions, professional associations, and organizations and malpractice carriers to recognize appropriate training programs. Toward that end, specific criteria have been adopted to establish credible certification course offerings. Standards and protocols establishing credible MUA certification training programs are recognized by the National Academy of MUA Physicians and the International Academy of MUA Physicians and are subscribed to by the accredited academic institutions offering postgraduate certification in MUA.

## REFERENCES


1. Chrisman, O.D., et al. A study of the results following rotary manipulation of the lumbar intervertebral disc syndrome. *J. Bone Joint Surg.* 1964: 46-A, 517.
2. Siehl, D. Manipulation of the spine under general anesthesia. *J. Am. Osteopathic Assoc.* 1963: 62, 881.
3. Kohlbeck, F., Haldeman, S. Technical assessment: Medication assisted spinal manipulation. *Spine J.* 2002 (July/Aug.): 2.
4. Kohlbeck, F., et al. Medication-assisted manipulation for low back pain. Paper presented at the World Federation of Chiropractic, Biennial Congress, May 2003.
5. Krumhansl, B.R., Nowacek, C.J. Manipulation under anesthesia. *Modern Manual Ther.* 1988: 777–786.
6. Mensor, R. Non-operative treatment, including manipulation for lumbar intervertebral disc syndrome. *J. Bone Joint Surg.* 1955: 5, 925–936.
7. Palmieri, N., et al. Chronic low back pain: A study of the effects of manipulation under anesthesia. *JMPT* 2002: 25(8).
8. Siehl, D., Bradford, W.G. Manipulation of the low back under general anesthesia. *J. Am. Osteopathic Assoc.* 1952: 52, 239–241.
9. Turek, S L. *Orthopaedics: Principles and Their Application*, 3rd ed. J.B. Lippencott, Philadelphia, 1984: 1495.
10. West, D., et al. Effective management of spinal pain in one hundred seventy-seven patients evaluated for manipulation under anesthesia. *JMPT* 1999: 22(5), 299–308.

# 2 The Scientific Basis of Manipulation Under Anesthesia

*Robert C. Gordon, Robert S. Francis, and Anthony B. Morovati*

## CONTENTS

# Basic Spinal Anatomy in Relation to MUA

*Robert C. Gordon*

The motion unit is made up of two segments of the vertebral column as they articulate with each other. One motion unit is regarded as extending from the midportion of the body of one unit to the midportion of the body of the unit below. Figure 2.1 illustrates this concept.[1–3]

## FUNCTIONS OF THE MOTION UNIT

In the cervical spine, the motion units are the most flexible and movable but, in turn, are the most unstable.[4,5] The cervical spine is both a static structural support and a mobile kinetic mechanism.[4–6] The motion units in the spine are basically alike in relation to the structural function. There is a size difference in the bodies and a posterior element difference, but motion units consist of two vertebral segments and depend on the integrity of their articulations as protection for the spinal cord and segmental element confluence. Two exceptions to the rule are the occipital–atlanto articular relationship and the atlas–axial relationship. These vertebrae are shaped differently and have considerably different functions than any other vertebrae in the spine.[4–6] Specifically, they are shaped for, and function for, the infinitely complex movements of the head and upper cervical spine.[4–7]

The anterior portions of the vertebral motion units are the bodies of the vertebrae that make up the supporting portion of the motion unit. The upper two vertebrae are different in that they are

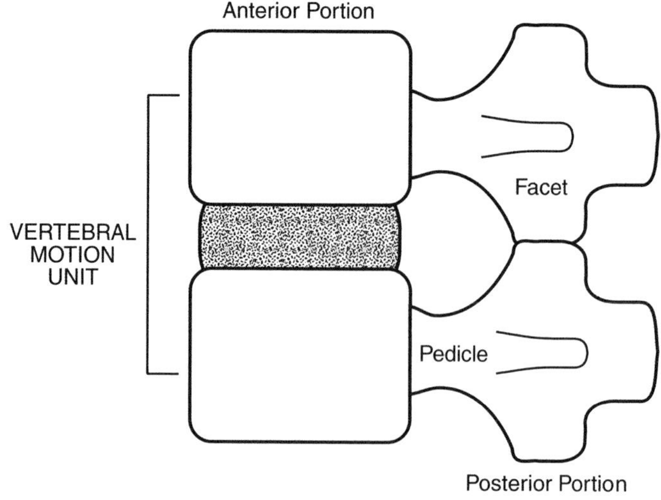


**FIGURE 2.1**  Basic vertebral motor unit.

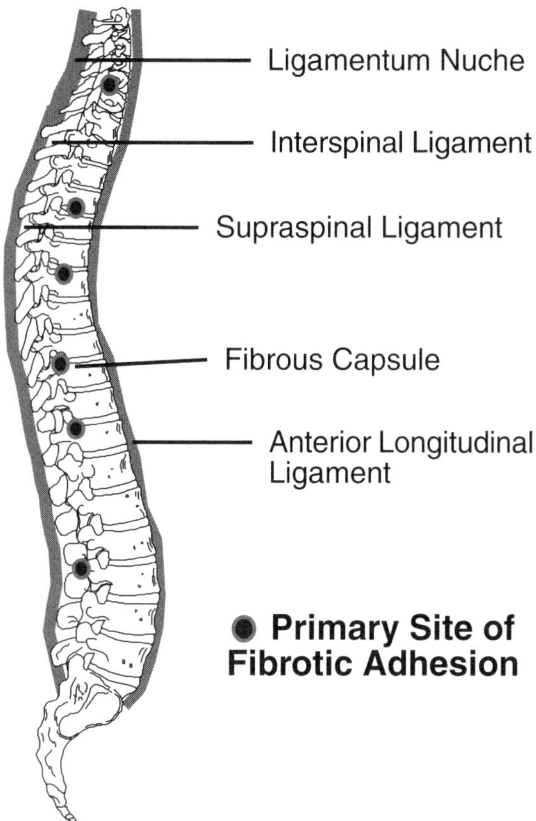


**FIGURE 2.2** Predominant sites of the spine for adhesion formation.

shaped for specific movement and do not have bodies, but instead serve as support for the skull and for gliding/guiding of the head on the cervical spine.[4]

The posterior portions of the motion units are true joints, called *facets*, which are lined with synovia and lubricated by synovial fluid within the joint capsule. Again, the upper two cervical vertebrae have different functions and so are different in biomechanical architecture. Movement of the *cervical spine* is basically confined to five vertebrae since the atlas functions principally with the occiput and the seventh cervical vertebra functions as a thoracic vertebra.[4,6]

The *thoracic spine* comprises the middle of the spinal column and is responsible for rotation and rib articulation. The motion units are basically the same but take on a slightly different shape than the cervical and lumbar spine in order to accommodate the biomechanical dynamics of the thoracic area of the spine. The articulations in the thoracic spine comprise both the posterior motion unit articulation and the rib articulation as well as the anterior disc area, which gives the thoracic motion unit the ability to function through rotation and creates biokinetic support for rib movement.[7-9] Lateral bending is not part of the function of the thoracic spine but instead comes from the relationship of the articulation in the lumbar spine. (See Figure 2.2.)[4,7]

In the *lumbar spine*, the vertebral motion units are the largest, with the articular facets shaped to accommodate lateral bending, a small portion of the rotational dynamics such as when lateral bending occurs, and flexion and extension of the spinal column. The posterior articulations change as the motion units progress from the upper lumbar vertebrae to the lower lumbar vertebrae. As they do, they allow for the motion required in that specific area of the spine.[1,3,7]

## THE FACET ARTICULATION AS IT PERTAINS TO MUA

The concern for the facet articulation with regard to the MUA procedure is fairly obvious. Since the facet articulations are one of the primary articular sites in the vertebrae column, it is the facet articulation that will be a primary site of the articular fibro-adhesion formation. It is definitely possible to form adhesions in the surrounding tissues of the articular joint capsules, but it will become evident as the MUA procedure is learned that reestablishing the integrity of the joint is a very important part of what is being accomplished.

If the facet articulations are misaligned or imbrication develops, the microtrauma or macrotrauma that causes the biomechanical aberration will cause an inflammatory reaction (which is discussed in the next section). As is shown in the breakdown from the vertebral column to the facet articulation, the base of the articulation is a primary site of adhesion formation.[10] The facet joint is typically a synovial joint containing synovial fluid, which certainly can become inflamed as the joint is moved out of alignment. The articular surfaces are hyaline cartilage and as such are significant areas of joint deterioration with resultant inflammatory reaction. The capsules of the facet articulation are usually thick and fibrous, and cover the dorsum of the joint. The ventral aspect of the capsule is made up of an extension of the ligamentum flavum. These are definitely sites of compromise should the facet misalign or imbricate, which can also cause a resultant painful stimulus. The inflammatory reaction is the precursor to adhesion formation, which is a protective mechanism that the body goes through as described in the next section. (See Figure 2.3.)

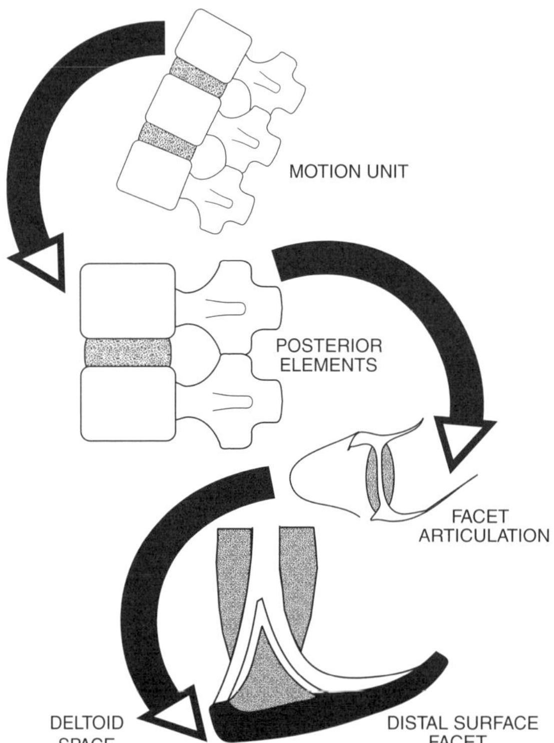


**FIGURE 2.3** Schematic representing spine–motor unit facet and distal end, called the deltoid space, where adhesions form.

## REFERENCES

1. Cailliet, R. *Low Back Pain Syndrome*, 2nd ed. F.A. Davis Co., Philadelphia, 1968: 3.
2. Cossette, J.W., Farfan, H.F., Robertson, G.H., Wells, R.V. The instantaneous center of rotation of the third lumbar intervertebral joint, *J. Biomechan.* 1971:4, 149–53.
3. Cox, J.M. *Low Back Pain, Mechanism, Diagnosis and Treatment*, 5th ed. Williams & Wilkins, Baltimore, 1985: 139–56, 257–90, 467–72.
4. Cailliet, R. *Neck and Arm Pain.* F.A. Davis Co., Philadelphia, 5th printing, 1972.
5. Foreman, S.M., Croft, A.C. *Whiplash Injuries, the Cervical Acceleration Deceleration Syndrome.* Williams & Wilkins, Baltimore, 1988: 1–72.
6. Jackson, R. *The Cervical Syndrome*, 4th ed. Charles Thomas, Pub., Springfield, IL, 1978: 5–60.
7. Gray, H. *Anatomy.* Running Press, Philadelphia, 1974: 224, 1086–96.
8. Kotlke, F.J. Therapeutic exercise to maintain mobility. In *Handbook of Physical Medicine and Rehabilitation*, Kotlke, F.J., Lehman, F. (eds.). W.B. Saunders, Philadelphia, 1971: 389–401.
9. McMahon, T.A. *Muscles, Reflexes, and Locomotor.* Princeton University Press, Princeton, NJ, 1984: 12–13, 72–74, 143–52.
10. Kirkaldy-Willis, W.H. *Managing Low Back Pain*, 2nd ed. Churchill-Livingstone, New York, 1988: 29–48, 49–75, 77–81, 287–96.

# Manipulation Under Anesthesia: Pathomechanics

*Robert S. Francis*

This section develops an overview for a spinal manipulative model that identifies the manipulative lesion for which MUA is most effective: the treatment of pathomechanics of the spine. This discussion conveys the role of the various factors comprising this model, which include the three-joint complex (intervertebral disc and two posterior motor units), resting length of musculature, articular neurology, the pressure hierarchy of the intervertebral foramen, and the role of synovial production and cavitation. These factors play an important role in moderating the source of back pain by restoring, improving, and maintaining mechanical integrity.

It has been well documented in the medical literature that chronic unresolved musculoskeletal conditions respond well to MUA. MUA is a procedure designed to restore the lost range of motion, flexibility, and viscoelasticity of the spine and extremities and to reduce scar tissue in soft tissues, peri- and intra-articular structures that results in articular dyskinesia. The restoration of motion and the reduction of scar tissue result in more flexibility and viscoelasticity of the paraspinal musculature and associated articulations, thereby increasing the functional capacity of the patient.

MUA is a procedure utilized in a selected patient population that has been recalcitrant to an adequate trial of conservative care in the office setting. MUA requires the use of nonparalyzing anesthesia (patients continue to breathe on their own during the procedure) toward an effort to provide relaxed skeletal musculature, enabling the manipulator to reduce fibroblastic proliferative tissue and restore articular motion without patient guarding and pain. Generally, pre-op medications include Versed and Fentanyl with Propofol used in the operating room without intubation to accomplish flaccid muscular relaxation. This is an outpatient procedure and is performed in an appropriate setting, making available access to monitoring and resuscitation equipment in a facility certified or licensed to offer a safe operative environment that can provide transfer capability to inpatient care.

Spinal manipulative therapy is designed to restore biomechanical integrity to areas of articular dyskinesia due to pathomechanical factors, including loss of joint mobility, fibroblastic proliferative

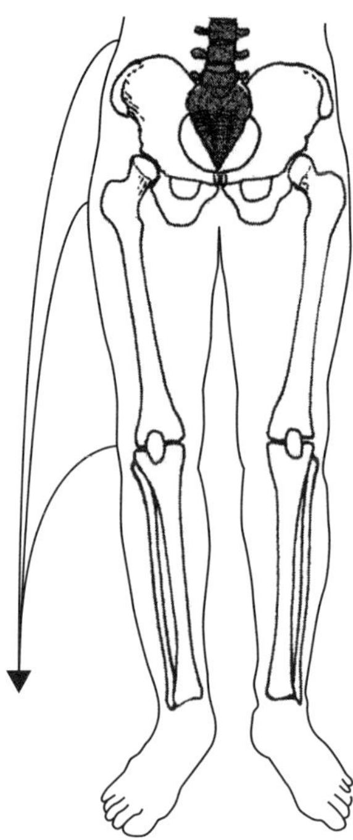

**FIGURE 2.4** Somatic pain stems directly from musculoskeletal structures of the lumbar spine.

changes of the supporting soft tissues resulting in decreased or lost flexibility/viscoelasticity, and neurological and vascular changes resulting from articular dyskinesia.

## THE SOURCE OF BACK PAIN

Not all back pain is necessarily due to disorders of the spine. Lumbar pain can be due to visceral or vascular disease in the abdomen or pelvis. Therefore, the assessment of lumbar pain must include an assessment of these possibilities. It is not within the scope of this text to address a review of systems other than the pathomechanical systems that become the treatment objective of the MUA procedure.

There are two types of pain based on physiological considerations: somatic and radicular. (See Figure 2.4.) Somatic pain stems directly from musculoskeletal structures of the lumbar spine. Radicular pain is caused by a disorder of the spinal nerves or the spinal nerve roots.

Any structure that has a nerve supply is potentially a source of pain. The structures in the lumbar spine that receive a nerve supply include the zygapophyseal joints, the ligaments of the posterior elements, the paravertebral muscles, the dura mater, the anterior and posterior longitudinal ligaments, and the intervertebral discs.

Kellgren demonstrated that low back pain could be induced by stimulation of the lumbar back muscles and interspinous ligaments. Steindler and Luck showed that certain forms of low back pain could be relieved, at least temporarily, by anesthetizing these same structures. It has been experimentally shown that stimulation of lumbar zygapophyseal joints could cause low back pain in normal volunteers and that back pain stemming from these joints could be relieved by fluoroscopically controlled blocks of their nerve supply. It has also been demonstrated experimentally with provocation discography that intervertebral discs can be a source of pain. The dura mater has also been shown to be able to cause back pain, with experiments demonstrating the dura mater/back pain relationship. Back pain was evoked by traction on the dural sleeves of lumbar nerves by pulling

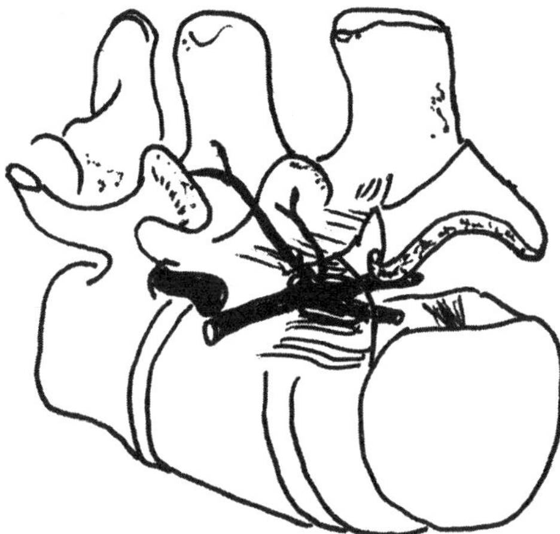

**FIGURE 2.5** Each joint receives multiple innervations from a dorsal ramus and two medial branches.

on sutures threaded through the dura at operation for laminectomy and, in another experiment, chemical irritation of the dura, in the form of injections of hypertonic saline, evoked back pain. All innervated structures of the back except the blood vessels have been shown experimentally to be capable of producing back pain. However, distension of epidural veins is thought to cause pain.

## ARTICULAR NEUROLOGY

The lumbar spine is used as a model to illustrate these mechanisms. It is the medial branch of the dorsal primary ramus that is of paramount clinical relevance due to its distribution to the zygapophyseal joints. The medial branches of the dorsal rami run across the top of their respective transverse processes and pierce the dorsal layers of the intertransverse ligament at the base of the transverse process. Each medial branch supplies the zygapophyseal joint above and below its course. Each zygapophyseal joint receives an additional innervation ventrally, from the dorsal ramus in front of the joint. Each joint therefore receives a multiple innervation: from a dorsal ramus and two medial branches. (See Figure 2.5.)

To achieve reduction in symptoms and decrease in pain, manipulation is utilized to recruit the neurological mechanism of collateral inhibition. Collateral inhibition is that part of the arthrokinetic reflex that inhibits the central transmission of pain through mechanoreceptor collateral fibers inhibiting the nociceptors in the posterior motor units of the spine and the zygapophyseal capsules.

The muscular distribution of the medial branches of the lumbar dorsal rami is very specific. Each medial branch supplies only those muscles that arise from the lamina and spinous process of the vertebra with the same segment as the nerve. (See Figure 2.5.) Therefore, the muscles arising from the spinous process and lamina of a vertebra are innervated by the medial branch of the dorsal ramus that issues immediately below that vertebra. This relationship indicates that the principal muscles that move a particular segment are innervated by the nerve of that segment. Often, diagnostic facet blocks, selective nerve root blocks, and facet challenges confirm segmental arthrogenic etiology for paravertebral muscle spasms.

The mechanoreceptors include kinesioreceptors, barroreceptors, and proprioceptors. As long as the mechanoreceptors' sensory input to the cord is within normal limits, a collateral fiber from each mechanoreceptor inhibits nociception and the central transmission of pain. (See Figure 2.6.)

However, when, for example, there is abnormal range of motion of the posterior motor units, kinesioreception (sensory input regarding normal or aberrant range of motion) is abnormal, the collateral fiber inhibiting nociception from the kinesioreceptor no longer inhibits the nociception.

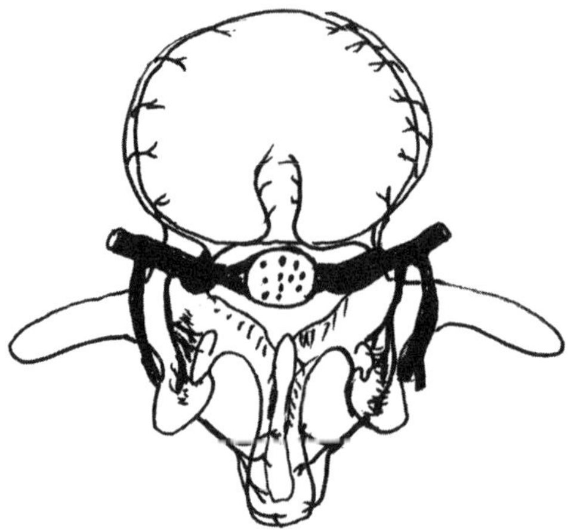

**FIGURE 2.6**

The threshold for depolarization of the nociceptor is thereby lessened, requiring fewer stimuli to depolarize the nociceptor causing pain.

If additional stimulation of abnormal sensory input occurs, such as a decrease in synovial fluid production due to lack of proper motion of the joint, the intra-articular pressure changes and the barroreceptor collateral inhibition is interrupted, thereby causing an even more sensitive state of depolarization of the nociceptor. If this condition persists, the lack of synovial fluid production due to lack of motion causes a settling or imbrication of the facets due to decreased intra-articular distention and development of intra-articular microadhesions. The proprioceptor collateral inhibition is interrupted due to abnormal stimulus from the orientation in space of the facets. With all three mechanoreceptors ceasing collateral inhibition of nociception, this thereby fully initiates the arthrokinetic reflex, causing a cascade of nociception resulting in a motor response to the segmental level from which the stimulus originated.

The nociceptor input is through the lateral spinothalamic tract, which carries pain and temperature. When fully depolarized, the nociceptor initiates an arthrokinetic reflex, resulting in a state of hypertonic paraspinal muscle splinting and pain.

Manipulation restores the mechanical integrity of the joint by increasing range of motion and disrupting microadhesions, thereby restoring kinesioreception and its collateral inhibition to nociception. This restoration of motion allows for increased stimulus to the synovial membrane, which produces synovial fluid in direct proportion to the mechanical stimulation it receives from motion of the joint. This in turn produces more synovial fluid and exchanges existing fluid in the joint. The barroreceptor in the joint senses increased pressure from intra-articular fluid and restores its corresponding collateral inhibition, thereby inhibiting the central transmission of pain through the nociceptors, resulting in a state of relative muscular relaxation.

Additional stimuli can initiate nociception, such as chemical noxious stimuli. With chronic low-grade inflammatory conditions, an inflammatory "soup" is created, replete with substance P, bradykinins, and prostaglandins causing irritation to nociceptors and initiating the arthrokinetic reflex, resulting in a state of hypertonicity of the segmental muscles. Chronic inflammation allows for microphage and fibroblast migration to the site, which further complicates the clinical sequelae. Proper motion of the joints allows for fluid exchange and nutrition to the joints, which prevents the accumulation of inflammatory noci-irritant mediators and fibroblastic substances. Proper motion restores the mechanoreceptor mechanism of collateral inhibition of pain. It is the mechanical input to the joint that is responsible for restoration of collateral inhibition, reduction of microadhesions, and the pain-free state.

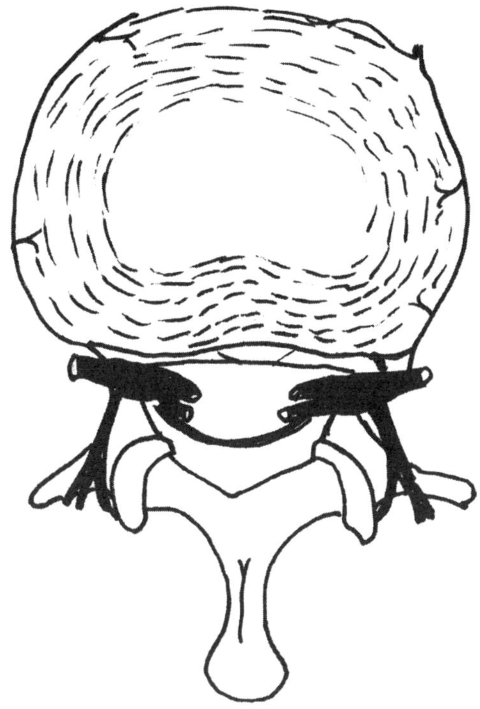

**FIGURE 2.7**

## PROPRIOCEPTIVE NEUROFACILITATION

Chronic pathomechanics is often accompanied by chronic muscular contractions or shortening, which further contributes to articular dyskinesia. It is essential to address the soft tissue component of articular dyskinesia for complete restoration of the pathomechanical lesion. Shortened musculature crossing the joint creates compressive forces across the joint, further compromising joint mechanics and contributing to the articular dyskinesia.

A longer resting length of the musculature often results post-SMT (spinal manipulative therapy). This is accomplished through the process of proprioceptive neurofacilitation (PNF). This occurs when the spindle cell mechanism in the belly of the muscle is stimulated to reset to a new resting length after the actin/myosin heads are gently stretched or pulled apart under anesthesia. (See Figure 2.7.)

While asleep, the sensory and motor mechanisms of the skeletal muscles are "turned off." The muscles are stretched to a new and longer resting length. Once awakened, this system is "turned back on," and the messages sent by the golgi tendon organ and received by the spindle cell are different than before the stretch, resulting in a longer resting length pursuant to the PNF effect.

Proprioceptive neurofacilitation of the golgi tendon organ and the spindle cell result in less tonic muscle contraction, reducing compressive forces across joints. Microadhesions present in the myofibrils contributing to contractures and decreased elasticity are also reduced by this stretching, resulting in a more viscoelastic, flexible, and functional musculature.

Benefits of MUA procedures include the reduction of peri-/intra-articular microadhesions in and about the posterior motor units, restoration of the pathomechanics in the three-joint complex (two posterior motor units and the intervertebral disc joint), increase in range of motion, flexibility and visco-elasticity of the soft tissues, a reduction of fibroblastic proliferation, and recruitment of collateral inhibition, thereby preventing pain.

The pain picture consists of biochemical and mechanical components. By only addressing the chemical component — for example, administering anti-inflammatory medications or epidural or facet injections — only one factor of pain production is addressed: the biochemical. Restoring mechanical integrity to the joint as well as biochemical components with manipulation provides more comprehensive healing by establishing proper mechanics of the joint, thus allowing for the exchange of fluid and the restoration of appropriate biochemical balance. These synovial fluid dynamics were well documented by Robert Salter, MD[27] (1999), in several landmark experimental studies demonstrating that fluid exchange and joint nutrition is dependent on proper motion of the synovial joint and that lack of proper motion accelerates degenerative changes. Salter showed that synovial joints produce synovial fluid directly proportionate to the amount of mechanical stimulation the synovial membrane receives through joint motion.

The cause of inflammation is commonly articular dyskinesia of the joint and is therefore the source of altered chemistry. Addressing the pathomechanical source with MUA ensures that total restoration of joint dynamics can be established. The manipulative results may also be enhanced with proper and judicial administration of injections.

## PRESSURE HIERARCHY OF THE INTERVERTEBRAL FORAMEN (IVF)

The intervertebral foramen (IVF) transmits significant structures, which must maintain a defined pressure hierarchy to function normally. These include the artery, capillaries, vein, and fascicles of the spinal nerve, and all are cushioned with adipose and connective tissue inside the IVF tunnel. The nerve roots are particularly susceptible to the consequences of vascular compression, particularly venous compression, because they lack lymphatics. Consequently, there are no alternative channels whereby exudated fluid can leave the roots. Intraneural and perineural edema can interfere with nerve conduction by exerting pressure on axons. Nerve root ischemia can be the result of long-standing edema or inflammatory exudate, which tends to organize, that is, convert to fibrous tissue.

This system of maintaining the pressure hierarchy of the intervertebral foramen is described as follows:

$$(P_a > P_c > P_v > P_f > P_t)$$

meaning the pressure in the artery must be greater than the pressure in the capillary, which must be greater than the pressure in the vein, which must be greater than the intrafascicular pressure of the spinal nerve, which finally in turn must be greater than the pressure of the "tunnel" or IVF itself.

The interstitial fluid inside the fascicle (endoneural fluid pressure) is greater than that of the surrounding tissues. The intrafascicular vascular bed extends along the whole length of the nerve and consists mainly of capillaries that communicate with the extrafascicular vessels through multiple anastomoses. When there is a pressure change at the IVF — for example, from decreased disc height — it affects first and most significantly the most distensible tissue in this system, which is the venous system. Due to its thinner vascular wall, the veins are more easily compressed than are the arteries and capillaries. Data obtained from studies of nerve roots subjected to graded, acute compression demonstrate that even low-pressure compression of the nerve roots (5–10 mmHg) can induce venous congestion in the intraneural microcirculation and up to 130 mmHg compression results in complete ischemia of the nerve root. Intraneural edema results in extravasation of serum albumin even at 50 mmHg. It has been shown that mechanical compression of nerve roots produces acute and chronic impairment of the blood supply and transport of nutrients to the nerve tissue. As a result of mechanical compression, waste product clearance from the nerve root tissue is also impaired. These alterations of the metabolic balance potentiate chronic tissue changes such as fibroblastic proliferation in and around the nerve root, which can result in clinical manifestations of epineural fibrosis.

Clinically, epineural fibrosis may mimic discogenic radicular pain due to the tethering of the existing nerve root, causing distinct dermatomal distribution of pain patterns. MUA can effectively reduce this scar tissue with the inclusion of specific fibrosis release procedures (FRP). The specific MUA stretching techniques of FRP is described elsewhere in this text and can be referred to in order to further enhance the understanding of epineural scar tissue reduction.

In summary, disturbance of the IVF pressure hierarchy can induce changes in microcirculation and nutrition of the nerve root. The permeability of the vasculature is increased, resulting in endoneural edema. This increases endoneural fluid pressure and migration of inflammatory mediators to the area stimulated by the extravasation of serum albumin, thus leading to a low-grade chronic inflammatory process of fibroblastic proliferation in and about the nerve root.

It is this fibroblastic proliferation, if allowed to persist, that alters the normal neuromechanics of the spine manifesting clinically as articular dyskinesia or aberrant spine pathomechanics.

## THE INTERVERTEBRAL DISC

Anatomically, the intervertebral disc (IVD) consists of two parts: the annulus fibrosis and the nucleus pulposus. The annulus is distinct at its periphery, and the nucleus is quite distinct at the center; however, there is no clear boundary between the nucleus and the annulus within the disc. The major components of the disc are proteoglycans and collagen, with proteoglycan content greater in the nucleus and collagen content greater in the annulus.

The nucleus is made up of glycosaminoglycans. When linked together in long chains, these become proteoglycans, which physiochemcially have the property of attracting and retaining water, a process called *water imbibition*. A normal healthy well-hydrated disc has a water imbibition ratio of 9:1. With aging and dessication, this ratio, which is so essential to the mechanical integrity of the IVD, decreases, resulting in reduced ability of the nucleus to attract and retain water and thus allowing for less deformation. It is this water imbibition property that gives the nucleus its visco-elasticity.

Biomechanically, the fluid character of the nucleus allows for deformation under pressure, but its volume cannot be compressed. When compressed, its fluid nature will deform, transmitting pressure in all directions like a balloon filled with water. Any change in the proteoglycan, and thereby water, content of the nucleus will inevitably alter the mechanical properties of the disc because the water content of the nucleus is a function of its proteoglycan content.

The annulus consists of collagen fibers arranged in 10/12 sheets of concentric rings called *lamellae* surrounding the nucleus. The fibers run alternately at about a 65° angle to the vertical in successive layers such that one lamella is oriented 65° to the right and the next layer 65° to the left. (See Figure 2.8.)

The annulus is much like a thick book, such as a telephone directory. When the book is folded into a cylindrical shape and stood on end, its weight-bearing capacity is significant so long as the

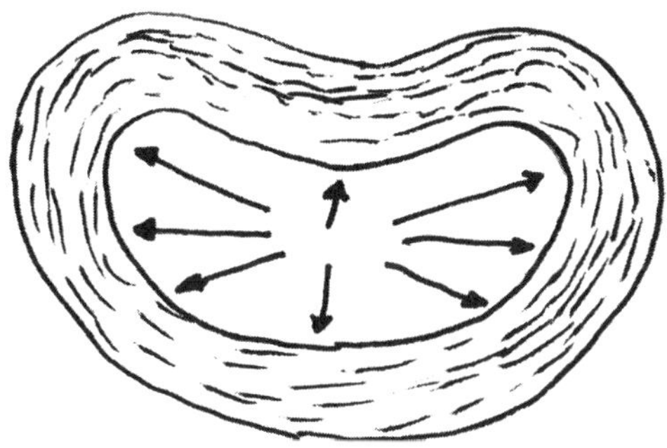

FIGURE 2.8

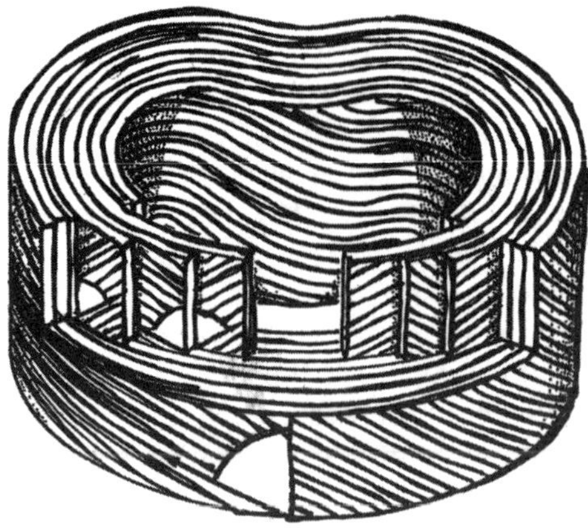

**FIGURE 2.9**

pages do not bend or buckle. However, sustained pressure would buckle this system without the nucleus providing its internal turgor due to its water content exerting pressure in all directions, 360° spherically, like a water balloon. (See Figure 2.9.) So with the phone book on end and a competent water balloon inside, this system can sustain tremendous axial loading as the nucleus supports the annulus. Prolonged axial loading, however, will tend to reduce the height of the nucleus as it loses water content due to constant axial loading. Intermittent pressure allows the nucleus to reimbibe water as pressure is alternately increased and decreased. With axial loading, the nucleus begins to deform the annulus, which tries to expand radially, thus stretching the lamellae outward. The tensile properties of the annular collagen resist the stretch and oppose the outward pressure.

This is much like a woven wicker toy, the Chinese finger trap, which is made up of alternating wicker fibers; once you insert your fingers tip to tip and attempt to pull them apart, the fibers tighten. If your fingers, while pulling apart, are twisted inside, the alternating wicker fibers tighten even further around your fingers, containing them tightly inside the "annulus" of the toy. So functions the annulus under traction and torsion. It tightens around the nucleus, opposing radial pressure of the nucleus, thus causing the nuclear pressure to increase and exert upward and downward pressure. This separates the vertebra above from the one below, further causing the lamella to tighten its concentric alternating rings of lamella as it is pulled from above and below — just as the finger trap toy does around the finger trapped inside when attempts are made to pull the fingers out.

This very mechanism is recruited during manipulation to reduce disc protrusions and herniations. It is the mechanism alluded to by James Cyriax,[4] who reported in his *Illustrated Manual of Orthopedics* that "the main purpose of manipulation is restoration of internal derangement of the disc."

There have been many studies on intradiscal pressure demonstrating different postures, and the concomitant pressure increases and decreases in the nucleus with various postures. Essentially, axial loading in the standing, sitting, or forward bending positions increases intradiscal pressure while recumbent side lying or supine positions decrease that pressure. Nuclear pressure decreases directly as a result of decreased axial loading or compression. These pressures can change from as much as 140 psi at the L5 nucleus in the seated position to as little as 25 psi at the L5 nucleus in the supine position so that the lateral decubitus position used for lumbar manipulation prior to the thrust procedure is actually a decompressive procedure. Then adding the traction and torsional effects of the annulus during manipulation, combined with the decreased nuclear pressure from the position of the patient, there is intradiscal pressure reduction at the nucleus, thus allowing water to enter the disc through its inherent imbibition property. This in turn follows the mechanism described earlier as the two functional units of the intervertebral disc support each other with hydration and tensile properties of visco-elasticity, resulting in a more functional intervertebral disc.

## CAVITATION

An audible "pop" often accompanies spinal manipulation. This is the process of *cavitation*. Cavitation ($PV = nrt$) occurs when the intra-articular pressure decreases. Volume and pressure are inversely proportionate. During SMT, the joint surfaces are separated, increasing the volume of the joint space and reducing the intra-articular pressure. The reduction in pressure causes a $CO_2$ gas bubble to come out of the synovial fluid. This causes the audible "pop" much the same as removing the bottle cap from a soda pop bottle (the pressure inside the bottle is reduced and $CO_2$ comes out of solution, making a popping noise).

This cavitation has been experimentally shown to increase joint space post-manipulation as the gas bubble distends the joint a slight degree. This distention, or internal autotraction, may be sufficient to reduce the pressure at the IVF, which can cause venous congestion and the clinical sequelae that manifest from chronic compression and inflammation at the IVF.

With even minimal facet distention, a reduction in intradiscal pressure is accomplished. As the water imbibition properties of the nucleus "drink" water, it allows the nucleus and annulus to function with greater integrity, as mentioned earlier. Salter's landmark work on synovial fluid production and exchange demonstrates the mechanism responsible for the facet joint dynamics seen in manipulation. The stimulation of the synovial membrane through manipulation allows simultaneous production and exchange of synovial fluid, maintaining and restoring the intra-articular pressure and fluid dynamics affecting collateral inhibition and thus preventing nociceptive depolarization, as described in the articular neurology section in this chapter.

Arthrogenic conditions and their attendant myofascial symptoms are among the most commonly treated with MUA. This can be a confounding presentation to the provider unfamiliar with facet syndrome. Facet syndrome is common, but because it is not demonstrable on plain film radiographic studies, it is frequently misdiagnosed as nerve compression syndromes, dismissed as myofascial pain, or, unfortunately, simply overlooked. It is known that this syndrome may produce pain in the legs, and the course of this referred pain may be in the buttocks, lateral or posterior thigh down to the knee, and occasionally outer calf, but rarely to the foot.

The differential diagnosis of discogenic versus arthrogenic pain is necessary to rule out space-occupying lesions. In the absence of space-occupying lesions nerve root tension signs may persist. This is almost always due to epineural fibrosis tethering the existing nerve root as described earlier. It is most effectively treated with a judicious combination of epidural steroid injection and MUA-FRP procedures. The innervation of the facet joints has been adequately described in this chapter. The mechanical intervention of MUA procedures in facet syndrome recruits those mechanoreceptor mechanisms responsible for collateral inhibition and the decreased input of the central transmission of pain while at the same time restoring the mechanical integrity of the posterior and intervertebral joints — the three-joint complex.

The restoration of intervertebral disc integrity by restoring the water imbibition ability of the nucleus pulposus is accomplished by the decreased intradiscal pressure accompanying the manipulation. The slight distention of the joints due to cavitation, and the gas bubble occupying more space inside the joint effectively "tractions" the vertebra for about one-half of a millimeter, as demonstrated by Sandoz. This allows for imbibition of water into the nucleus from the adjacent vertebral bodies, allowing it to distend and reinforce the annulus fibrosis as described earlier. The two functional units of the intervertebral disc, the nucleus and the annulus, are then allowed to function as a unit to provide the visco-elasticity and tensile properties necessary to the competent disc.

The appropriate functioning of the three-joint complex is necessary to maintain the pressure hierarchy of the IVF. The pressure hierarchy of the IVF prevents the venous congestion at the site of the existing nerve root, thereby disallowing accumulation of the inflammatory edematous "soup" constituents responsible for epineural fibrosis and mimicking nerve root tension signs of a space-occupying lesion.

MUA has a definite place in the clinical armamentarium of the physical medicine practitioner. The basic science studies described in this chapter and the clinical application of that information provide an enduring status for MUA procedures in the broad spectrum of clinical interventions for chronic pain patients.

## REFERENCES


1. Bogduk, N., Engel, R.M. The menisci of the lumbar zygapophyseal joints, *J. Anatomy* 135, 795–809, 1982.
2. Bogduk, N., Jull, G. The theoretical pathology of acute locked back: a basis for manipulative therapy, *Manual Medicine* 1, 78–82, 1985.
3. Chen, H.I., Granger, H.J., Taylor, A.E. Interaction of capillary, interstitial and lymphatic forces, *Circ. Res.* 39, 245–54, 1976.
4. Cyriax, J. *Textbook of Orthopaedic Medicine*, Vol. 1, 8th ed. Bailliere Tindall, London.
5. Dorman, T. *Diagnosis and Injections Techniques in Orthopedic Medicine*. Williams & Wilkins, Baltimore, 1991.
6. Francis, R. Spinal manipulation under general anesthesia: a chiropractic approach in a hospital setting. *ACA J. Chiropr.* 1989: 12, 39–41, 1989.
7. Francis, R. Manipulation under anesthesia, *Am. Chiropr.* 24, 26–27, 1991.
8. Francis, R. *Guidelines for Chiropractic Quality Assurance and Practice Parameters: Proceedings of the Mercy Center Conference*, commission member, Aspen Publishers, New York, 1992.
9. Francis, R. Spinal manipulation under anesthesia: A review of chiropractic training programs and protocols, *Am. Chiropr.* 27, 37, 1995.
10. Francis, R. Postgraduate and continuing education courses: September. Pasadena (TX): Texas Chiropractic College [cited 2002 Oct 01].
11. Francis, R., Beckett, R.H. Spinal manipulation under anesthesia, *Adv. Chiropr.*, 1, 325–40, 1994.
12. Giles, L.G.F. Lumbosacral zygapophyseal joint inclusions, *Manual Med.* 2, 89–92, 1986.
13. Giles, L.G.F. and Taylor, J.R. Inter-articular synovial protrusions, *Bull. Hosp. Joint Dis.* 42, 248–55, 1982.
14. Giles, L.G.F. and Taylor, J.R., Innervation of human lumbar zygapophyseal joint synovial folds, *Acta Orthopaedica Scand.* 58, 43–46, 1987.
15. Gordon, R., Rogers, R., West, D., Matthews, R., and Miller, R., Manipulation under anesthesia: an anthology of past, present and future use, Chapter 26 in *Pain Management, a Practical Guide for Clinicians*, 6th ed., Weiner, R., ed., CRC Press, New York, 2002.
16. Haldeman, S., The neurophysiology of spinal pain syndromes, in Haldeman, S., ed., *Modern Development in the Principles of Chiropractic*, Appleton-Century Crofts, New York, 1980, 119–42.
17. Kellgren, J.H., On the distribution of pain arising from deep somatic structures with charts of segmental pain areas, *Clin. Sci.*, 4, 35–46, 1939.
18. Korkala, O., Gronblad. M., Liesi, P., and Karaharju, E., Immunohistochemical demonstration of nociceptors in the ligamentous structures of the lumbar spine, *Spine* 10, 156–57, 1985.
19. Kramer, J., Kolditz, D., and Gowin, R., Water and electrolyte content of human intervertebral disc under variable load, *Spine* 19, 69–71, 1985.
20. Low, P., Marchand, G., Knox, F., and Dyck, P.J., Measurement of endoneurial fluid pressure with polyethylene matrix capsules, *Brain Res.* 122, 373–77, 1977.
21. Murphy, R.W., Nerve roots and spinal nerves in degenerative disk disease, *Clin. Orthop.* 129, 46–60, 1977.
22. Myers, R.R., Murakami, H., and Powell, H.C., Reduced nerve blood flow in edematous neuropathies — A biochemical mechanism, *Microvasc. Res.* 32, 145–51, 1986.
23. Olmarker, K., Rydevik, B., and Holm, S., Edema formation in spinal nerve roots induced by graded, experimental compression. An experimental study on the pig cauda equina, *Spine* 14, 569–73, 1989.
24. Olmarker, K., Rydevik, B., Hansson, T., and Holm, S., Compression-induced changes of the nutritional supply to the porcine cauda equina, *J. Spinal Disord.* 3, 25–29, 1990.

25. Pedersen, H.E., Blunck, C.F.J., and Gardner, E., The anatomy of lumbosacral posterior rami and meningeal branches of spinal nerves: with an experimental study of their function, *J. Bone Joint Surg.* 38A, 377–91, 1956.

26. Rydevik, B. and Norborg, C., Changes in nerve function and nerve fibre structure induced by acute, graded compression, *J. Neurol. Neurosurg. Psychiatr.* 43, 1070–82, 1980.

27. Salter, R B., *Textbook of Disorders and Injuries of the Musculoskeletal System, 3rd ed.,* Lippincott, Williams & Wilkins, Baltimore, 1999.

28. Sandoz, R., Physical mechanisms of effect of spinal adjustment. Ann. Swiss Chiro. Assoc; 6:91; 1976.

29. Steindler, A. and Luck, J.V., Differential diagnosis of pain low in the back: allocation of the source of pain by the procaine hydrochloride method, *JAMA* 110, 106–12, 1938.

30. Sunderland, S., *Nerves and Nerve Injuries*, 2nd ed., Churchill Livingstone, New York, 1978.

31. Sunderland, S., The nerve lesion in the carpal tunnel syndrome, *J. Neurol. Neurosurg. Psychiatr.* 39, 615–26, 1976.

32. Taylor, J.R. and Twomey, L.T., Innervation of the lumbar intervertebral discs, *Med. J. Aust.* 2, 701–2, 1979.

33. Urban, J. and Maroudas, A., The chemistry of the intervertebral disc in relation to its physiological function, *Clin. Rheum. Dis.* 6, 51–76, 1980.

34. White, A.A. and Panjabi, M.M., *Clinical Biomechanics of the Spine*, Lippincott, Philadelphia, 1998.

35. Wiberg, G., Back pain in relation to the nerve supply of the intervertebral disc, *Acta Orthop. Scand.* 19, 211–21, 1947.

36. Wyke, B., The neurology of low back pain, in *The Lumbar Spine and Back Pain*, 2nd ed., Jayson, M.I.V., ed., Pitman, Tunbridge Wells, 1980, 265–339.

37. Yoshizawa, H., O'Brien, J.P., Thomas-Smith, W., and Trumper, M., The neuropathology of intervertebral discs removed for low back pain, *J. Pathol.* 132, 95–104, 1070–82, 1980.

# The Myofascial Component and Predetermining Factors to Consider in MUA

*Anthony B. Morovati*

Having been involved with MUA for the last 14 years, I have witnessed firsthand the many successes that this program has to offer. It is an invaluable procedure that, if used correctly, can lead to great results. However, the most important aspect of MUA is proper patient selection and diagnosis. Having performed numerous procedures and having followed up with the patients post procedure, it is self evident that MUA is valuable in the management of spinal conditions which fit the diagnosis.

In volume I of Janet Travell's text,[11] *Myofascial Pain and Dysfunction, the Trigger Point Manual* (1983), a foreward by Rene Cailliet, MD, formerly the professor and chairman of the Department of Rehabilitative Medicine at USC, and also the director of Department of Rehabilitation at Santa Monica Hospital notes that:

> The medical education of today and even the continued medical education efforts currently employed do not sufficiently instruct the clinician in functional anatomy, surface anatomy, kinesiology, and the techniques of evaluating this musculoskeletal aspect of the human body. Trauma is too simply considered to be the evidence of eternal contact, but it is not documented as postural stress, occupational, unphysiologic postures, or faulty mechanical activities of everyday living. Yet, these are important in the full evaluation and management of myofascial pain syndromes. Examination of the patient today is also so dependent upon machines and equipment, that the use of touch, palpation, and manual examination of joints, muscles and ligaments remains a lost art.

In the second foreword in Janet Travell's text[11] Parker E. Mahon, DDS, PhD, professor and chairman, Department of Basic Dental Sciences, University of Florida, Gainesville, FL, states: "Such factors as nutritional deficiencies, endocrine imbalances, chronic infection, allergy, psychological stress, nerve entrapment, congenital skeletal abnormalities, and trauma to muscle are often overlooked when these unfortunate patients are examined and treated."

I was fortunate enough to have attended several of Dr. Janet G. Travell's lectures, as well as participating in several modules in myofascial pain management and treatment. I must say without any hesitation that these techniques have enhanced my practice tremendously since the early 1990s when I began practicing. I believe that as DCs, if we address these methods in conjunction with our chiropractic methods, we will have approached the patient in a truly holistic manner, and will achieve outcomes that are unimaginable. The following is a brief review of principles.

## BACKGROUND AND PRINCIPLES

*Myo* = muscle. *Fasciae* = connective tissue. *Myofascial pain*, therefore, is muscle and connective tissue pain, or pain that arises from muscle and connective tissue.

*Muscle:* Voluntary (skeletal) muscle is the largest single organ of the human body, and accounts for 40% or more of body weight. "Bardeen" quoted the *Basle/Nomina Anatomica* as recognizing 347 paired and two unpaired muscles for a total of 692 muscles. Not counting heads, bellies, and other parts of muscles, the nomina anatomica reported by the International Anatomical Nomenclature Committee under the Berne Convention lists 200 paired muscles, or a total of 400 muscles. Any one of these muscles can develop myofascial trigger points that refer pain and other distressing symptoms usually into a remote location. Yet, the muscles receive little attention in modern medical school teaching and medical textbooks. Contractible muscle tissues are extremely subject to wear and tear of daily activities, but it is the bones, joints, bursa, and nerves on which physicians concentrate their attention.

*Prevalence:* Myofascial trigger points are extremely common and become a distressing part of nearly everyone's lives at one time or another. Latent trigger points that may cause some stiffness and restricted range of motion are far more common than active trigger points.

*Severity:* The severity of symptoms from myofascial trigger points range from painless restriction of motion due to latent trigger points, so common in the aged, to agonizing incapacitating pain caused by very active trigger points. Patients who have had other kinds of severe pain, such as that due to a heart attack, broken bones, or renal colic, say that the myofascial pains and trigger points can be just as severe. Despite their painfulness, myofascial trigger points are not directly life-threatening, but their painfulness can and often does devastate the quality of life.

*Cost:* Unrecognized myofascial headaches, shoulder pain, and low back pain that have become chronic are major causes of industrial lost time and compensation applications. Bonica[1] pointed out that disabling chronic pain costs the American people billions of dollars annually. Low back pain alone costs the people of California over $200 million. Analgesics to relieve chronic pain are costly and a significant cause of nephropathy. A considerable portion of chronic pain due to myofascial trigger points can be relieved by their diagnosis and appropriate treatment. When the myofascial pain is not recognized, such as a mimicking of cardiac pain by trigger points in the pectoral muscles, the symptoms are likely to be diagnosed as neurotic, adding frustration and self-doubt to the patient's misery.

Common terms for myofascial trigger points (usually synonymous terms) include the following:

- Muscular rheumatism
- Myalgia
- Myolgelosis
- Interstitial myofibrositis
- Myofascial pain syndrome
- Myofascitis
- Trigger points
- Myofascial pain dysfunction syndrome
- Fibrositis

*Trigger point* is defined as a focus of hyperirritability in a tissue that when compressed is locally tender and, if sufficiently hypersensitive, gives rise to referred pain and tenderness, and sometimes to referred autonomic phenomena and distortion of proprioception. Trigger points can be classified as myofascial cutaneous, fascial, ligamentous, and periosteal. There are two basic types of trigger points: (1) Active, which cause pain and dysfunction; and (2) latent, which do not cause pain but do cause dysfunction.

## Clinical Characteristics of Trigger Points

Trigger points often cause pain, decreased range of motion, restricted strength, or endurance. Trigger points also:

- Refer pain peripherally, as in the infraspinatus trigger point, which is located in the infraspinatus muscle and refers pain distally into the arm and forearm
- Can be centralized, such as in the biceps muscle, where the trigger points are in the belly of the muscle, and refer pain in the central zone of pain
- Can be localized, where the pain basically is overlapped in the area of the trigger point, such as in the multifidi muscles of the spine
- Common causes of myofascial trigger points (perpetuating factors) may include mechanical, genetic, chemical/nutritional and psychological factors.

## Common Causes of Myofascial Trigger Points (i.e., Perpetuating Factors): Mechanical Stressors

### Structural Inadequacies

The term *structural inadequacies* refers to such genetic or acquired factors as lower leg length inequality, small hemipelvis, short upper arms, and long second metatarsal.

1. Signs of lower leg length inequality include the following:
   - Outer canthus of the eye to the corner of the mouth.
   - The patient stands on the lower leg with the long leg in front diagonally or with bent knee.
   - The arm on the short leg side hangs away from the body.
   - The gluteal fold is lower on the short leg side.
   - There is an increased skin fold in the flank on the short leg side, or concaved side.
   - PSIS is fixated.
   - There is 90% flexion at the hips secondary to sacral leveling.
   - Height of greater trochanter in obese patients.
   - When the patient is asked to swing each leg back and forth, the short leg will swing more easily, and the pelvis will have to be shifted on the side with the long leg.

- Scoliosis (functional versus structural).
- Inferior angle of scapula for height difference; this is especially important in head, neck, and shoulder pain patients.

2. Signs of small hemipelvis that can cause scoliosis are:
   - Patients lean and sit on small side.
   - Patients cross the small hemipelvis leg over the other side to balance out.
   - Placing a lift on the small "hemi" side decreases drop appearance when patient sits.

3. Signs of long second metatarsal (according to Dudley J. Morton,[13] MD) include the following:
   - The lateral part of the heel and the medial part of the big toe are worn from overburden of structural abnormality.
   - Dorsoplantar radiographs and weight bearing will give most accurate and reliable techniques for measurements of metatarsals.
   - Even if the sesamoid bone is posteriorly displaced in relation to the second metatarsal, patients may have symptoms.
   - Correction can be made by using "Kirofelt" shoe inserts.

Surprisingly, trigger points in the lower extremity muscles can react with tense muscles of the head and neck to restrict range or motion. By inactivation of trigger points caused by Morton's foot configuration (described above), one may at once increase a trigger point restricted intercisal opening of the jaw by 20%–30%.

4. Signs of short upper arms include the following:
   - Elbows measured are above the iliac crest.
   - Stresses levator/trapezius/scaleni, and shortens muscles on the leaning side.
   - Patient leans to one side to support the upper torso, which causes shortening of the quadratus lunborum (QL) on the same side.

## Postural Stressors

1. Misfitting Furniture
   - Chair, home, auto, office
   - Tables
2. Poor Posture
   - Unphysiologic work surface
   - Reading and writing at eye level
   - Prolonged unilateral repetitive action
   - Rounded shoulders, i.e., hypertonic pectoralis
   - Standing on head causes head to counter weight, therefore, reversal of cervical lordosis and lumbar spine reversal of lordosis
   - Physical disabilities
   - Ergonomics
3. Abuse of Muscles
   - Poor body mechanics
   - Sudden stressful movement
   - Repetitive movement
4. Immobility
   - Lack of movement, especially when muscle is in the shortened position
   - Dental malocclusion, bruxism, and emotional tension, which can interact to overload the masticatory and neck muscles
   - Jerkiness of movement, sudden starts and stops

**Other Mechanical Stresses**

1. Constriction of Muscle
   - Bag over shoulder
   - Bra strap
   - Tight shirt collar
   - Tight belt
   - Edge of chair too high, compressing hamstrings

## COMMON CAUSES OF MYOFASCIAL TRIGGER POINTS (I.E., PERPETUATING FACTORS): CONTINUED GENETICS

Genetics plays a major role in structural inadequacies, as well as chemical and psychological inadequacies. These are covered in detail in Volume I, Chapter 4, of Janet G. Travell and David Simons' textbook of myofascial pain and dysfunction.[12] However, some of these inadequacies, such as eye/hand dominance, can be categorized in either biomechanical, ergonomic, and genetic perpetuating factors.

Eye/hand dominance merely means if you are left-handed and right-eye dominant, you twist the head more to accommodate a perpendicular view to the right hand, thus stressing the sternocleidomastoid. This would in turn be a mechanical stress, perpetuating trigger points and causing symptoms.

Note that if the short leg is 1 cm or less, it usually causes a "C"-shaped scoliosis, that is, a low shoulder on the opposite short leg side. If the short leg is 1.3 cm or greater, the shoulder on the same side of the short leg sags. If the short leg is 1.3 cm or greater, the patient may not have any symptoms for life. Three basic deviations can occur together or independently:

- Short leg
- Sacral tilt
- Angulation of lumbar spine

## COMMON CAUSES OF MYOFASCIAL TRIGGER POINTS (I.E., PERPETUATING FACTORS): NUTRITIONAL/CHEMICAL INADEQUACIES

A patient with a serum level at the low end but within normal limits may show no metabolic evidence of deficiency. Yet the levels may be inadequate for optimal health. Myofascial pain syndromes are aggravated by inadequate levels of at least vitamins B1, B6, B12, folic acid, and vitamin C. These inadequacies apparently increase the irritability of myofascial trigger points by several mechanisms, such as impairment of the energy metabolism needed for contraction of muscles and increased irritability of the liver system.

Common symptoms of nutritional deficiencies include:

- Watery stool/occasional diarrhea could be due to folate deficiency.
- Constipation could be due to a hypothyroid condition and a decreased vitamin B1 level.
- Excessive flatus could be due to diet or decreased normal flora.
- Restless leg could be due to folic acid deficiency.
- Hypoglycemia (episodic) could be due to sudden myofascial pain.

Diet is determined not only by what patients eat, but how they have prepared it. For example, exposure of food to heated trays and flourescent light causes rapid degeneration and loss of vitamin C and some B vitamins.

## Deficiency

Inadequacy becomes a deficiency when effects due to impaired function of essential enzymes are grossly apparent. This is determined by laboratory serum levels; however, they are not reliable. In my practice, laboratory analysis is used to obtain a functional intracellular analysis of the patient's vitamin state.

## Dependence

*Dependence on nutrition* means the need for substances to survive. One can suffer from congenital deficiencies.

## Insufficiency

Insufficiency may result from:

- Inadequate ingestion
- Impaired absorption
- Inadequate utilization
- Increased metabolic requirements
- Increased excretion
- Increased body destruction

In 1995 Robert Gerwin,[4] MD, performed a study on patients with myofascial pain syndrome. He showed that the most common causes are iron deficiency, folic acid deficiency, vitamin B12 deficiency, and hypothyroidism. In the elderly, decreased absorption is partly due to folate deficiency.

## Prevalence of Unrecognized Hypovitaminosis

In a randomly selected municipal hospital population, 105 of 1200 patients (88%) had abnormally low levels of one or more of 11 vitamins. Over half the patients were low in two or more vitamins. Serum folate was low in 45% of the patients. This was the most common vitamin deficiency. Despite the low blood levels, there was a history of inadequate dietary intake in only 39% of the patients with hypovitaminosis. Moreover, hypovitaminosis was clinically apparent in only 38% of the entire group.

Toxicity of vitamin A may cause bone and joint pain and severe, throbbing headaches. Folic acid is the only vitamin of the B complex vitamins in which megaconsumption may lead to toxicity.

### Thiamine (Vitamin B1)

1. *Inadequacy*: These patients are more prone to trigger points, nocturnal calf cramps, mild dependent edema, constipation, fatigue, and decreased vibratory perception in relation to neurofiber length. Patients may experience tinnitus, which is relieved by a combination of thiamine (vitamin B1) and niacin (vitamin B2).
2. *Requirements*: Vitamin B1 requirements for older persons are 0.5 mg/1000 Kcal of energy expended, with a minimum of 1 mg/day.
3. *Source*: Sources of vitamin B1 include lean pork, beans, nuts, and certain whole grains. Kidney, liver, beef, eggs, and fish also have a good amount.

### Pyridoxine (Vitamin B6)

Pyridoxine (vitamin B6) plays a role in energy metabolism and in nerve function. It is critical for the synthesis and/or metabolism of nearly all neurotransmitters, including norepinephrine and serotonin, which strongly influence pain perception.

Vitamin B6 is a complex formed from three distinct, chemically different compounds: pyridoxol (an alcohol), pyridoxal (an aldehyde), and pyridoxamine (an amine). These dietary precursors are phosphorylated in the liver to the active coenzymes, pyridoxal phosphate, and pyridoxamine phosphate.

Pyridoxal is critical in lipid metabolism and pyridoxal phosphate deficiency causes myelin degeneration in humans. Pyridoxal phosphate deficiency also causes:

- Anemia
- Hormonal imbalance expressed as growth retardation
- Reduced absorption and storage of cobalamin
- Increased excretion of vitamin C
- Blocked synthesis of nicotinic acid (niacin)
- Shortcomings in both anaerobic and aerobic metabolism
- Microcytic hypochromic anemia that fails to respond to iron

Pyridoxal plays an essential role in the following pathways:

- Hemoglobin synthesis.
- Neurotransmitter synthesis and/or metabolism, such as dopamine, norepinephrine, serotonin, tyramine, tryptamine, taurine, histamine, aminobutyric acid (GABE), and indirectly acetylcholine. Serotonin is derived, with pyridoxal phosphate, from 5-hydroxytryptophan.

*Pyridoxine insufficiency and deficiency*: Pyridoxine insufficiency and deficiency rarely occur alone, but usually are seen with deficiency of the other B complex vitamins. Pyridoxine insufficiency may play a role in carpal tunnel syndrome (CTS); however, research results are mixed at this time.

*Requirement and sources*: The current Recommended Daily Allowance (RDA) is 2 mg/d. Vitamin B6 is highly conserved in the body. Excretion of vitamin B6 and its metabolites rapidly adjusts to changes in the intake of the vitamin. The vitamin B6 requirement rises roughly in proportion to the increase in protein intake and with age.

Vitamin B6 is widely distributed in nature but not in large amounts. The most available sources of the vitamin include liver, kidney, the white meat of chicken, halibut, tuna, English walnuts, soybean flour, navy beans, bananas, and avocados. Helpful sources are yeast, lean beef, egg yolk, whole wheat, and milk.

Fresh milk contains 0.14 mg/8 oz serving. Very little is destroyed in milk during processing, but much is lost when milk is exposed to sunlight for more than a few minutes.

Animal sources of vitamin B6 are less susceptible to loss of the vitamin because of cooking or preserving than are plant sources.

*Causes of deficiency*: In addition to inadequate dietary intake, tropical sprue and alcohol interfere with its absorption. The requirement for vitamin B is increased by oral contraceptives, pregnancy and lactation, excessive alcohol consumption, antitubercular drugs, corticosteroids, hyperthyroidism, and uremia.

Oral supplementation of at least 10 mg/d of vitamin B6 is strongly recommended for those taking oral contraceptive.

During pregnancy and lactation, the requirement for pyridoxine is markedly increased. Obstetricians have used supplemental pyridoxine to combat the nausea and vomiting of early pregnancy for many years. Travell found that one or two intramuscular injections of 100 mg of pyridoxine may promptly terminate these common distressing symptoms of early pregnancy. Vitamin B6 therapy also has provided effective prophylaxis against motion sickness in nonpregnant individuals, both adults and children.

Pyridoxine deficiency is aggravated in alcoholics by

- A reduced dietary intake of the vitamin through substitution of alcohol for food
- Impaired absorption of the natural dietary forms of vitamin B6
- Interference with the conversion of vitamin B6 to the active phosphorylated form by both the alcohol and liver disease

Corticosteroid use increases the need for pyridoxine. Hyperthyroidism increases the need for pyridoxine. Pyridoxine deficiency often occurs in both dialyzed and undialyzed uremic patients.

*Therapy*: Pyridoxine is available over the counter in 10-, 25-, and 50-mg tablets and in larger amounts by prescription. Parenteral pyridoxine hydrochloride is supplied in vials of 10 ml and 30 ml in concentration of 100 mg/ml. A single intramuscular injection of 100 mg of pyridoxine effectively raises the serum level of the vitamin.

A B 50 vitamin supplement contains 50 mg of pyridoxine and is an ample daily dose to protect nearly all individuals from pyridoxine insufficiency. That supplement can be taken indefinitely as an inexpensive form of health insurance.

Doses of 500 mg/d given chronically (6 months or longer) produce a peripheral sensory neuropathy and ataxia. Doses over 100 mg/d are unnecessary. Doses as low as 200 mg/d have produced a sensory neuropathy and constitute a warning against the use of such pharmacologic doses of the vitamin.

*Cobalamin (Vitamin B12) and Folic Acid and their Role in Myofascial Pain Syndromes*

Cobalamin and folic acid are considered together because their metabolism and function are intimately linked. These two essential enzyme cofactors are required:

- For DNA synthesis
  - In erythropoiesis
  - In rapidly dividing cells such as gastrointestinal cells
- For fatty acid synthesis, which is critical for nerve myelin formation

Vitamin B12 and folate insufficiency and deficiency states can be seen in chronic myofascial pain syndromes. However, there is no clear-cut explanation of how they play a role.

A lack of these vitamins reduces blood cell production. The blood cells transport oxygen to muscles, oxygen that is essential for their energy metabolism. A severe local energy crisis exists in the region of the dysfunctional endplates of trigger points. The crisis releases substances that sensitize the local nociceptors, causing pain and local tenderness. This increased sensitization feeds back to increase acetylcholine release from the nerve terminal, further aggravating the trigger point dysfunction.

The role of both vitamin B12 and folic acid on nerve function raises the possibility that these vitamins produce central or peripheral nerve dysfunction that predisposes to altered nerve/muscle junction or motor endplate dysfunction. Vitamin B12 inadequacy or deficiency causes a myelopathy as well as peripheral neuropathy that is less common than that seen with vitamin B12 deficiency. Neuropathy is associated with increased trigger point irritability.

*Functions*: Cobalamins serve numerous essential metabolic functions, including:

1. DNA synthesis (making folate cobalamin essential for normal growth and tissue repair)
   - Regeneration of intrinsic folate, which in turn plays a role in DNA synthesis
   - Transport of folate to and from its storage in cells
   - Fat and carbohydrate metabolism
   - Protein metabolism
   - Reduction of sulfhydryl groups
   - Folic acid functions in DNA synthesis and is critical for the development of the brain and essential for its normal function after birth.

*Cobalamin insufficiency* could lead to

- Nonspecific depression
- Fatigability
- Increased susceptibility to myofascial trigger points
- Exaggerated startle reaction to unexpected noise or touch

*Folate insufficiency* is the most common vitamin inadequacy and causes the following symptoms:

- Increased muscular irritability and susceptibility to myofascial trigger points
- Becoming tired easily, sleeping poorly, and having feelings of discouragement and depression
- Frequently feeling cold and having a reduced basal temperature, similar to that observed in hypothyroid patients

*Cobalamin deficiency* has the greatest impact on the cord and peripheral nerves, whereas folate deficiency is more likely to be associated with mental disorders that affect the intellect.

Deficiency of cobalamin (vitamin B12) can cause

- Megaloblastic anemia (pernicious anemia)
- Neurologic dysfunction leading to degeneration of the spinal cord, loss of vibratory and position sense, weakness and spasticity, as well as peripheral neuropathy
- Gait ataxia and spasticity with weakness producing neuromuscular stress, further predisposing to myofascial trigger point formation
- Diarrhea, sore tongue, and other gastrointestinal (GI) complaints reflecting the disturbance of DNA synthesis
- Constipation
- Fatigue, syncope, personality change, and memory loss
- Dementia, visual loss, and psychosis

*Folic acid deficiency*: Symptoms of folic acid deficiency are as follows:

- Fatigue
- Diffuse muscular pain
- Restless legs
- Megaloblastic anemia
- Depression
- Peripheral sensory loss
- Diarrhea

A disproportionately high percentage of psychiatric patients are folic acid deficient.

*Dependence*: Impairment of one of the metabolic pathways that requires cobalamin or folic acid results in a need for more than the usual amount of the vitamins.

*Sources*: The primary source of cobalamins is from bacteria found in soil, sewage, water, intestine, or rumen. Herbivorous animals depend entirely on microbial sources for their cobalamin. The vitamin is not found in vegetable food sources and is available to humans only from animal food products or supplements. Brewers yeast does not contain cobalamin unless grown on a special cobalamin-containing medium.

Dietary sources of folate are leafy vegetables (foliage), yeast, liver and other organ meats, fresh or fresh frozen uncooked fruit or fruit juice, and lightly cooked fresh green vegetables such as broccoli and asparagus. Although folate is readily available, it is highly susceptible to oxidative destruction due to processing and preparation.

*Causes of insufficiency and deficiency*: There is a complicated chain of events that needs to occur before cobalamin is absorbed into the portal venous blood. Ingested cobalamins have to be freed from their polypeptide linkages in food by gastric acids and gastric intestinal enzymes. Then the freed cobalamin forms complexes with the intrinsic factor produced by GI cells, which then attaches to protein receptors on the villi of the terminal ileum. In the presence of ionic calcium and a pH of about 6, the cobalamin passes through the mucous membrane into the portal venous blood. There it must join the transport protein transcobalamin II, which carries it to the liver.

Causes of insufficiency and deficiency of cobalamin include the following:

- Drug interactions that may reduce serum cobalamin levels.
- Folic acid deficiency, which causes interference in metabolic steps, leading to cobalamin deficiency.
- Drugs, including neomycin, colchicine, *p*-aminosalicylic acid, and slow-release potassium cause insufficiency.
- Chloride, biguanide therapy, and ethanol, which cause malabsorption of cobalamin.
- Ingestion of large doses of vitamin C for long periods.
- Decreased gastric acid and gastric intestinal enzymes cause deficiency

Folic acid deficiency can be caused by:

- Advanced age
- Pregnancy and lactation
- Dietary indiscretion
- Drug abuse, most commonly of alcohol

*Therapy*: Individuals on limited diets of animal foods are at high risk for vitamin B12 deficiency as it is only derived from animal products. Initial replacement of vitamin B12 is by intramuscular administration of 1000 μg of cyanocobalamin weekly. Monthly injections thereafter will usually maintain adequate blood levels of the vitamin. Oral administration should be 500–1000 μg.

As far as folic acid replacement and maintenance are concerned, it is imperative to test vitamin B12 levels before administering folic acid, as high doses of folic acid will aggravate the neurological deficits of vitamin B12. Folic acid will reduce elevated homocysteine levels associated with folic acid deficiency. Reduction of homocysteine levels to the point that there is no increased mortality from cardiac and cerebral thrombosis requires 700–1000 μg (hence 1 mg).

Folic acid absorption is impaired by the simultaneous ingestion of antacids. In Gerwin's experience,[4] fatigue and sleep disturbance improve after 2–4 weeks of folate replacement therapy and reduction in the irritability of myofascial trigger points takes 4–6 weeks.

It is wise to routinely prescribe adequate amounts of vitamin B12 and folic acid together, not just one. They are both water-soluble vitamins, inexpensive, available without prescription, and can be taken orally as a 500-mg tablet of vitamin B12 and a 1-mg tablet of folic acid daily.

### Ascorbic Acid (Vitamin C)

Vitamin C prevents post-exercise soreness or stiffness and prevents capillary fragility.

### Functions

Functions served by vitamin C include the following:

- Collagen synthesis (collagen provides firmness to vessel walls).
- Degradation of amino acids.
- Synthesis of two neurotransmitters.
- It is the most active reducing agent in living tissue.

- Provides a ready source of hydrogen atoms since it is easily oxidized, protecting vital tissues from oxidation damage.
- Helps terminate bouts of diarrhea due to food allergy.
- Decreases toxicity and TrP irritability caused by chronic infection.

### Insufficiency and Deficiency

Smokers, alcoholics, older people, infants fed primarily on cow's milk, food faddists, and psychiatric patients tend to be deficient in vitamin C.

In the U.S. the basic recommended daily allowance is 200 mg/d.

Excellent sources of ascorbic acid that contain more than 100 mg/100 g of raw food are broccoli, brussels sprouts, collard, kale, turnip greens, guava, sweet peppers, and oranges. Individuals with poor health, or under a great deal of stress, require higher doses of the vitamin.

Women taking estrogen or oral contraceptive agents require a 3–10-fold increase as well.

### Dietary Minerals and Trace Elements

Iron, calcium, potassium, and magnesium are needed for normal muscle function, and a deficiency in these increases the irritability of myofascial TrPs.

Iron is essential part of the hemoglobin and myoglobin molecules that transport oxygen to and within the muscle fibers.

Calcium is essential to muscle for the release of acetylcholine at the nerve terminal and for the excitation-contraction mechanism of the actin and myosin filaments.

Potassium is needed for rapid repolarization of the nerve and muscle cell membranes following action potential.

Magnesium is essential for the contractile mechanism of myofilaments.

### Iron

Iron plays the following roles in relation to TrPs:

- Energy production and oxygenation that affects the ability of muscle to meet its energy demands.
- Regulation of hormonal functions like thyroid hormone that again plays a critical role in energy metabolism.
- Iron plays a role in body temperature regulation that may affect both body temperature and the perception of coldness that is often seen in persons with chronic myofascial pain.
- Essential for oxygen transport.
- Required for enzymatic reactions that have to do with tissue respiration, oxidative phosphorylation, porphyrin metabolism, collagen synthesis, and neurotransmitter synthesis and catabolism.

Iron deficiency occurs in several stages:

- Depletion of tissue stores of iron that is detected by serum ferritin levels
- Depletion of essential iron stores associated with metabolic and enzymatic activity
- Deficient erythropoiesis that leads to iron deficiency anemia

Detection of iron insufficiency before anemia develops is most important, because decreased work capacity and impaired energy metabolism may produce a total body incipient "energy crisis" that predisposes to myofascial TrP formation, yet is easily correctable.

Serum ferritin levels assess tissue iron stores. Normal serum ferritin levels are as high as 300 ng/ml. When they reach 20 ng/ml, depletion of tissue stores occurs. Levels of 30–50 ng/ml indicate a need for replacement of iron stores.

*Sources*

Heme iron is easily absorbed, whereas nonheme iron is poorly absorbed. Vitamin C enhances the absorption of nonheme iron. Calcium and phytates can inhibit nonheme and heme iron absorption by 50%. Phytic acids are components of cereal and grains. Vitamin C can overcome the effect of dietary inhibitors to a significant degree.

*Causes of Insufficiency and Deficiency*

Causes of iron insufficiency and deficiency include the following:

- Insufficient dietary intake to replace menstrual blood loss.
- Gastric irritation with microscopic blood loss due to nonsteroidal anti-inflammatory drugs.
- Pernicious anemia.
- Moderate exercise reduces iron stores but increases iron absorption.

*Treatment*

The recommended dosage is 150 mg of iron taken twice daily, or once daily if necessitated by constipation or gastric irritation. This supplement is not to be taken with calcium and dairy, but with vitamin C to increase absorption. Folic acid in a 1-mg dosage lessens the symptom of gastric irritation. Once the serum ferritin level reaches 30–40 ng/ml, a small daily supplement of 12–15 mg (which is commonly found in most multivitamin/mineral preparation) is sufficient. Iron supplementation should always be monitored to avoid excessive iron storage and hemochromatosis. Iron overload can lead to hemochromatosis, ischemic heart disease, and poorer outcome after stroke.

*Calcium*

Optimum calcium intake is as follows:

| | |
|---|---|
| Adolescents and young adults | 1200–1500 mg/d |
| Women ages 25–50 | 1000 mg/d |
| Postmenopausal women on hormone replacement | 1000 mg/d |
| Post menopausal women not on hormone replacement | 1500 mg/d |
| Adult men | 1000 mg/d |

Vitamin D is essential for optimal absorption of calcium.

Calcium is of great interest in myofascial pain responses at the nociceptor cell level through voltage-gated calcium channels.

Calcium supplements have the same bioavailability as calcium supplied by drinking milk.

*Potassium*

The recommended daily allowance for potassium is at least about 2 g. Potassium deficiency aggravates myofascial TrPs, and disturbs function of smooth muscle and cardiac muscle.

Foods rich in potassium are bananas, citrus fruits, potatoes, green leafy vegetables, wheat germ, lentils, nuts, dates, and prunes.

*Magnesium*

Magnesium is the second-most abundant cation in intracellular fluid and is a cofactor for over 300 cellular enzymes to energy metabolism.

Magnesium (Mg) deficiency is unlikely to occur for purely dietary reasons but rather is more likely to occur as a result of malabsorption, fluid and electrolyte losses, renal dysfunction, or malnutrition. Symptoms of Mg deficiency include neuromuscular hyperexcitability with Chvostek and Trosseau signs and seizures, and also weakness and fasciculation. Mg deficiency is often complicated by secondary hypokalemia, which aggravates muscular weakness. Likewise, hypocalcemia is commonly seen in moderate to severe Mg deficiency. Neither the hypokalemia nor the hypocalcemia can be corrected until the low Mg is corrected.

The recommended dietary intake of Mg is 4.5 mg/kg body weight, or about 250–350 mg/d for adults. The optimal Ca/Mg ration is 2:1; otherwise, Mg absorption will be reduced.

## Therapeutic Approach to Nutritional Deficiencies

If a patient fails to respond to a specific myofascial therapy or obtains only temporary relief, vitamin deficiencies must be ruled out as a major contributing cause.

Treatment for either folate deficiency or cobalamin (vitamin B12) deficiency should not be pursued without establishing the level of, or supplementing, the other vitamin. This is due to the fact that their symptoms overlap so widely and they interact so strongly that treatment of one may mask or precipitate a deficiency of the other.

A full evaluation of the total vitamin status of the patient has the following issues and drawbacks:

- The signs and symptoms of vitamin deficiency are overlapping and nonspecific.
- There are individual variations in the daily requirement.
- Multiple causes of inadequacy exist.
- Expense of laboratory tests is high.
- High standards of performance are needed to ensure meaningful results that are reliable.

As a result, complementing the diet is a cost-effective form of health insurance. The following supplementation should be considered:

A complete balance multivitamin/mineral supplement is the best alternative. R.J. Williams in the *Physicians Handbook of Nutritional Science*,[13] recommends ingesting the RDA of water-soluble vitamins several times during the day but below any possible toxic levels. Fat-soluble vitamins, particularly vitamin A, should be taken below toxic levels. The supplement should include close to a recommended daily allowance of the essential minerals.

Another approach is to supplement B vitamins with a balanced mixture of the B-complex rather than individual supplementation. If rapid results are needed, 45 intramuscular injections may be given in addition to oral supplements as follows in a mixed injection:
  - 100 mg each of vitamin B1 and B6
  - 5 mg of folic acid
  - 1 mg of vitamin B12
  - 2 mg of procaine

Finally, vitamin C 500 mg in a timed-release preparation can be given daily. Vitamin C is poorly stored and its dietary intake is commonly inadequate.

## Metabolic and Endocrinological

Hypometabolism, or thyroid inadequacy, describes the condition of someone whose serum levels of thyroid hormones are in the low euthyroid or just below the normal to standard deviation limits. These patients are more susceptible to myofascial TrPs. Commonly cited manifestations of hypothyroidism and hypometabolism are

- Muscle pain
- Stiffness
- Weakness

- Muscle cramps
- Cold intolerance
- Patients who are thin, nervous, and hyperactive
- Constipation more likely than diarrhea
- Dry, rough skin

*Measurement of Thyroid Function*

The newest thyroid function test is the more sensitive thyrotropin (sTSH) assay as reviewed by Klee and Hay. Linear changes in free thyroxin (FT4) concentrations away from an individual's "set-point" for thyroxine result in logarithmic changes in thyrotropin secretion.

Elevated sTSH indicates a primary hypothyroidism or inadequate thyroid hormone replacement therapy. A very low sTSH level of less than 0.1 mlU/L indicates hyperthyroidism, either exogenous or primary.

Free thyroxine (FT4) measurement gives an indication of the severity of the thyroid dysfunction. FT4 is elevated in hyperthyroidism and is low in hypothyroidism. Free triiodothyronine (FT3) is useful in the assessment of hyperthyroidism, and is appropriate assessed when sTSH is low and FT4 is normal.

STSH determinations are not affected by renal or hepatic disease or by estrogen therapy. Pituitary tumors can sometimes produce TSH, and cause hyperthyroidism. Pituitary failure causes secondary hypothyroidism; the low sTSH is accompanied by low FT4. Klee and Hay recommend the following steps in assessing thyroid function: use of a second-generation TSH test that can measure to 0.1 mlU/L of accuracy. If sTSH is normal, no further testing need be done. If sTSH is elevated, which is an indication of hypothyroidism, then both FT and microsomal antibody tests are done to assess the severity of the condition. If sTSH is low, which is an indication of hyperthyroidism (less than 0.3 mlU/L), the FT4 levels are obtained once again to assess the severity of the condition. If FT4 levels are normal, then FT3 is measured. If sTSH is below 0.1-mlU/L, a third-generation sTSH is performed. Laboratories can do this "thyroid cascade"on the initial sample of blood, thereby providing a rapid turnaround time and minimizing patient discomfort and inconvenience.

*Drugs That Can Cause Hypothyroidism*

Drugs in this category are

- Anticonvulsant drugs (phenytoin and carbamazepine)
- Phenobarbital
- Long-term lithium use
- Excess inorganic iodine
- Antiarrhythmic agent amiodarone
- Asthma drug combination elixophyllin-KI

## Hypoglycemia

Hypoglycemia aggravates myofascial TrP activity and reduces or shortens the response to specific treatment. Two kinds of hypoglycemia are generally recognized: fasting and postprandail. However, they both present with the same symptoms.

*Symptoms of Hypoglycemia*

Increased epinephrine causes sweating, trembling, shakiness, a fast heart rate, and a feeling of anxiety. Activation of SCM TrPs may cause headache and dizziness.

Severe hypoglycemia can cause visual disturbances, restlessness, impaired speech, impaired thinking, and sometimes syncope. These symptoms are due to hypoxia.

*Fasting Hypoglycemia*

In a normal person, fasting does not cause hypoglycemia as the liver releases glucose in response to the production of epinephrine from the adrenal medulla. However, for the adrenal medulla to produce epinephrine, it needs stimulation from the anterior pituitary. Liver disease can also impair this mechanism.

*Post-Prandial (Reactive) Hypoglycemia*

Symptoms occur 2–3 h after ingestion of a meal rich in carbohydrates. Large amounts of carbohydrates cause overstimulation of the pancreas and release of excess insulin. The insulin triggers a compensatory epinephrine response. Post-prandial hypoglycemia lasts 15–30 min until it is terminated by the liver's response to an increased epinephrine level.

This type of hypoglycemia is associated with high anxiety levels and is most likely to occur during periods of emotional stress.

When a glucose tolerance test is performed, the results may be more accurate if the patient is active rather than resting in the intervals between blood samples as this stimulation is closer to real life circumstances.

*Fasting Hypoglycemia*

Fasting hypoglycemia appears many hours after eating and tends to persist. It is due to an identifiable organic disease process.

*Post-Prandial Hypoglycemia*

Post-prandial hypoglycemia is secondary to mild diabetes and is most likely to occur between the third and fifth hours of a glucose tolerance test. Diagnosis requires demonstration of the hypoglycemia while the symptoms are present.

*Treatment of Hypoglycemia*

Treatment includes the following:

- Eating small, balanced meals
- Exercise to reduce anxiety
- Elimination of caffeine, alcohol, and nicotine as they stimulate the release of adrenaline

## Gouty Diathesis

Myofascial TrPs are aggravated in patients with hyperuricemia or gout due to an unknown reason. Gout is a disorder of purine metabolism. Elevation of uric acid > 7.0 mg/dl in men and > 6.0 mg/dl in women is an indication of gout. A definite diagnosis of gout is made by identifying uric acid crystals in fluid aspirated from inflamed tissue.

*Psychological Factors*

A number of psychological factors can contribute to perpetuation of myofascial TrPs. Most important, the physician must be careful not to assume that the psychological factors are primary. However, some of the following psychological aspects should be considered:

- Hopelessness
- Depression
- "Good Sport" syndrome
- Psychological and behavioral aspects leading to primary and secondary gain

*Chronic Infection and Infestations*

The following can aggravate myofascial TrPs:

- Persistent viral disease (especially herpes simplex)
- Chronic focus of bacterial infection
- Infestations by certain parasites

The mechanism of aggravation is unknown.

### Other Factors

#### Allergic Rhinitis

Many patients with active myofascial TrPs, who also have active symptoms of allergic rhinitis, have been found to respond only temporarily to specific myofascial therapy. Allergic rhinitis is characterized by episodic sneezing, rhinorrhea, obstruction of the nasal passages, conjunctival and pharyngeal itching, and lacrimation.

#### Impaired Sleep

Impaired or interrupted sleep occurs with greater frequency in patients with more severe myofascial pain syndromes. Moldofsky and Scarisbrick[14] found muscle tenderness and a sense of physical tiredness in the morning in healthy university students when the slow wave non-REM (rapid eye movement) sleep had been disrupted throughout the night. This is a vicious cycle. The painful muscles interrupt sleep, and disrupted sleep can make the muscles more painful.

Anxious and tense patients have trouble falling asleep. Depressed patients are likely to awaken during the night. When during the night does the patient awaken? This information helps to identify the cause. Was the patient chilly or in pain? What was the sleeping position? The position helps to identify what TrPs may be responsible for pain. How does the patient get back to sleep again? Is the lack of sleep at night compensated for by sleep during the day?

#### Treatment

Treatment includes the following:

- Warm bath and/or a glass of milk before retiring.
- Electric blanket or setting thermostat to a level to prevent chills.
- Proper pillow positioning. When neck and shoulder muscles are involved the corner of the pillow can be tucked between the ear or chin and the shoulder to prevent tilting of the head and neck.

## Nerve Impingement

Studies are strongly suggestive that the presence of radiculopathy activates TrPs in the muscles of the involved extremity corresponding to the level of root involvement. The situation is clouded by the fact that TrPs activated and satellites of the original pain of radiculopathy may refer pain in patterns that mimic the radicular pain.

The two conditions may appear as one in the post-disc syndrome but in reality are separate entities. These patients continue to experience pain following a well-performed and truly needed laminectomy. They suffer from continuing activity of myofascial TrPs in muscles that refer pain in much the same distribution as that of the previous radicular pain. Recurrent disc herniation and postoperative scar tissue formation with root compression must be identified and treated, but even in these cases, the pain often comes from myofascial TrP. In the lumbar disc syndrome involving the S1 root, TrPs in the hamstring muscles are commonly the cause of the ongoing pain.

Recognition and inactivation of myofascial TrPs that remained following a successful laminectomy for nerve root compression has provided complete and lasting relief in many patients.

*Screening Laboratory Tests*

The following tests are valuable in the detection of perpetuating factors in patients with chronic myofascial pain.

*Hematologic Profile*

The erythrocyte sedimentation rate (ESR) is normal in uncomplicated MPS. A normal ESR eliminates the possibility of a chronic bacterial infection. When elevated, it is nonspecific and may indicate other conditions such as polymyositis, polymyalgia rheumatica, rheumatoid arthritis, or cancer.

A decreased erythrocyte count, low hemoglobin, and/or microcytosis indicates anemia, which tends to make the muscles hypoxic and increases TrP irritability.

Iron deficiency is identified by a low serum ferritin level.

Anemia can be caused by a folate and/or cobalamin deficiency, each of which additionally increases TrP irritability. An increased corpuscular volume of > 92 fl is suspicious. As it rises from 95 to 100 fl, the likelihood of a folate or a cobalamin deficiency increases.

Eosinophilia may be due to an active allergy or to infestation with an intestinal parasite, such as E. hitoytica or a tapeworm.

An increased proportion of mononuclear cells (> 50%) may occur because of low thyroid function, or due to active infectious mononucleosis or acute viral infection.

*Blood Chemistry Profile*

Increased serum cholesterol can result from decreased thyroid function. Low serum cholesterol may reflect folate deficiency. Elevated levels of uric acid occasionally results in gout. Low serum total calcium suggests a calcium deficiency, but for determination of the adequacy of available calcium a serum ionized calcium measurement is needed. Low serum potassium can cause muscle cramps and perpetuation of TrPs. Elevated fasting blood sugar deserves investigation to rule out diabetes.

*Vitamin Determination*

Serum levels of vitamins B1, B3, B6, B12, folic acid, and vitamin C are enormously valuable in the management of patients with MPS. Values in the lower quartile of normal are highly suspect as perpetuators of myofascial TrPs.

*Thyroid Tests*

TSH measures the adequacy of hormone production by the thyroid gland. When the TSH is low, low T4 levels will identify pituitary failure. The third-generation sTSH test and T3 will evaluate hyperthyroidism, whereas sTSH and free T4 are used to assess the adequacy of thyroid replacement.


## REFERENCES


1. Bonica, J.J., Preface. In *Advances in Neurology*, edited by J.J. Bonica, vol. 4. Raven Press, New York, 1974, p. vii.
2. Cailliet, R., *Low Back Pain Syndrome*, 3rd ed., F.A. Davis Company, Philadelphia, 1977.
3. Cailliet, R., *Soft Tissue Pain and Disability*, F.A. Davis Company, Philadelphia, 1977.
4. Gerwin, R.D., Gevritz, R., Chronic myofascial pain: Iron insufficiency and coldness as risk factors. *J Musculoskeletal Pain* 3:120, 1995.
5. Jensen, I., Nygren, A., Gamberale, F. et al., Coping with long-term musculoskeletal pain and its consequences: is gender a factor? *Pain* 57:167–72, 1994.
6. Kirkaldy-Willis, W.H., Bernard, T.N. Jr., *Managing Low Back Pain*, 4th ed., Churchill Livingstone, New York, 1999.
7. Mense, S., Simmons, D.G., *Muscle Pain: Understanding Its Nature, Diagnosis, and Treatment*, Lippincott Williams & Wilkins, Philadelphia, 2001.
8. Rachilin, E.S., *Myofascial Pain and Firbomyalgia: Trigger Point Management*, Mosby, St. Louis, MO, 2002.

9. Simmons, D.G., Myofascial Pain Syndrome: one term but two concepts. A new understanding (editorial), *J. Musculoskeletal Pain* 3(1):7–13, 1995.

10. Travell, J.G., Simmons, D.G., *Myofascial Pain and Dysfunction: The Trigger Point Manual*, Williams & Wilkins, Baltimore, 1983.

11. Travell, J.G., Simmons, D.G., *Myofascial Pain and Dysfunction: The Trigger Point Manual, Volume 1. Upper Half of Body,* Williams & Wilkins, Baltimore, 1983.

12. Travell, J.G., Simmons, D.G., *Myofascial Pain and Dysfunction: The Trigger Point Manual, Volume 2. The Lower Extremities*, Williams & Wilkins, Baltimore, 1992.

13. Morton, D.J., *The Human Foot: Its Evolution, Physiology and Functional Disorders.* Columbia University Press, New York, 1935.

14. Moldofsky, H., Scarisbrick, P., England, R., Smythe, H. Musculoskeletal Symptoms and non-REM Sleep Disturbance in Patients with "Fibrositis Syndrome" and Health Subjects. *Psychosom. Med.* 37:341–351, 1975.

# 3 Mechanisms of Spinal Pain and Pain Modulation

*James Giordano and Thomas Schultea*

## CONTENTS



## INTRODUCTION

Clinical consideration of back pain syndromes becomes more meaningful upon appreciation of both the epidemiologic and medico-economic impact of such disorders. Recent reports estimate that pain and resultant debilitation from spinal pathologies represent the leading cause of occupational disability among Americans aged 45 or younger,[1] with greater than $16 billion spent in therapeutic intervention(s).[2] A beguiling issue in the management of spinal pain pathologies is the nature of both the provocative disorder and the clinical course of the resultant pain syndrome. Often, the clinical picture is somewhat clouded in that the nature and/or extent of the organic lesion (or apparent lack thereof) is inequitable to the frequency, intensity, and duration of the pain presentation. Thus, while the dogmatic approach of a) assessing and isolating the offending pathology, b) identifying contributory mechanisms and their extent, and c) therapeutically addressing those mechanisms to facilitate recovery and resolution may often be (initially) applied, the relationship of [a] to [b] in the spinal pain patient may not always be linear, clear, or both. This can result in therapeutic inadequacy, diminution of patient compliance, and ultimately inadequate outcomes.

### MECHANISMS OF SPINAL PAIN

### Structural Considerations

In part, the difficulty may be due to the fact that heterogeneous structures and mechanisms can be directly (and indirectly) contributory to spinally generated pain. The nature of the vertebral segments

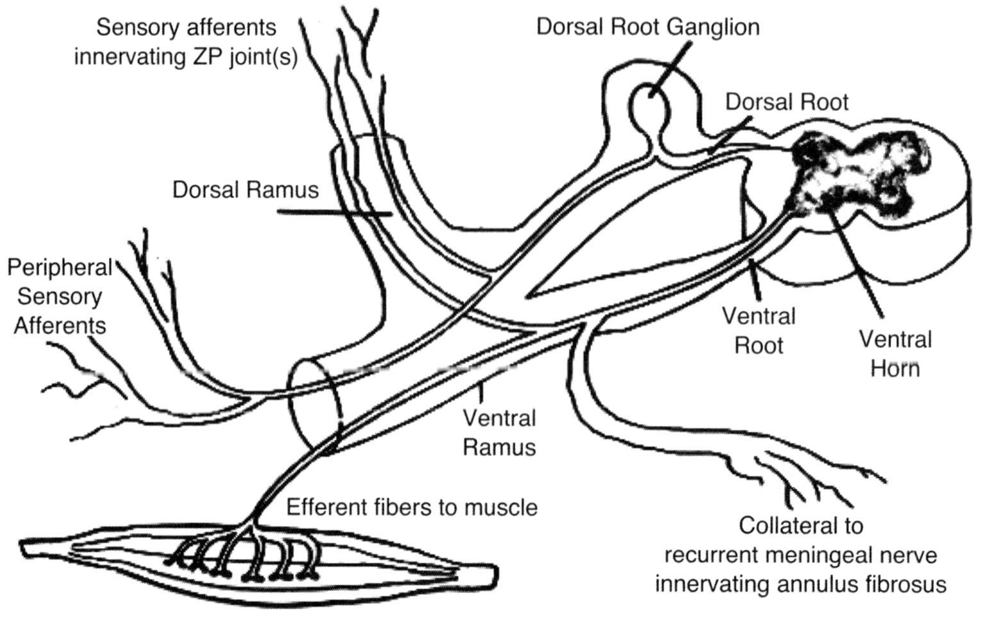


**FIGURE 3.1** Schematic diagram of representative spinal nerve illustrating dorsal and ventral rami and their respective subdivisions and innervations. Details are provided in text. Note that structures are not drawn to scale. (Adapted from Edgar, M.A., Ghadially, J.A., Innervation of the lumbar spine, *Clin. Orthop.* 115:35–41 [1976].)

(i.e., vertebral bodies and processes, zygapohyseal joints, intervertebral discs, ligamentous, tendinous and synovial soft tissue components, as well as the supportive and associated musculature) is such that pathologic change to one component of the system may activate both afferent and efferent neural pathways to affect other components and produce multifocal pain. These structures are heterogeneously innervated by nociceptive and nonnociceptive afferent fibers. Knowledge of this innervation is critical to understanding the causative and correlative effects that insult to components of the system may incur upon nociceptive processing.

At the spinal cord, fibers from the dorsal and ventral zones converge into rootlets that aggregate at the intervertebral foramena (IVF) into the common, or mixed, spinal nerves. The spinal nerves are encased in the sleeves of the dural roots, which are affixed to the perimeter of the IVF by fibrous attachments. At this level, both the epineurium and arachnoid remain continuous with the connective attachments of the dural roots within the IVF. Subsequently, the spinal nerve(s) proceed distally and separate into the dorsal and ventral rami, each containing both sensory and motor fibers. The dorsal ramus divides into two primary divisions. Of these, the medial branch bifurcates into ascending and descending divisions to innervate the capsular and intra-articular zones of the superior and inferior zygapophyseal joints, at each spinal segment, respectively.[3] The medial branch innervates the interspinous ligaments and the interspinalis and mutifidi muscles as well. The lateral branch innervates structures that course laterally to the apophyseal plane, including the longissimi and iliocostalis muscles and thoracolumbar fascia. In the lumbar spinal areas, the lateral branch of the dorsal rami continue through the iliocostalis and longissimi to become the (cutaneous) cluneal nerves subserving afferent input from the lumbar paraspinal region, buttocks, hips, and superior thighs. (See reference 4 for review; refer to Figure 3.1.)

The ventral ramus gives rise to the sinuvertebral, or recurrent meningeal, nerve. This nerve is joined by the gray ramus communicantes of the sympathetic chain in the innervation of posterior longitudinal ligament, periosteum of the posterior border of the vertebral bodies, ventral aspect of the spinal dura mater, epidural and basivertebral vasculature, and the posterolateral aspect of the annulus fibrosus of the intervertebral discs,[5] although Bogduk[6] has reported that the lateral aspect of the annulus fibrosus is primarily innervated by fibers of the ventral ramus directly (see Figure 3.2).

## Receptors and Primary Afferent Typology

It becomes obvious that pathologic events occurring in any or all of the innervated structures could be sufficient to generate afferent discharges of sufficiently high threshold to produce pain sensation(s). These are summarized in Table 3.1.

The question arises as to what events on a cellular or tissue level are capable of generating pain in these innervated structures. Critical to the initiation of the afferent signal is the type and characteristics of the transductive receptors and primary afferents that are present in the tissue(s) involved. The receptors in spinal tissues are heterogeneous; Ruffini-type spray endings are localized within the ZP (zygapophyseal) joint capsules and interspinous and longitudinal ligaments.[7] Together with intraligamentous and tendinous Golgi tendon-type receptors, these specialized structures form the endings of A-beta (and some A-alpha) type afferents, transducing and sensitive to relatively low-threshold inputs of torsion, pressure, and positional distortion. Vater-Paciniform corpuscular endings on A-beta afferents, also sensitive to positional change, are found within the intervertebral joints.[8] Free nerve endings also innervate the majority of spinal structures.[9] Frequently associated with A-beta afferents, the free nerve ending serves as a mechanoreceptor that is engaged by low-moderate intensity torsion and/or compression of the innervated tissue, evoking a rapid discharge capable of some spatial and temporal summation.[10] Characteristically, these receptors and primary afferents do not subtend painful sensations, and their response output is greatest in the low-threshold range. However, it should be noted that if the stimulation is sufficiently intense in either magnitude or duration, the summative capacity of A-beta fibers can engage amplified output of post-synaptic neurons (primarily of the Wide Dynamic Range type) in spinal laminae I and IV to incur noxious sensation.[11]

Free endings are also associated with nociceptive A-delta and C-fibers. A variety of stimuli are capable of directly acting at these endings to produce depolarizing responses in the afferent nociceptive fiber(s). Of note are those substances that are liberated or produced as a consequence of membrane disruption or insult. A rise in $H^+$ ion (and resultant lowering of local pH) and elevation of free interstitial calcium ($Ca^{2+}$) and sodium ($Na^+$) can directly alter the polarity of free nerve endings and initiate a depolarizing response. Biochemical substrates, such as phospholipase-A2, prostaglandins, histamine, and peripheral serotonin, released from insult to the annulus fibrosus are also stimulatory.[12,13] Both ionic alterations and the production of pro-inflammatory and pro-nocisponsive substances are consequences of insult to ligamentous, muscular, and connective tissues (as well as the annulus) of the vertebral segments.[14,15] There is also evidence to suggest that local concentration in $H^+$ ion occurs as a consequence of even short-term neural ischemia.[16] Thus, in addition to provocation caused by inflammatory events, compressive or irritative insult can also release these substances to act at free endings of A-delta and C-fiber afferents of the spinal innervation to contribute to the initiation and development of pain. This latter point is of particular interest in that inflammatory pathologies may evoke afferent discharges to engage compensatory efferent output, resulting in reactive spasm in the ipsi- or contralaterally innervated spinal musculature.[17,18] Similarly, such pathologic events may induce compensatory recruitment of spinal muscular activity to produce aberrant mechanics of posture and gait, resulting in distortion at one or more IVF segments to induce compressive insult and secondary pain provocation at additional spinal nerves.[19,20] Table 3.2 presents those structures that have been empirically demonstrated to be specific foci for the generation of spinal pain. The pathomechanical basis involved of spinal pain is more fully addressed by Francis elsewhere in this volume (Chapter 2).

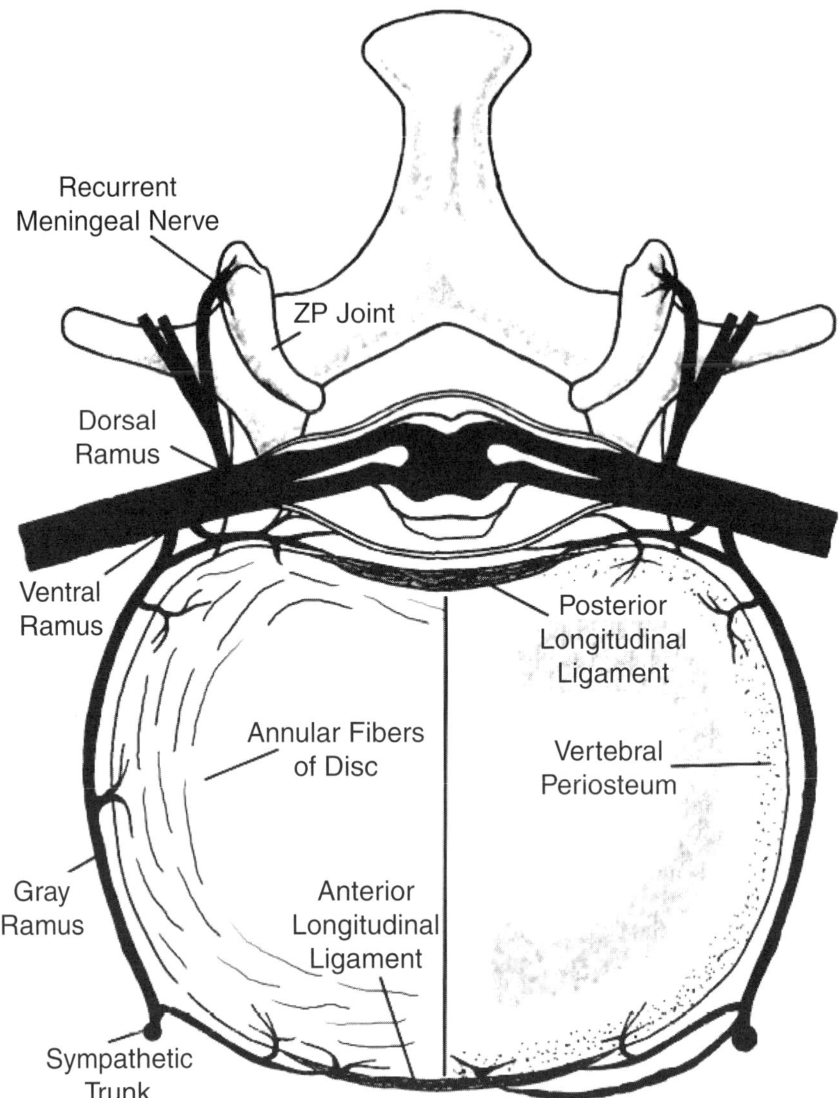


**FIGURE 3.2** Horizontal section of lumbar vertebral segment illustrating innervation of vertebral structures by components of the dorsal and ventral rami. Of note is the innervation of the zygapophyseal joint process(es) by the medial branch of the dorsal ramus. The intervertebral disc is illustrated in the left-hand section of the vertebral segment to illustrate innervation by the recurrent meningeal nerve and sympathetic components of the gray ramus communicantes. The intervertebral disc has been dissected from the right-hand section of the vertebral segment to reveal the underlying periosteum that is innervated by both the medial branch of the dorsal ramus (vertebral arch) and the recurrent meningeal nerve (posterior vertebral body). Refer to Table 2 and text for further detail.

**Primary Nociceptive Afferents**

*A-Delta Fibers*

A-delta fibers are small, myelinated fibers with rapid conduction velocities (5–30 m/sec). The relative majority of A-delta fibers innervating spinal tissues are mechanosensitive. These are activated by high-threshold mechanical input (e.g., stretch, pressure, etc., caused by physical trauma or extraphysiologic deviations of movement or posture), with a relatively linear and asymptotic

**TABLE 3.1**

| Type | Accessory Structure(s) | Location | Function |
|---|---|---|---|
| Free nerve end | None | Found in all basic tissues | Nociception, thermoreception, and mechanoreception |
| Pacinian corpuscle | Concentric rings of epithelial cells interlaced with fluid | Subcutaneous and other connective tissues | Rapidly adapt for response to vibration |
| Ruffini ending | Spindle-shaped capsule traversed with longitudinal collagen fibers | Subcutaneous and other connective tissues | Slowly adapt for response to squeezing |
| Meissner's corpuscle | Elongated capsule surrounding layers of epithelial cells | Dermal papilla of hairless skin | Rapidly adapt for response to touch |
| Neuromuscular spindle | Encapsulated, modified small diameter striated muscle cells | Intertwined among striated muscle cells | Conduct muscle stretch to the CNS |
| Neurotendonous organ | Encapsulated, small diameter collagen fibers | Within tendons at the myoneural junction | Conduct tendon stretch to the CNS |

**TABLE 3.2**
**Possible Sites of Spinal Pain Generation**

| Structure | Innervation |
|---|---|
| Zygapophyseal joints | Medial branch, dorsal ramus |
| Periosteum of vertebral arch | Medial branch, dorsal ramus |
| Spinous and transverse ligaments | Medial branch, dorsal ramus |
| Ligamentum flavum | Medial branch, dorsal ramus |
| Deep paraspinal musculature | Medial branch, dorsal ramus |
| Intermediate and superficial musculature | Lateral branch, dorsal ramus |
| Skin | Lateral branch, dorsal ramus (cuneal nerve) |
| Periosteum of posterior vertebral body | Recurrent meningeal nerve |
| Posterior annulus fibrosus of disc | Recurrent meningeal nerve |
| Internal and basivertebral veins | Recurrent meningeal nerve |
| Anterior dura mater | Recurrent meningeal nerve |
| Posterior longitudinal ligament | Recurrent meningeal nerve |
| Anterior/lateral annulus fibrosis | Sympathetic trunk and gray ramus |
| Anterior longitudinal ligament | Sympathetic trunk and gray ramus |

response pattern to increasing intensities of input.[21,22] In deep spinal tissue proximal to vertebral structures, there is a minority of thermosponsive A-delta fibers, engaged by noxious heat in excess of 45°C and cold temperatures below 10°–20°. Both mechano- and thermosensitive A-delta fibers have small, punctate receptive fields; rapid firing rate; and brief on–off characteristics that appear to subserve the acute, well-defined sensory qualities attributable to A-delta–mediated pain.[21]

*C-Fibers*

Unlike A-delta fibers, C-fibers are unmyelinated (with resultant slower conductance velocities in the range of 0.25–1.5 m/sec), with broad, overlapping receptive fields. C-fibers are polymodally responsive, stimulated by high-threshold mechanical, thermal, and chemical input. C-fibers also can be cross-sensitized, primarily by chemical stimulation, to respond to lower threshold (frequently nonnoxious) mechanical and/or thermal input. C-fiber responses are spatially and temporally summative, and often are accompanied by significant volleys of independent, durable afterdischarges.[23] Characteristically, C-fibers are engaged by the consequences of tissue disruption, and reflect a reaction to substantive tissue injury. However, it should be noted that once sensitized, C-fiber activity can occur spontaneously, even in the absence of a discriminable organic insult. Similarly, with continued activation, C-fibers may release their principal peptide neurotransmitter, Substance-P (Subs-P), antidromically from their free endings into the tissues innervated.[24] A potent vasodilator, this retrogradely released Subs-P promotes local microedema and extravasation of several biochemical mediators of the inflammatory and nociceptive response (e.g., prostaglandins, bradykinin, serotonin, cytokines) to produce neurogenic inflammation (see Figure 3.3).[25]

Such neurogenic inflammation could occur as a consequence of any stimulus that provokes ongoing C-fiber–mediated activity, including micro- or macrotears of the annulus fibrosus (thus releasing products of the arachidonic acid cascade onto C-fiber free endings),[12] compressive irritation or ischemia (caused by disruption or distortion of the IVF or extrusion of discal material onto nerve),[13,14] and/or trauma and inflammation of the innervated tissue (e.g., ligamentous tears, erosive or distortive arthroses of the ZP joint(s)[13–20] (see Table 3.2).

## Neurochemistry of Spinal Pain Transmission

The chemistry of synaptic transmission between primary spinal nociceptive afferents and second-order, post-synaptic neurons of the spinal dorsal horn is also contributory to the properties of A-delta- and C-fiber–mediated pain. Both A-delta and C-fibers release the 11 amino acid peptide Subs-P that post-synaptically binds to neurokinin-1 (NK-1) receptors. With persistent activation, NK-1 receptors can engage second-messenger–mediated activity of several protein kinases to affect both transcriptional and translation processes within the second-order neurons. The alteration of functional and structural proteins in these neurons may facilitate synaptic efficacy and "remodel" the organization of these repetitively active nociceptive circuits.[26]

In addition to Subs-P, C-fibers also release the excitatory amino acid glutamate that initially binds to post-synaptic AMPA (alpha amino 3-hydroxy–5-methyl isoxazole proprionic acid) receptors, to produce a rapid, excitatory response. With continued release of glutamate, AMPA-receptor activity induces a change in intracellular $Na^+$ concentration to alter magnesium-dependent activation of a second binding site, the NMDA (N-methyl D-aspartate) receptor. Prolonged activation of NMDA receptors can lead to enhancement of $Ca^{2+}$-dependent neuronal excitation and may be responsible for a component of spontaneous activity within the spinal pain pathway.[27]

The relevance of this neurochemistry is that the cascade of events leading to sensitization and spontaneous activity within the nociceptive neuraxis (i.e., neurogenic pain) may be divertable through early and prudent intervention. This could be achieved using pharmacologic agents that specifically target these substrates and/or by the use of nonpharmacologic techniques that are aimed at subverting the pain process early in its generation.

### Second-Order Afferents

Both A-delta and C-fiber afferents project to the superficial dorsal horn of the spinal cord and synaptically contact two populations of second-order afferents. The first, nociceptive-specific (NS) neurons, are explicit to the nomenclature, specific for the processing of pain. These are primarily located in Rexed's laminae I and II, with a smaller number found in lamina V.[28] NS neurons function to localize and discriminate properties of the pain stimulus (e.g., bodily region, stimulus type and perhaps intensity; see reference 29). The second type of spinal afferent is the wide dynamic range (WDR) neuron. Located in lamina I, II, V, and VI, these cells also receive input from nonnociceptive (A-beta) afferents.[30] Direct stimulation of WDR units alone produces sensations of flutter, pressure, itch, and vibration that vary in intensity from mild to noxious, and it appears that WDR cells

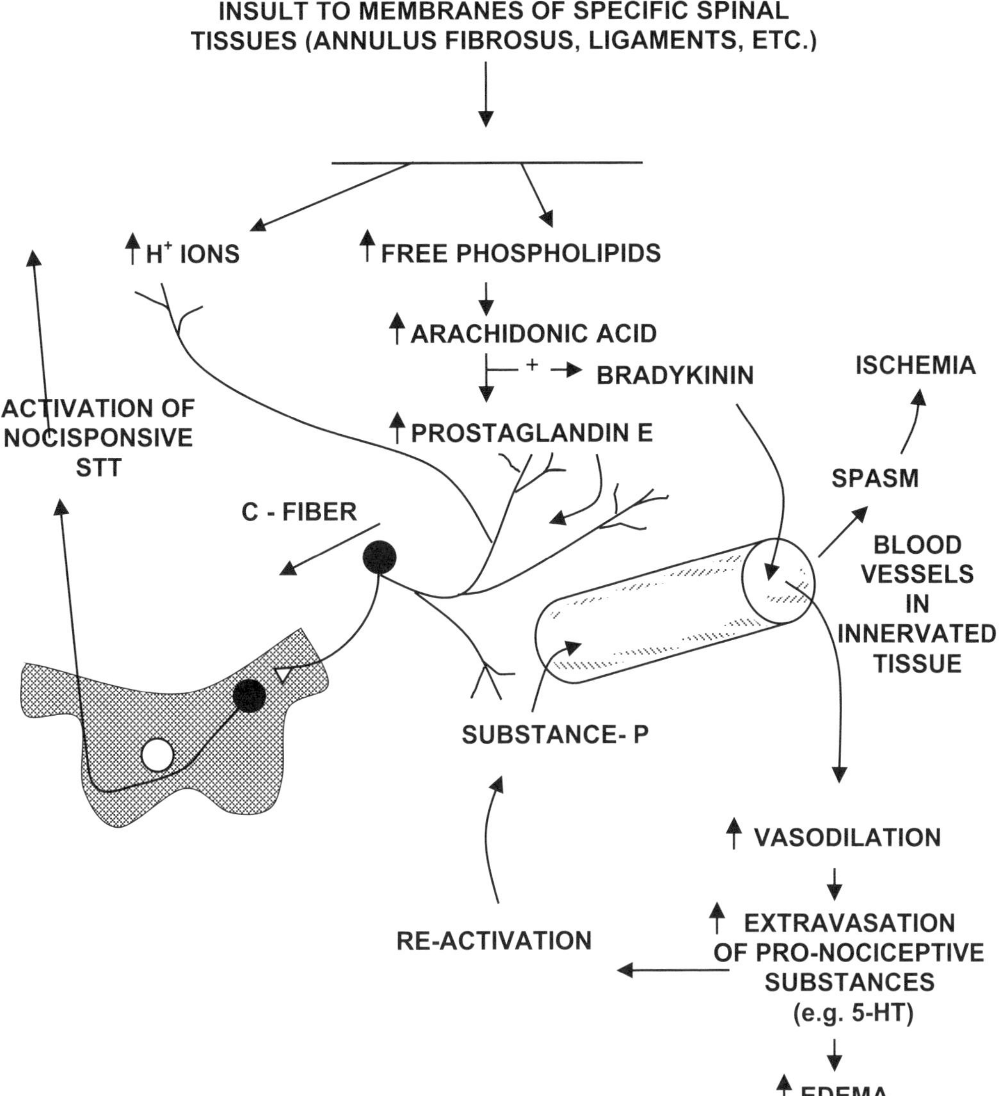


**FIGURE 3.3** Schematic diagram of processes involved in neurogenic inflammation. Insult to membranes of spinal structures causes the release of free phospholipids that induce activity of phospholipase A2 (PLA2) to catalyze the formation of arachidonic acid. Products of the arachidonic acid cascade catalyzed by induced-cyclooxgenase-2 include the unstable prostaglandins, which together with bradykinin are vasodilatory to the local vasculature. In addition, PLA2, bradykinin, and H⁺ ion are directly stimulatory to C-fiber afferents innervating the tissue. Activated C-fibers antidromically release Substance-P into the peripheral microenvironment, exerting potent vasodilatory effects, promoting the extravasation of pro-inflammatory and pro-nociceptive substances such as blood-borne serotonin (5-HT) and thus potentiating the inflammatory-pain cycle (details in text).

function to discriminate stimulus intensity along a sensory continuum from innocuous to painful. Characteristically, the greater the intensity of the stimulus, the greater the number and duration of the WDR units' firing.[31] Thus, although WDR neurons are capable of responding to noxious stimuli, it appears that the quantitative and qualitative responses of both NS and WDR units are important for the complete sensory experience of pain. Additionally, the prolonged activation of WDR units by C-fibers often contributes unusual sensations (e.g., itch, tingling, etc.) to the overall constellation of chronic and neurogenic pain.[23]

## Ascending Pain Pathways: Anterolateral System

The anterolateral column contains neo- and paleospinothalamic ascending pathways, both of which are relatively specific for the transmission of pain impulses. The predominance of the neospinothalamic tract (NSTT) is activated by Aδ-fiber afferents of dorsal root ganglia neurons, which synapse directly with neurons of Rexed's lamina IV & V (nucleus Proprius) primarily, but also apparently neurons of Rexed's lamina I (dorsomarginal nucleus). To a lesser extent, C-fibers terminate on interneurons of lamina II and those interneurons synapse with laminae I and V. Second-order neurons for pain found in these laminae decussate in the anterior white commissure and ascend contralaterally to primarily the caudal part of the ventral posterior lateral nucleus (VPLc) of the thalamus.[31,32] The neospinothalamic tract is mildly somatotopically organized such that the lateral part contains stimuli from sacral and lumbar receptors and the medial part contains stimuli from thoracic and cervical receptors. The posterior portion of the tract contains primarily pain fibers while the anterior part contains primarily thermal fibers. This tract serves to relay properties of stimulus modality (i.e., heat, cold, pressure, irritation, pain, tickling). In contrast, the paleospinothalamic tract (PSTT) projects to several nonthalamic regions that are involved in processing and modulating the pain signal. The PSTT can be further divided into spinothalamic, spinoreticular, and spinotectal pathways based on the anatomical sites to which the specific ascending fibers project.[33]

The PSTT is activated by C-fiber afferents of dorsal root ganglia neurons and projects to the thalamus, but unlike the NSTT, neurons of the PSTT terminate in the midline and intralaminar thalamic (nuclei centralis lateralis and medialis dorsalis) nuclear groups. This heterogeneous projection within the thalamus may subserve a sensory integrative function that imparts additional qualitative and quantitative characteristics to the incoming pain sensations and may subsequently activate regions of the cortex in sensory processing and evoke behavioral responses.

The spinoreticular pathway is activated by C-fiber afferents of dorsal root ganglia neurons and projects to sites within the brain-stem reticular formation, including the raphe nuclei and the medullary and pontine reticular formation nuclei (reticularis gigantocellularis and para gigantocellularis). These brain-stem nuclei respond to PSTT input by altering the synthesis and release of serotonin (5-HT) and norepinephrine (NE), respectively. Discrete 5-HT and NE pathways project to numerous areas of the central nervous system, where they modulate a variety of physiologic and behavioral functions. 5-HT and NE circuits that descend in the spinal cord modify afferent pain signals. Ascending 5-HT and NE pathways project to numerous regions in the brain. In the hypothalamus, 5-HT and NE synergistically regulate neuroendocrine functions. 5-HT and NE pathways to limbic and forebrain structures work in concert to mediate mood, emotion, and cognition.

The spinotectal (Spinomesencephalic) pathway is activated by C-fiber afferents of dorsal root ganglia neurons and projects to the midbrain superior colliculus (SC) and periaqueductal gray (PAG) area. Neurons of the superficial layer of the SC contribute to an extrageniculate visual pathway, terminating on the pulvinar thalamic nucleus, and participate in turning the eyes toward the site of pain. Nerve cells of PAG surrounding the cerebral aqueduct are rich in opioid peptides and receptors. This site appears to be primary for the initiation of opioid-mediated pain control, as PSTT activation of these neurons can evoke a release of several opioid peptides and amplify serotonergic and noradrenergic pain modulation at descending pathways in the spinal cord. There are also connections with the midbrain central gray area, hypothalamus, and limbic forebrain. It is thought that activation of these neural axes is responsible for the aversive and frightening emotional responses that often accompany chronic pain.[34,35]

Together, the NSTT and PSTT provide connections to the thalamus and extra-thalamic nuclei that modify the effects of the pain signal and initiate perceptual responses to pain that are directed by emotion, memory, and cognition.

## Mechanisms of Endogenous Pain Modulation

The interaction between painful stimuli emanating from several possible spinal structures (refer to Table 3.2) and the sensory experience of these events is mediated by heterogeneous systems that are capable of modulating pain at various levels of the neuraxis. Efferent opioid, monoaminergic, and hormonal systems function to selectively modify activity in pain transmitting pathways. The early work of Melzack and Wall[36] proposed that these systems function as a series of neurological "gates" in the transmission of painful impulses within the spinal cord, spinothalamic tracts and at supratentorial levels.

The therapeutic goal is to either 1) reduce the transmission of noxious afferent impulses by directly affecting the factors that provoke nocisponsive discharges and/or 2) to engage one or more of the antinociceptive efferent systems to amplify endogenous pain modulation. Clinically, this may become increasingly difficult as the frequency, duration, and intensity of multiple nocisponsive inputs increase and the efficacy of these modulatory mechanisms becomes inadequate. Thus, progressive activation of these nociceptive afferent pathways by suprathreshold noxious stimulation and/or sensitization of afferent substrates can overcome gating mechanisms and thereby fortify the pain signal leading to the initiation and maintenance of chronic (i.e., Type II) or neurogenic (i.e., Type III) spinal pain syndromes.

### Supraspinal Mechanisms

### Midbrain Periaqueductal and Periventricular Gray Mechanisms

The midbrain periaqueductal (PAG) and periventricular gray (PVG) regions are rich in opioid neurons. These neurons receive input from the paleospinothalamic tract, as well as other, supraspinal sites (see Figure 3.4). Activation of these neurons evokes the release of leucine- and methionine-enkephalins; alpha-, beta- and gamma-endorphins, and a unique family of opioids known as the nociceptins (previously called the orphanins). Opioid neurons of the PA/PVG project to the hypothalamus and form reciprocal connections with the terminals of the spinothalamic tract.[37] Opioids modulate hypothalamic neuroendocrine function, and can regulate levels of the hormonal precursor molecule, pro-opiomelanocortin (POMC). This is produced and released at the hypothalamic median eminence, and is the substrate from which corticotropic hormone and endorphin species are enzymatically cleaved. This appears to be an important mechanism through which changes induced by pain (and stress) in opioid chemistry are capable of exerting broad effects on endocrine status, immune reactivity, and physiologic status.[38]

Of major interest, however, are the connections between the midbrain gray and the brain stem. An inhibitory polysynaptic circuitry exists through which serotonin (5-HT) and norepinephrine (NE) neurons of the brainstem are tonically regulated by inhibitory gamma amino-butyric acid (GABA)-containing interneurons from the posterior midbrain gray. Opioid neurons of the PAG/PVG form synaptic contacts with these GABA neurons; nociceptive impulses from the paleospinothalamic tract evoke the release of opioids from the PAG/PVG that act at mu receptors on GABA interneurons, thereby suppressing GABA release, disinhibiting output of brain-stem monoaminergic systems and ultimately potentiating the release of 5-HT and/or NE from descending spinal pathways in a centrifugal analgesia (see reference 39; as discussed below).

In addition to spinal input to the midbrain gray, projections from the cortex, several limbic structures, and the hypothalamus to the PA/PVG have been identified.[40] These strongly support a role for cognitive, emotive, and homeostatic influences on centrifugal pain control (refer to Figure 3.4).

### Descending Bulbospinal Modulation

Nociceptive fibers of the paleospinothalamic tract project to several sites in the brain stem that function in pain control. Cell bodies of monoaminergic neurons that produce 5-HT are located in the medullary raphe nuclei; NE neurons are located in the pontine gigantocellular/paragigantocellular (NRGC/NRpG) nuclei (also known as the loci ceruleus and subceruleus, respectively). Axonal projections from these nuclei descend in the dorsal spinal cord within a discrete pathway known

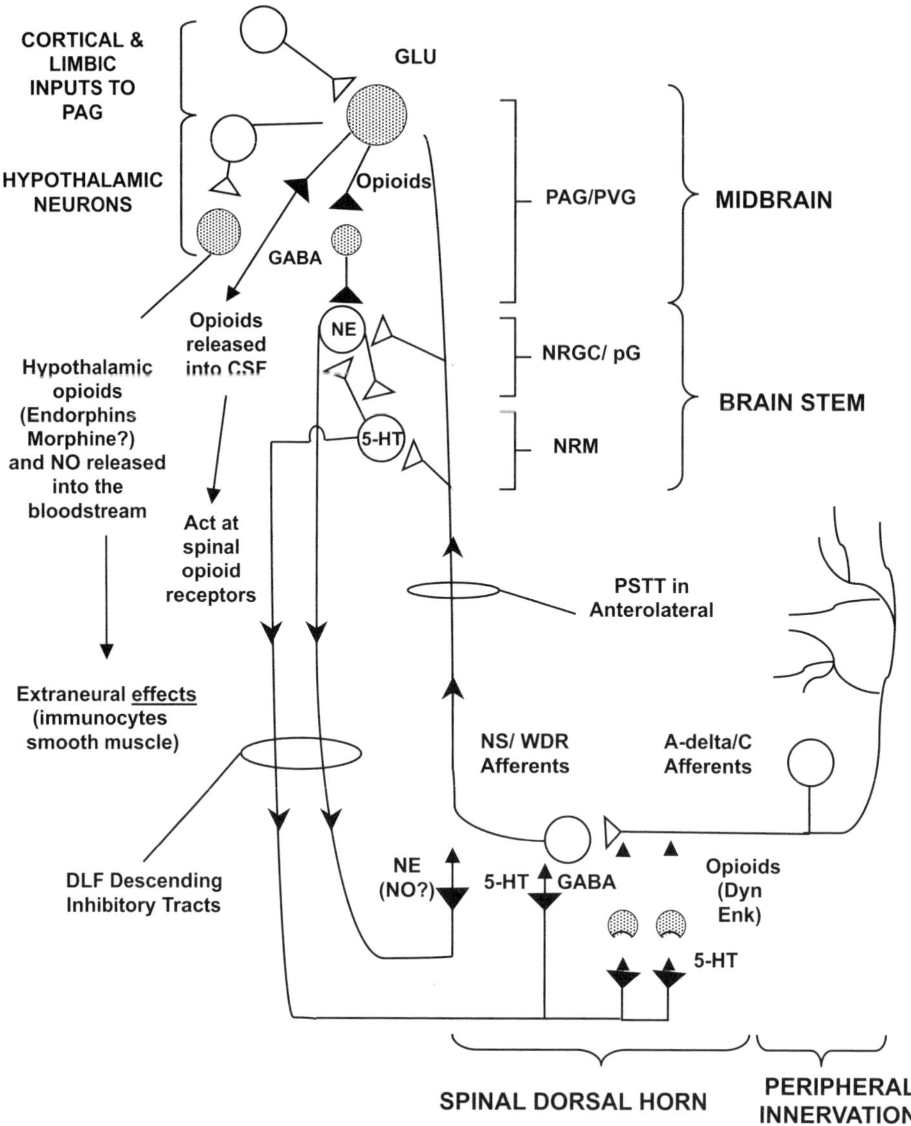


**FIGURE 3.4** Diagrammatic depiction of substrates involved in supraspinally mediated pain modulation. Fibers from the PSTT project to the brain-stem serotonergic nucleus raphe magnus and noradrenergic cerulear nuclei (NRGC/NRpG). Fibers from these sites descend in the dorsolateral funiculi to form synaptic contact upon primary- and second-order nocisponsive afferents in the superficial dorsal horn of the spinal cord. Serotonergic tracts also activate populations of inhibitory opioid and GABAergic spinal interneurons to suppress nociceptive transmission. The output of these brain-stem nuclei can be centrifugally facilitated by opioid mechanisms from the midbrain periaqueductal and periventricular grey (PAG/PVG) regions. Hypothalamic and cortical/limbic influences on the midbrain gray can potentiate centrifugal pain modulation. Additionally, opioid peptides (perhaps including endogenous morphine) released from the PAG/PVG and hypothalamus can exert pain modulatory and physiologic effects through neural and extra-neural action via the CSF or bloodstream, respectively. *Abbreviations:* DLF = dorsolateral funiculus; Dyn = dynorphin; Enk enkephalin; GABA = gamma aminobutyric acid; GLU = glutamate; 5-HT = serotonin; NE = norepinephrine; NO = nitric oxide; NRGC/pG = cerulear/subcerulear nuclei; NRM = nucleus raphe magnus; NS/WDR = nociceptive specific/wide dynamic range second-order neurons; PAG/PVG = periaqueductal/periventricular gray; PSTT = paleospinothalamic tract. (Note: Open connections represent excitatory synapses; shaded connections represent inhibitory synapses.)

**TABLE 3.3**
**Supraspinal Substrates of Pain Modulation**

| Anatomic Site | Neurochemistry |
| --- | --- |
| Midbrain periaqueductal/periventricular gray | *Opioids*: Facilitation of bulbospinal analgesia and centrifugal noxious inhibitory control |
| | Direct release of opoids into CSF |
| Raphe nuclei: Descending raphe-spinal system | *Serotonin (5-HT)*: Inhibition of primary- and second-order afferents directly and through engagement of inhibitory spinal interneurons. |
| NRGC/NRpG: Descending ceruleo-spinal system | *Norepinephrine (NE)*: Direct inhibition of primary and second-order afferents |
| | *Nitric oxide (NO):* Possible facilitation of NE and/or opioid-mediated inhibitory effects |

as the dorsolateral funiculus, and form multiple synaptic contacts with neurons in laminae I, II, IV, and V of the dorsal horn. These contacts include terminals of primary afferents (primarily C-fibers), cell bodies of second-order NS and WDR neurons, and opioid and GABAergic interneurons.[41] While the release of NE appears to inhibit the firing of primary- and second-order afferents directly, 5-HT released within the dorsal horn appears to both directly reduce nocisponsive afferent discharges and may engage opioid- or GABA-mediated inhibition (see reference 42; refer to Figure 3.4).

There appears to be some stimulus-specificity involved in the differential engagement of 5-HT or NE-based pain modulation, although stimulus intensity and duration may also play a role in determining whether one or both descending systems are activated.[43,44] Our recent investigations indicate that moderate mechanical stimulation (of both A-delta and C-fibers, as well as moderate to high velocity stimulation of A-beta mechanoreceptor afferents) evokes a substantive discharge of NE bulbospinal neurons. In addition, studies suggest that nitric oxide (NO) may be released (or co-released) from noradrenergic terminals.[45,46] Although the exact function of NO remains unknown, there is speculation that it may facilitate NE effects, regulate the production and release of pro-inflammatory cytokines, and may modulate opioid-receptor mediated (antinociceptive and perhaps immunologic) effects on a molecular level.[46] The substrates involved in centrifugal and bulbospinal analgesia are presented in Table 3.3.

## Spinal Mechanisms

### Segmental Pain Modulation

Significant pain processing occurs at the focal and/or segmental levels within the spinal cord. Initially, the neurophysiologic characteristics of nocisponsive A-delta and, subsequently, C-fibers serve as a barrier to prevent transmission of noxious stimuli that is less than their firing threshold value. Thus, stimuli that cannot sufficiently generate a response in high-threshold nociceptive afferent fibers do not activate the pain circuitry and are not interpreted as pain. Such local modulation is limited, however, as the extent and duration of tissue insult increase. This becomes an important factor in chronic, or Type-II pain, in which the tissue damage is sufficient to produce chemical substrates in concentrations that evoke continued C-fiber activation.

One of the primary substrates in spinal pain processing is dynorphin interneurons that are located in the superficial laminae of the dorsal horn. These form reciprocal synaptic contacts with A-delta and C-fiber primary afferents, as well as contacting NS and some WDR second-order units. Dynorphinergic neurons are activated by Subs-P, glutamate, and calcitonin gene related peptide (CGRP) released from primary afferents, both by direct polysynaptic contact and by perfusion of these chemicals into the local neural microenvironment. Dynorphin acts at post-synaptic kappa

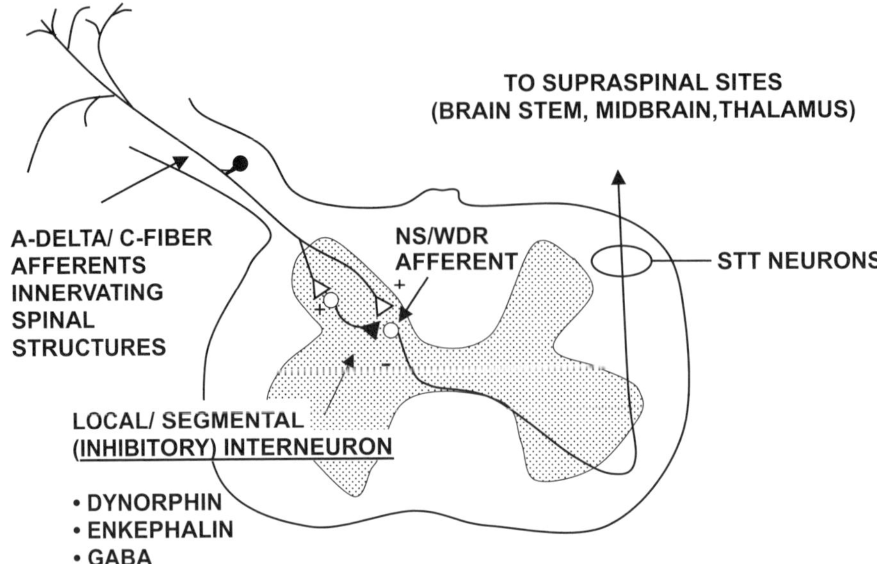



**FIGURE 3.5** Local/segmental pain modulation mediated by activation of opioid or GABAergic interneurons in the dorsal horn of the spinal cord. Pools of enkephalinergic, dynorphinergic and GABAergic interneurons are driven by afferent A-delta and C-fibers and can suppress firing of second-order NS and WDR neurons of the STT. These interneurons may also be engaged by descending serotonergic fibers from the raphe-spinal pathway (refer also to Figure 3.4; details in text). *Abbreviations:* GABA = gamma aminobutyric acid; NS = nociceptive specific neurons; STT = spinothalamic tract; WDR = wide dynamic range neurons. (Note: Open connections represent excitatory synapses; shaded connections represent inhibitory synapses.)

opioid receptors located on primary C-fiber afferents and second-order neurons, to inhibit their firing.[47] Multiple synaptic contacts in the dorsal horn also exist between enkephalin containing neurons and second-order nocisponsive afferents. Enkephalin acts at mu and delta opioid receptors on NS and WDR neurons to produce segmental or transsegmental analgesia.[48] Additionally, enkephalins, and perhaps endorphins, released into the cerebrospinal fluid (CSF) from opioid neurons of midbrain PAG and PVG may diffuse from the CSF to act at delta and mu receptors, respectively, to inhibit transmission in nocisponsive neurons.[49,50]

Interneurons that release the inhibitory transmitter GABA are also located in the dorsal spinal cord, and modulate the transmission of nociceptive signals at both primary- and second-order afferent neurons.[51] The amino acid glycine may be co-released from GABA and/or dynorphin neurons to facilitate this inhibition (refer to Figure 3.5). Table 3.4 summarizes the anatomic and chemical basis of spinal pain modulation.

Previous work from our group has shown that these dynorphin, enkephalin, and GABAergic spinal interneurons can be also be driven by 5-HT released at the terminals of descending bulbospinal fibers projecting from the raphe nuclei, as previously described (see reference 42; see also Figure 3.5).

*Dorsal Columnar Mediation*

Discussion of mechanisms that exert pain modulatory effects within the spinal neuraxis must also address the role of mechanoreceptor stimulation of the dorsal columnar/medial lemniscal pathway. Low- and moderate-threshold mechanosponsive A-beta afferents appear to exert suppressive control over certain populations of WDR and NS second-order afferents that are driven by A-delta and, to a lesser extent, C-fibers.[52] There is some overlap of the synaptic fields of A-beta type mechanoreceptors with inhibitory interneurons that form synaptic contacts with spinothalamic tract neurons.[53] Brief, low-level mechanoreceptor activation can engage these interneurons to suppress second-order

## TABLE 3.4
## Spinal Substrates of Pain Modulation

| Anatomic Site | Neurochemistry |
| --- | --- |
| Interneurons in superficial dorsal horn | Dynorphin: Kappa opioid receptor-mediated inhibition of primary- and second-order afferents. |
| Interneurons in superficial dorsal horn | Enkephalin(s): Mu- and delta opioid receptor mediated inhibition of second-order afferents. |
| Interneurons in superficial dorsal horn | GABA: Inhibition of second-order afferents. |

*Note:* These interneurons can be driven by A-delta/C-fiber activation in recurrent inhibition and/or can be stimulated by serotonin (5-HT), released from raphe-spinal efferents, that acts at 5-HT3 receptors on these interneurons.

STT cell firing within the dorsal horn.[54] In addition, both the dorsal columnar/medial lemniscal pathway and STT project to the ventroposterolateral, ventromedial, and pulvinar thalamic areas.[54]

### Ascending Pain Pathways: Posterior System

Mechanoreceptor A afferent fibers enter the vertebral canal in the medial dorsal root and form collaterals that terminate in 1) the inferior medulla, and 2) the dorsal horn of the spinal gray. Collaterals destined for the medulla ascend in the posterior funiculus (posterior column) to terminate in the nucleus gracilis and cuneatus. Axons of second-order neurons located in these nuclei decussate as internal arcuate fibers to form the contralateral medial lemniscus, which ascends through the central pons and midbrain to the caudal part of the ventral posterior lateral nucleus (VPLc) of the thalamus. Axons from VPLc terminate in the primary somesthetic cortex, Brodmann's areas 3,1, and 2, and are responsible for modality perception. Collaterals to the dorsal horn terminate in primarily in lamina IV.

Following inflammation, upregulation of nerve growth factor in the inflamed tissue results in transcription changes in A fiber neurons, which begin producing substance P and CGRP (substances usually only produced by C and A delta fibers). In addition, A collaterals, which normally terminate in lamina IV of the dorsal horn, may invade lamina II, where they interact with second-order pain pathway neurons. Lamina II neurons now receive nonnoxious stimuli, which may be misinterpreted as noxious resulting in allodynia.[55,56]

VPL axons may share intranuclear as well as internuclear collaterals with the intralaminar and midline nuclei of the thalamus, creating the possibility for thalamic misinterpretation of nonnoxious stimuli and resulting in stimuli conducted in the posterior funiculus being interpreted as painful.[57,58]

Further, it has been reported that a pathway in the medial part of the posterior column conveys nociceptive signals from pelvic visceral organs.[59,60] The precise location of this pathway has not been determined. However, the possible existence of such a pathway seems to be supported by recorded symptoms related to transection of the spinothalamic tract resulting in anesthesia of the body wall but not the viscera.[33]

### Hormonal Mechanisms

While the neural mechanisms represent critical components of pain control, several hormonal systems are also capable of exerting powerful pain modulatory effects. Hypothalamic corticotropin releasing factor (CRF) and pituitary adrenocorticotropic hormone (ACTH) have both been shown to produce a moderate level of analgesia. A component of this analgesia is opioid dependent, suggesting that part of the action of ACTH may be to mediate the stress response while another might involve feedback induction of synthesis and release of its parent metabolite, pro-opiomelanocortin (POMC).[61] This would lead to the increased production of substances (i.e., ACTH and opioids) that mediate enhanced responses to both stress and pain.[62] A role for centrally released NO has been postulated in this neuroendocrine axis as well. Nitric oxide levels in the hypothalamic median eminence steadily increase with exposure to opioids (following activation of the PA/PVG) and norepinephrine (e.g., released through NE brainstem-hypothalamic circuitry consequential to pain and perhaps moderate mechanoreceptor-induced activation of the brainstem). Nitric oxide induces vasodilation within the median eminence, leading to increased hypothalamic neurosecretion of CRF, which acts at the pituitary to release ACTH.[63] This pattern may be phasic, with changing levels of ACTH affecting adrenally mediated stress responses (i.e., during the rise phase) and evoking production of analgesic (and immunomodulatory) opioids through POMC induction (i.e., during the trough phase). Both acute and chronic pain can induce sympathetic neural activation, both by engaging sympathetic innervation of spinal structures and by evoking a more generalized autonomic response.[64] Such sympathetic stimulation of chromaffin cells of the adrenal medulla evokes the release of enkephalins directly into the bloodstream to produce analgesia mediated by multiple subtypes of mu and delta opioid receptors heterogeneously distributed throughout both the central and peripheral nervous systems and in several nonneural tissues.[65]

The differential activation of one or more of these analgesic systems may rely, at least in part, on the type of stimulus (e.g., characteristics of the pain stimulus or intensity, frequency or duration of mechanoreceptor activity), its quality and quantity, as well as its somatotopic location (e.g., lumbar, thoracic, or cervical segments of the spine, as well the possibility for peripherally evoked engagement).[43]

The involvement of the pain transmitting and modulating neuraxes provides a vital link between the sensory, perceptual, and emotive experiences of pain and may serve as a critical domain for the body/brain–mind interaction. As we come to recognize the functional relationships that exist between afferent systems, efferent modulation, and the factors that influence them, we develop enhanced insight to the role of different therapeutic approaches to clinical pain intervention. The complexity of this physiology underscores the need for multidisciplinary, integrative models of intervention that employ diverse therapeutic techniques to engage the multiplicity of systems that may subserve a particular patient's pain.

## ACKNOWLEDGMENT

The authors are grateful to Sherry Loveless for technical and graphic artistic assistance on this project.

## REFERENCES

### MECHANISMS OF SPINAL PAIN

1. Borenstein, D., Epidemiology, etiology, diagnostic evaluation and treatment of low back pain, *Curr. Opinions Rheumatol.* 10: 104–06 (1998).
2. Burton, A.K., Spine update: back injury and work loss: biomechanical and psychosocial influences, *Spine* 22(21): 2575–80 (1997).
3. Wyke, B., The neurology of low back pain. In M. Jayson (Ed.), *The Lumbar Spine and Back Pain*, 4th ed., New York, Churchill Livingstone, 1987, 155–60.
4. Edgar, M.A., Ghadially, J.A., Innervation of the lumbar spine, *Clin Orthop.* 115: 35–41 (1976).
5. Porterfield, J.A., DeRosa, C., *Mechanical Low Back Pain*, Philadelphia, WB Saunders, 1991, p 23–30.
6. Bogduk, N., The innervation of the lumbar spine, *Spine*, 8, 286–93 (1983).
7. Gardner, E., Martin, J.H., Jessell, T.M., The bodily senses. In E.R. Kandel, J.H. Schwartz, T.M. Jessel (Eds.), *Principles of Neural Science*, 4th ed., New York, Elsevier, 2000, p. 430–50.
8. McLain, R.F., Mechanoreceptor endings in human cervical facet joints, *Spine* 19 (5): 495–501 (1994).

9. Cavanaugh, J.M., Kallakuri, S., Ozaktay, A.C., Innervation of the rabbit lumbar intervertebral disc and posterior longitudinal ligament, *Spine* 20(19): 2080–85 (1995).

10. Snell, R,S., *Clinical Anatomy for Medical Students*, 2d ed. Boston, Little, Brown Co., 1987, p. 91–148.

11. Adriaensen, H., Gybels, J., Handwerker, H.O., VanHees, J.. Response properties of thin myelinated (a) fibers in human skin nerves. *J. Neurophysiol.* 49: 111–22 (1983).

12. Marshall, L.L., Trethewie, E.R., Curtain, C.C., Chemical radiculitis, *Clin. Orthop.* 129: 61–67 (1977).

13. Chen, C., Cavanaugh, J.M., Ozaktay, A.C. et al., Effects of phospholipase A2 on lumbar nerve root structure and function, *Spine* 22 (10): 1057–64 (1997).

14. Bashline, S.D., Bilott, J.R., Ellis, J.P., Meningovertebral ligaments and their putative significance to low back pain, *J. Manipulative Physiol. Ther.* 19 (9): 592–96 (1996).

15. Rydevik, B.L., The effects of compression on the physiology of nerve roots, *J. Manipulative Physiol. Ther.* 15(1) 62–66 (1992).

16. Bartels, E.M., Fairbank, J.C., Winlove, C.P. et al., Oxygen and lactate concentrations measured *in vivo* in the intervertebral discs of patients with scoliosis and back pain, *Spine* 23 (1): 1–8 (1998).

17. Indahl, A., Kaigle, A.M., Reikeras, O. et al., Interaction between the porcine lumbar intervertebral disc, zygapophyseal joints and paraspinal muscles, *Spine* 22 (21): 2834–40 (1997).

18. Christie, H.J., Kumar, S., Warren, S.A., Postural aberrations in low back pain, *Arch. Phys. Med. Rehabil.* 76: 218–24 (1995).

19. Sugawara, O., Atsuta, Y., Iwahara, T. et al., The effects of mechanical compression and hypoxia on nerve root and dorsal root ganglia: An analysis of ectopic firing using an *in vitro* model, *Spine* 21 (18): 2089–94 (1996).

20. Perl, E.R., Characterization of nociceptors and their activation of neurons in the superficial dorsal horn: first steps for the sensation of pain. In L. Kruger and J.C. Liebeskind (Eds.), *Advances in Pain Research and Therapy*, vol. 6, New York, Raven 1984, p. 23–51.

21. Perl, E.R., Sensitization of nociceptors and its relation to sensation. In J.J. Bonica, D. Albe-Fessard (Eds.), *Advances in Pain Research and Therapy,* vol. 1, New York, Raven, 1976, p. 17–28.

22. Torebjork, H.E., Ochoa, J., Pain and itch from C fiber stimulation, *Soc. Neurosci. Abstr.* 7: 228 (1981).

23. Weinstein, J., Neurogenic and non-neurogenic pain and inflammatory mediators, *Orthop. Clin. North Am.* 22 (2): 235–45 (1991).

24. Baldamente, M.A., Dee, R., Ghillani, R. et al., Mechanical stimulation of dorsal root ganglia induces increased production of substance P: A mechanism for pain following nerve root compromise? *Spine* 12 (6): 552–55 (1987).

25. Urban, M., Gebhart, G.F., Central mechanisms in pain, *Med. Clin. North Am.* 83: 585–67 (1999).

26. Dickenson, A.H., NMDA receptor antagonists as analgesics. In H.L. Fields, J.C. Liebeskind (Eds.), *Progress in Pain Research*, vol 1. Seattle, IASP Press, 1994, p. 173–76.

27. Mense, S., Light, A.R., Perl, E.R., Spinal terminations of subcutaneous high threshold mechanoreceptors. In A.G. Brown, M. Rethelyi (Eds.), *Spinal Cord Sensation*, Edinburgh, Scotland, Scottish Academic Press, 1981, p. 79–86.

28. Price, D.D., Dubner, R., Neurons that subserve sensory discriminative aspecys of pain, *Pain* 3: 307–10 (1977).

29. Kumazawa, T., Perl, E.R., Differential excitation of dorsal horn marginal and substantia gelatinosa neurons by primary afferent units with fine A-delta and C-fibers. In Y. Zotterman (Ed.), *Sensory Functions of the Skin in Primates*, vol 27, Oxford, Pergammon Press, 1976, p. 67.

30. Willis, W.D. Kenshalo, D.R., Leonard, R.B., The cells of origin of the primate spinothalamic tract, *J. Comp. Neurol.* 188: 543–50 (1979).

## ASCENDING PAIN PATHWAYS: ANTEROLATERAL SYSTEM

31. Albe-Fessard, D., Levante, A., Lamour, Y.. Origin of spinothalamic tract in monkeys, *Brain Res.* 65: 503–9 (1974).

32. Apkarian, A.V., Hodge, C.J., Primate spinothalamic pathways: I. a quantitative study of the cells of origin of the spinothalamic pathway, *J. Comp. Neurol.* 288: 447–73 (1989).

33. Parent, A., *Carpenter's Human Neuroanatomy*, 9th ed. Baltimore, Williams & Wilkins, 1996.

34. Antonetty, C.M., Webster, K.E., The organization of the spinotectal projection: an experimental study in the rat, *J. Comp. Neurol.* 163: 449–65 (1975).

35. Basbaum, A., Jessel, T.M., The perception of pain. In E.R. Kandel, J.H. Schwartz, T.M. Jessell (Eds.), *Principles of Neural Science*, 4th ed., New York, McGraw-Hill, 2000, p. 472–90.
36. Melzack, R., Wall, P.D., Pain mechanisms: a new therapy, *Science* 150: 971–79 (1965).
37. Behbehani, M.M., Fields, H.L., Evidence that an excitatory connection exists between the periaqueductal gray and nucleus raphe magnus mediates stimulation produced analgesia, *Brain Res.* 170: 85–93 (1979).
38. Akil, H., Madden, J., Patrick, R.L., Barchas, J.D., Stress-induced increase in endogenous opioid peptides; concurrent analgesia and its partial reversal by naloxone. In H. Kosterlitz (Ed.), *Opiates and Endogenous Opioid Peptides*, Amsterdam, Elsevier-North Holland, 1976, p. 63–70.
39. Fields, H.L., Brainstem mechanisms of pain modulation. In L. Kruger, J.C. Liebeskind (Eds.), *Advances in Pain Research and Therapy*, vol. 6, New York, Raven, 1984, p. 241–52.
40. Han, J.S., A mesolimbic neuronal loop of analgesia. In M. Tiengo, J. Eccles, A.C. Cuello, D. Ottoson (eds.), *Advances in Pain Research and Therapy*, vol. 10, New York, Raven, 1987, p. 219–34.
41. Basbaum, A., Fields, H.L., The origin of descending pathways in the dorsolateral funiculus of the spinal cord of the cat and rat: Further studies on the anatomy of pain modulation, *J. Comp. Neurol.*, 187: 513–32 (1979).
42. Giordano, J., Analgesic profile of centrally administered 2-methylserotonin against acute pain in rats, *Eur. J. Pharmacol.*, 199: 223–26 (1991).
43. Giordano, J., Barr, G.A., Possible role of spinal 5-HT and mu- and kappa-opioid-mediated analgesia in the developing rat, *Devel. Brain Res.*, 33: 121–26 (1988).
44. Satoh, M., Akaike, A., Nakazawa, T., Takagi, H.. Evidence for involvement of separate mechanisms in the production of analgesia by electrical stimulation of the nucleus reticularis paragigantocellularis and nucleus raphe magnus in the rat, *Brain Res.*, 194: 525 (1980).
45. Stefano, G., Fricchione, G., Slingsby, B., Benson, H.. The placebo effect and relaxation response: neural processes and their coupling to constitutive nitric oxide, *Brain Res. Rev.* 35: 1–19 (1999).
46. Welters, I., Fimiani, C., Bilfinger, T., Stefano, G., NF-kB, nitric oxide and opiate signalling, *Med. Hypotheses*, 54: 263–68 (1999).
47. Botticelli, L., Cox, B., Goldstein, A., Immunoreactive dynorphin in mammalian spinal cord and dorsal root ganglion, *Proc. Natl. Acad. Sci. USA* 78: 7783–86 (1981).
48. Hayes, A., Skingle, M., Tyers, M., Antinociceptive profile of dynorphin in the rat, *Life Sci.* 33 (Suppl. 1): 657–60 (1983).
49. Zieglgansberger, W., Tulloch, I.F., The effects of methionine- and leucine-enkephalin on spinal neurons in the cat, *Brain Res.*, 167: 53–61 (1979).
50. Yaksh, T.L., Gross, K.E., Lee, C.H., Studies on the intrathecal effects of B-endorphin in primates, *Brain Res.* 241: 261–69 (1982).
51. Hunt, S.P., Kelly, J.S., Emson, P.C. et al., An immunohistochemical study of neuronal populations containing neuropeptides or gamma aminobutyrate within the superficial layers of the rat dorsal horn, *Neuroscience* 6: 1883–89 (1981).
52. Rustinoni, A., Hayes, N.L., O'Neill, S., Dorsal column nuclei and ascending spinal afferents in macaques, *Brain* 102: 95 (1979).
53. Ruda, M.A., Bennett, G.J., Dubner, R., Neurochemistry and neurocircuitry in the dorsal horn, *Progress. Brain Res.* 66: 219–25 (1986).
54. Dong, W.K., Ryu, H., Wagman, I.H.,Nociceptive responses of neurons in the medial thalamus and their relationship to spinothalamic pathways, *J. Neurophysiol.*, 41: 1592 (1978).

## ASCENDING PAIN PATHWAYS: POSTERIOR SYSTEM

55. Ribbers, G.M., Geurts, A.C., Stam, H.J., Mulder, T., Pharmacologic treatment of complex regional pain syndrome I: a conceptual framework, *Arch. Phys. Med. Rehabil.*, 84: 141–46 (2003).
56. Baba, H., Doubell, T.P., Woolf, C.J., Peripheral inflammation facilitates A-beta fiber-mediated synaptic input to the substantia gelatinosa of the adult rat spinal cord, *J. Neurosci.* 19: 859–67 (1999).
57. McAllister, J.P., Wells, J., The structural organization of the ventral posterolateral nucleus in the rat, *J. Comp. Neurol.* 197(2): 271–301 (1981).
58. Liu, X.B., Warren, R.A., Jones, E.G., Synaptic distribution of afferents from reticular nucleus in ventroposterior nucleus of the cat thalamus, *J. Comp. Neurol.* 352(2): 187–202 (1995).

59. Hirshberg, R,M,, Al-Chaer, E.D., Lawand, N.B., Westlund, K.N., Willis, W.D., Is there a pathway in the posterior funiculus that signals visceral pain? *Pain* 67(2–3): 291–305 (1996).

60. Kamogawa, H., Bennet, G.J., Dorsal column postsynaptic neurons in the cat are excited by myelinated nociceptors, *Brain Res.* 364(2): 386–90 (1986).

61. Lewis, J.W., Chudler, E.H., Cannon, J.T., Liebeskind, J.C., Hypophysectomy differentially affects morphine and stress analgesia, *Proc. West. Pharmacol. Soc.* 24: 323–26 (1981).

62. MacLennan, A.J., Drugan, R.C., Hyson, R.L. et al., Corticosterone: a critical factor in an opioid form of stress-induced analgesia, *Science* 215: 1530–32 (1982).

63. Prevot, V., Rialas, C., Croix, D. et al., Morphine and anandamide coupling to nitric oxide-stimulated GnRH and CRF release from the rat median eminence: neurovascular regulation, *Brain Res* 790: 236–44 (1998).

64. Jinkins, J.R., Whittemore, A.R., Bradley, W.G., The anatomic basis of vertebrogenic pain and the autonomic syndrome associated with lumbar disk extrusion, *Am. J. Roentgenol.* 152: 1277–89 (1991).

65. Lewis, J.W., Tordoff, M.G., Sherman, J.E., Liebeskind, J.C., Adrenal medullary enkephalin-like peptides may mediate opioid stress analgesia, *Science* 217: 557–59 (1982).

# 4 The Core of the MUA Procedure: Tissue Injury Repair Sequence and Fibrous Release with Manipulation

*Robert C. Gordon*

## CONTENTS



### HOW FIBROTIC ADHESIONS FORM

An inflammatory response follows injury, and the injury can be macrotrauma or microtrauma in nature. When the trauma occurs, the capillary system is compromised and oxygen is temporarily terminated to the area, called *hypoxia*. As the body continues to respond to the injured area, surrounding areas will also suffer from hypoxia.

The body's response to this hypoxia is necrosis at the cellular level, which causes macrophages, granulocytes, and mast cells to attack the trauma area. This attack causes a capillary flush and the release of exudate from the damaged tissue, which causes the swelling that comes right after trauma. The trauma causes direct hemorrhage of capillaries and edema formation, which is the swelling. Macrophages and granulocytes form histocytes, which begin the tissue repair and regeneration, and begin to transform into collagen fibers or tissue-rebuilding blocks. Some of these cells also form fibroblasts, which start to build the damaged area by filling in any lost tissue. These fibroblasts develop into the adhesions or scar tissue. The damaged area now starts a remodeling phase, which can take up to one year to repair.[1, 2]

Restriction of joint motion occurs during the inflammatory cycle at three different levels: 1) during the initial swelling when fluids are trying to return the oxygen to the damaged area, 2) during the edema and hemorrhage phase when the capillaries are rebuilding and flushing the area to get rid of dead tissue and toxins, and 3) during the formation of the fibrotic adhesions.

If these three phases are not dealt with immediately, fluid accumulation and fibrotic scarring occur and joint restriction is extended. This, in turn, causes the fibrotic adhesions to become more and more embedded in an abnormal pattern where they form.

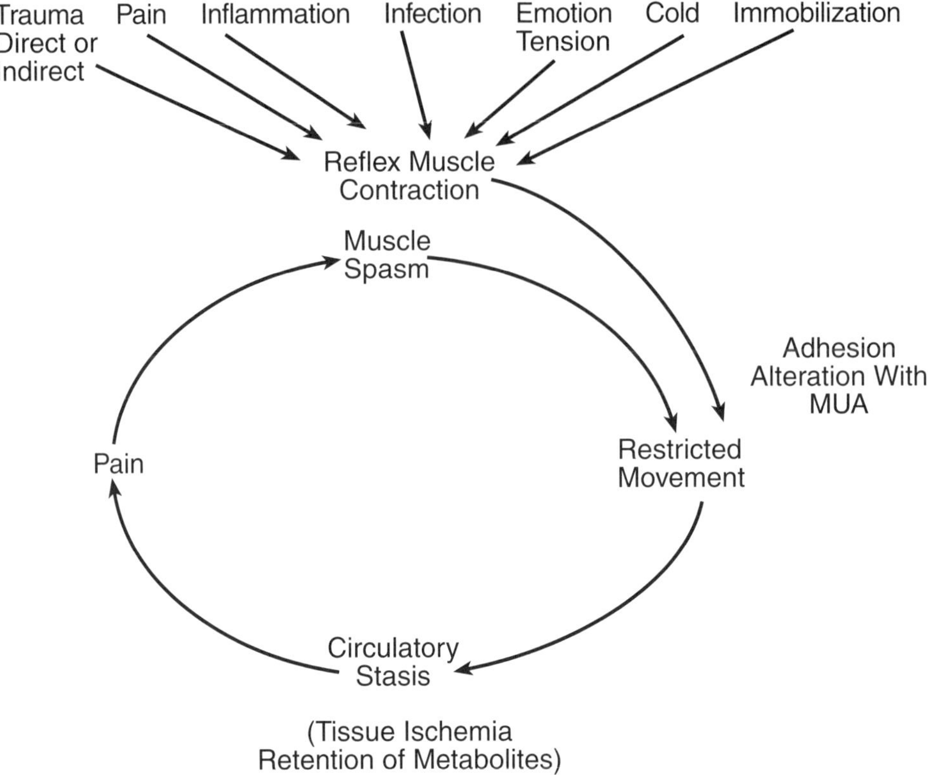


**FIGURE 4.1** Schematic of the self-perpetuating cycle of muscle spasm. Altering adhesions affects the cycle of pain and spasm when performing MUA.

When we use the MUA program to alter the fibrotic adhesions, we are interrupting the remodeling phase and retraumatizing (on a microtrauma level) the area, changing the design pattern of the collagen (fibrotic adhesions). The importance of keeping these adhesions from reforming the restrictive designs previously mentioned is what makes or breaks the MUA procedure.

The core of the MUA procedure is the changing of the adhesion designs back into a more normal pattern (toward areolar type tissue) in the muscle fibers or the capsules surrounding the joints. In order to do this, the MUA is done at a predetermined rate (using linear forces) at the discretion of the doctor. Physical therapy must then follow the procedure and progress into range of motion exercise and rehabilitation to prevent these abnormal adhesion designs from reforming in an abnormal fashion. (See Figure 4.1.)

## MUSCLE PHYSIOLOGY AND THE FIBROSUS RELEASE PROCEDURE AS IT PERTAINS TO MUA

One of the most important phases of the MUA technique is the stretching portion of the procedure. The stretching and myofascial release component elements of the MUA procedure are referred to as *fibrosus release*. In Chapter 12, the distinctive movements that comprise the fibrosus release part of the MUA procedure are explained. The stretching of the muscles, joints, and joint capsules creates the biophysiological atmosphere for change to occur when static flexibility becomes dynamic flexibility. By changing the physiological integrity of the muscle, elongation occurs, which causes the articular areas to return to more normal movement.[3,4]

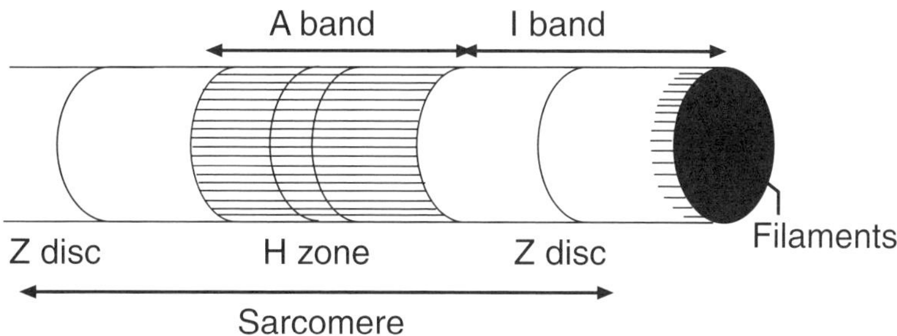



**FIGURE 4.2** Contractile portion of the microbril that allows the proper "sliding" action during muscle movement affected by the MUA technique.

In order to understand this concept further, it becomes necessary to briefly discuss the contractile components of the muscle.

Muscles do not maintain the same shape or size even bilaterally in the same person.[2, 5, 6] Each has a characteristic all its own in the area where it is to accomplish its function. There are also differences in type of muscles, as we all know.

In this section, we will only discuss striated muscle, which is the muscle of the skeletal system. Muscle has several layers, all of which have specific functions that control the neurophysiological response when the upper motor centers are stimulated to respond to movement. (Refer to Chapter 2.)

The central portion of the whole muscle is called the belly of the muscle. The belly of the muscle then, in turn, is comprised of smaller compartments that are called fascicule. Each fasciculus is then comprised of 100 to 150 muscle fibers. Muscle fibers contain smaller units called myofibrilis. The myofibril is the contractile unit of the muscle and is composed of smaller protein fibers, myofilaments, which are called actin and myosin. These "sarcomeres" are the action components of the muscle fiber, and it is the action of the actin and myosin that when neurologically stimulated cause contraction.[2,6,7]

It is this microfilament contractile component that I wish to discuss that relates to the scientific foundation for why MUA works. The myofibrils are seen as light and dark areas in the muscle fibers. The chief contractile unit of the muscle fiber is within these light and dark areas. The entire light and dark area is made up of Z bands (dark) and I bands (light); A bands (dark); and M bands (light) in between the dark. This entire area from Z disc to Z disc is called the sarcomere. (Refer to Figure 4.2.)

It is within the sarcomere (Z disc to Z disc) that the myofilaments (actin and myosin) contract. The sarcomere is referred to as the contractile unit of the muscle fiber.[7]

A muscle fiber is physiologically able to shorten and elongate depending on the response the body demands. In the shortened state, sarcomeres are lost by the muscle fibers, and when elongation occurs, sarcomeres are added by the muscle fiber (myofilaments).[2,6–8]

It is the body's ability to elongate the muscle fiber at the myofilament level that makes it possible to accomplish the return to more normal flexibility that occurs during the MUA procedure.

The mechanism by which muscles contract, relax, or elongate is not completely understood at the present time. However, the current accepted theory is the interdigitation, or sliding, of the myofilament theory.

When maximumly contracted, a sarcomere may shorten to as much as 50% of its normal size. When passively stretched, it may extend to as much as 120% of its normal length.[6,7,8] This is accomplished by a change in permeability of the myofilament at the time of the activation of the stretch reflex (the neurological stimulus). When this occurs, the myosin attaches to the actin by

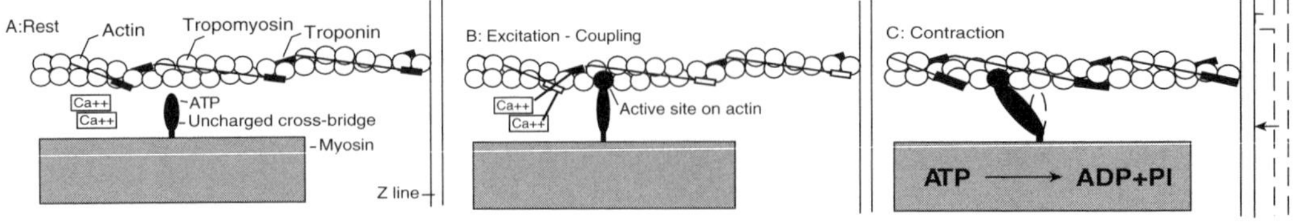


**FIGURE 4.3** Schematic of a muscle contraction from rest to contraction. This diagram also represents the response from contraction to rest necessary to achieve MUA results.

way of a cross-bridge, and by chemical attraction, the fibers slide inward, or outward depending on the function desired. (See Figure 4.3.)

The importance of this as we discuss MUA is that we hypothesize that fibro-adhesions form between the muscle fibers, and when these adhesions are present they do not permit normal muscle contraction. A myofilament or sarcomere could be in a shortened state during muscle contracture or muscle splinting, and the muscle fiber would not be performing at its optimum length.

By using the relaxation technique or placing the body under a twilight sedative/hypnotic, the MUA practitioner is able to mechanically/passively elongate the myofibril, engage dormant sarcomeres to the myofilament, and alter the fibro-adhesions between the muscle fibers.

By progressive stretching, the muscle fiber goes from a disuse, elastic-shortened state to an elastic phase and finally to the disuse-plastic deformans phase of muscle fiber stretch. The final phase can be permanent as long as continued therapy is maintained throughout the post-MUA physical therapy and rehabilitation. This exchange from disuse elastic range to disuse-plastic deformans range can be felt by the practitioner during MUA by a subtle "give" in the stretching process. This is not tearing the muscle fiber, but instead we hypothesize that this is disassociating the actin and myosin and moving the muscle fibers from a shortened "disuse" physiological state, to a more normal elastic range. If this stretching is maintained during post-MUA therapy, this "dormant" elastic range is changed and helps return the normal range of motion back to the muscle fiber and, in turn, to the joint.

It takes a very short period of time to rebuild the fibro-adhesions. By continuing the stretching of the muscles that have been worked with under anesthesia, the fibro-adhesions form a new design that is more in line with the integrity of the muscle fiber, thus allowing considerably more flexibility in the muscle, the joint, and the joint capsule in the area of involvement. This remodeling of the fibro-adhesion within the muscle fiber is in large part why, if done correctly, and followed with the proper post-MUA therapy and -rehabilitation program, the MUA technique works so well.

## HYPOTHESIS FOR NEUROLOGICAL CONDUCTION OF ACTION POTENTIAL AND MUSCLE CONTRACTION DURING AND FOLLOWING THE MUA PROCEDURE

Whenever a muscle is stretched, the stretch reflex mechanism is initiated. Stretching a muscle lengthens both the muscle fibers (i.e., extrafusal fibers, as we have already alluded to) and the muscle spindles (i.e., intrafusal fibers). The consequent deformation within the muscle spindle results in the firing of the stretch reflex, which contracts the muscle.[7,8]

However, when a sedative/hypnotic is introduced, the stretch reflex is interrupted or slowed down. Internuncial neurons are depressed, which act on the alpha motoneurons, and muscle contraction is temporarily interrupted.[9,10] It is feasible to assume that when the MUA procedure is being completed, and stretching of muscle occurs to alter fibro-adhesions, secondary reflex which causes immediate protective muscle reaction splinting to occur is slowed down. This can be both good and bad regarding this technique. It allows you as the treating physician to stretch the muscle fibers and use the force of passive stretch to alter the aberrant fibrous tissue that has accumulated in the muscle fibers. With a sedative/hypnotic, the patient is in a relaxed state, but since no analgesic is used, the patient does recognize pain and will let the practitioner know by various sounds that there is discomfort. Because of this, the primary care practitioner who is performing the procedure and the first assistant must be extremely aware of normal ranges of motion, and only attempt to reproduce normal ranges. If the practitioner progresses beyond the patient discomfort level, the muscle fiber itself could tear since the normal golgi tendon organ protective response is also temporarily slowed by using this technique.

Resistance to the stretching is usually due to two factors — muscle shortening as a result of contracture and abnormal fibrous tissue that has accumulated. It is the practitioner's responsibility to know when these areas have been reached, and what the mechanism is that is causing restriction. Consideration should be taken to visualize tendon appearance, such as with extreme contracture and muscle shortening and anatomical function, so that tearing of tissues does not occur. (A quick movement stretch [ballistic] would be contraindicated.) This is so the golgi tendon response is overcome and gentle linear force stretching is allowed which prevents potential tearing. When the MUA has been completed, and the patient is receiving post-MUA therapy, the practitioner should be aware of changes that have occurred and use the changes to continue working with the muscle fiber and articulation. The body will now respond, however, with the normal secondary protective reflexes, and contractures need to be prevented to an area that has undergone MUA, by using continued mild to moderate stretching within the first three to five days following MUA and especially on the same day as the MUA. Remember the remodeling of the fibro-adhesion at the end of the inflammatory cycle begins in 24–48 h, if not acted on.[2] The post-MUA therapy is completed to continue with the process of fibrous tissue breakdown, and is done with concern that tissue repair works in harmony with this remodeling process and not in discourse with this process. Of significant importance is the body's apparent neuromuscular reeducation that takes place with the MUA.

In every instance that I have seen treated, and followed up on, the patient's muscle has demonstrated considerable renewed range of motion and flexibility. If the post-MUA stretching is the same as the stretching accomplished with the MUA, the patient's muscle continues to respond well. If, however, I place the patient in a position they were not in during the MUA and try to administer therapy, there appears to be muscle resistance to the body position. This only seems to hold true for the days during the actual MUA procedure and three to five days following the MUA.

There appears to be a correlation between the patient having the MUA procedure completed in the supine, or side lying position, and trying to accomplish similar stretching maneuvers in other positions. Ettema and Huijing briefly address this concept when they speak of the muscle elasticity called series elastic elements and its relation to the surrounding aponeurosis in context with what they call angular compliance.[11]

Accordingly, shortened muscle fibers and specifically the myofilament cross-bridge effect are influenced by what they term contraction dynamics. If the stretch is a linear force with sustained or constant pressure exerted, the muscle lengthens in direct proportion to the exertion of the force applied. If angular compliance or short bursts of pressure are exerted, the cross-bridge is not affected, but only the aponeurosis is stretched, and the myofilament (actin and myosin) are not responsive.[11] This tends to suggest that the muscle fiber is being neurologically induced to respond to an action. Since the practitioner is guiding that action, it is feasible to contend that the muscle is being reeducated under anesthesia, and that during therapy in the office when the same stretch is being completed post-MUA, the muscle will continue to conform to the response requested under anesthesia simply because the cross-bridge function was guided into a new configuration.

Since this is new and deserves continued study, we cannot be positive that this concept is actually occurring, but since some research has been done with elements of the hypothesis and because this research is pointing in this direction, we can consider this concept to have merit.[11,12] (See Figures 4.4 and 4.5.)

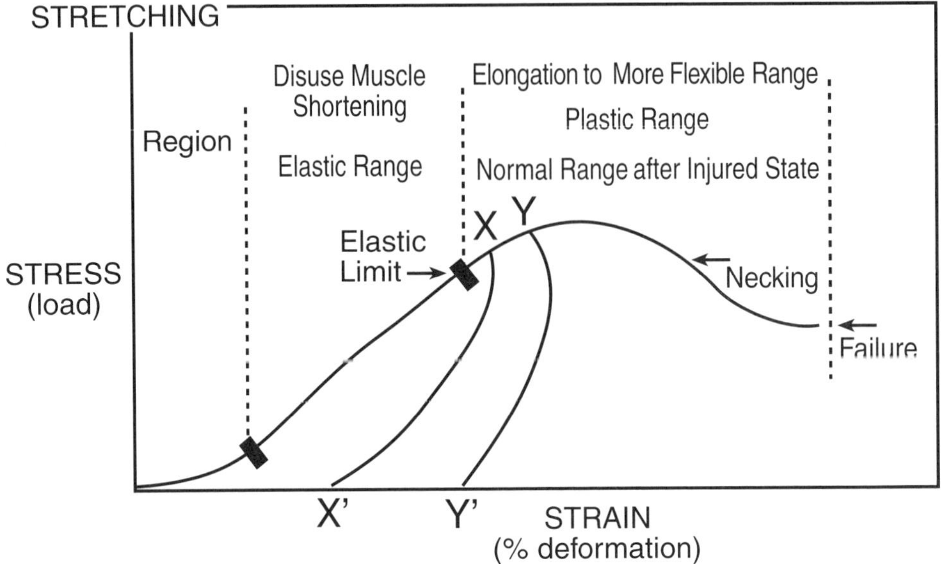


**FIGURE 4.4** Stress–strain curve.

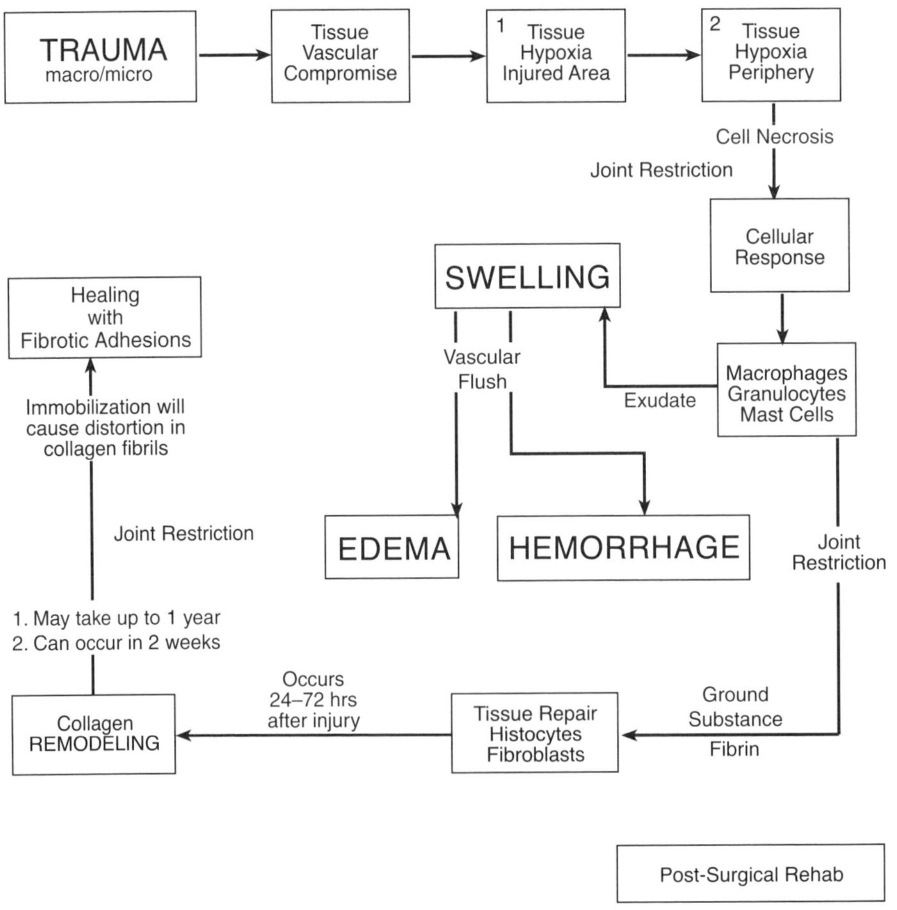


**FIGURE 4.5** The inflammatory cycle.

## TRACTION STRETCHING WITH MUA

Traction stretching, or sustained linear force stretching, is an integral part of the MUA procedure. When the patient is in the relaxed state of twilight sedation, the muscles that support the spinal areas of involvement are able to be tractioned into full elongation.

A muscle that has been traumatized has become inflamed, and as such, has undergone the changes in the inflammatory cycle.

In the case of the muscle fiber, the fibro-adhesions will be laid down in a matrix between the muscle fibrils over time from disuse and as a result of the trauma to the muscle. This abnormal fibrous tissue causes the muscle to stay shortened in length. Since the muscle is also probably not used properly, the length of the muscle is also affected by disuse.

Guyton speaks of the muscle fibrils as made up of filaments called actin and myosin, which are capable of sliding inward and outward in an interlocking mechanism as the muscle lengthens and shortens.[2,13] When there is disuse of a muscle from either immobilization or muscle splinting or contracture, the muscle does not have its full capacity to contract and relax.[8]

Since muscle is connected to bone even though layered, a joint that is inflamed and immobile will not move through its normal articular range because the muscles that make that happen have shortened from disuse. Fibro-adhesions form in these areas of disuse as a protective mechanism for the purpose of preventing tears should the patient move quickly and abnormally lengthen a muscle that has been in a contracted state for prolonged periods of time.[2,6,8,14]

When we use the stretching techniques prior to adjusting the anesthetized patient, we are altering the adhesions in the muscle fibrils and attempting to elongate the muscle. In this way, the joint can be taken to its full end range so that the adhesions in the joint and joint capsules are also capable of being altered.

If we did not use the stretching technique, the muscle fibril would be forced to work in a shortened state, causing the joint to be restricted and remain only slightly movable during adjustment. Complete muscle response from stretching a myofibril to this end range will allow the anesthesized muscle to better respond to articular motion from a low velocity-impulse thrust.

This is why multiple MUAs are necessary in many cases before final joint adhesions are altered. There are multiple mechanical functions required for spinal movement just as there are multiple impulses that create these movements. If the MUA is to benefit the patient, many of the adhesions that have formed in the muscles, joints, and joint capsules must be altered so that normal movement is allowed to return. (See Figures 4.6, 4.7, and 4.8.)

## STRESS–STRAIN CURVE

The stress–strain curve is comprised of the following.

1. **Elastic range:** Initially the strain is directly proportional to the ability of the material to resist the force. The tissue returns to its original size and shape when the load is released.
2. **Elastic limit:** The point beyond which the tissue will not return to its original shape and size.
3. **Plastic range:** The range beyond the elastic limit extending to the point of rupture. Tissue strained within this range will have permanent deformation.
4. **Yield strength:** The load beyond the elastic limit that produces permanent deformation within the tissue. Once the yield point is reached, there is sequential failure of the tissue with permanent deformation (remodeling), and the tissue passes into the plastic range of the stress-strain curve. The deformation may be from a single load or the summation of several subcritical loads.[15]
5. **Ultimate strength:** The greatest load the tissue can sustain. Once the maximum load is reached, there is increased strain (deformation) without an increase in stress.

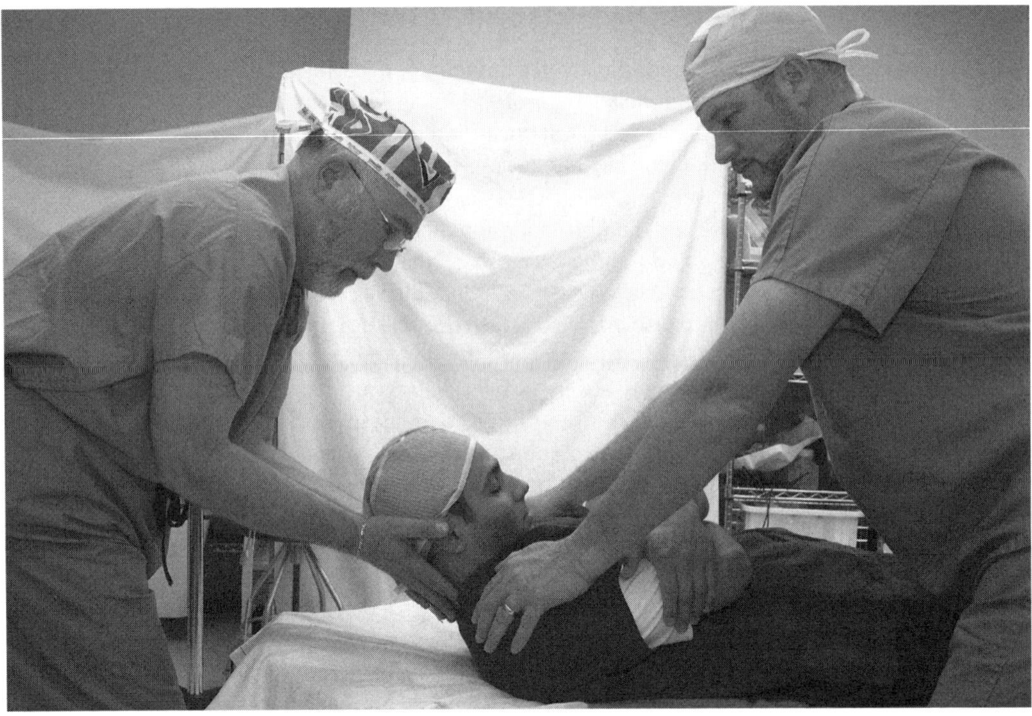

**FIGURE 4.6**

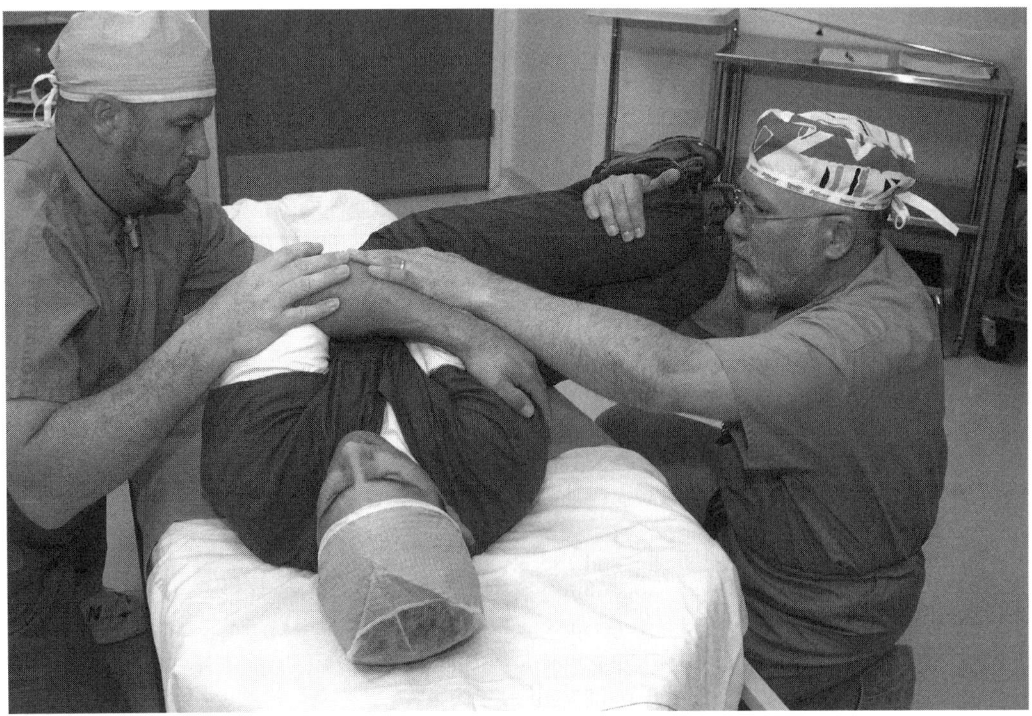

**FIGURE 4.7**

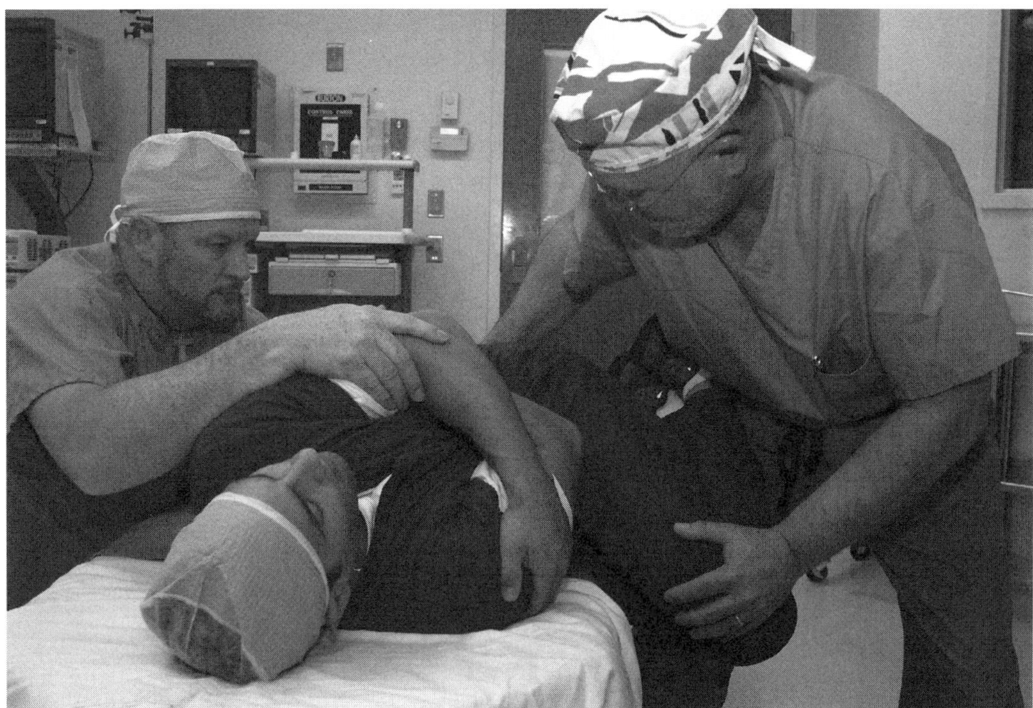

**FIGURE 4.8**

6. **Necking:** The region where there is considerable weakening of the tissue; less force is needed for deformation, and failure rapidly approaches.
7. **Breaking strength:** The load at the time the tissue fails.
8. **Failure:** Rupture of the integrity of the tissue.

Influences on the stress–strain curve include the following.

1. **Resilience:** The ability to absorb energy within the elastic range as work is accomplished. Energy is released when the load is removed and the tissue returns to its original shape.
2. **Toughness:** The ability to absorb energy within the plastic range without breaking (failing). If too much energy is absorbed with the stress, there will be rupture.
3. **Creep:** When a load is applied for an extended period of time, the tissue elongates, resulting in permanent deformation or failure. It is related to the viscosity of the tissue and is therefore time dependent. Deformation depends on the amount of force and the rate at which the force is applied. Creep occurs with low-magnitude load, usually in the elastic range, over a long period of time. The greater the load, the more rapid the rate of creep, but not in proportion to strain; therefore, a lesser load applied for a longer period of time will result in greater deformation. Increased temperature increases creep and therefore distensibility of the tissue.[4,8,16]
4. **Structural stiffness:** Tissue with great stiffness will have a higher slope in the elastic region of the curve, indicating there is less elastic deformation with greater stress. Contractures and scar tissue have greater stiffness, probably due to a great degree of bonding between collagen fibers and their surrounding matrix.

5. **Heat production:** Energy is released as heat when stress is applied. It is depicted by the area under the curve (hysteresis loop) in the plastic range. As the tissue is heated, it more easily distends.

6. **Fatigue:** Cyclic loading of the tissue may cause failure below the yield point. The greater the applied load, the fewer numbers of cycles are needed for failure. A minimum load is required for this failure; below the minimum load an apparent infinite number of cycles will not cause failure. This is the endurance limit. Examples of fatigue are stress fractures and overuse syndromes. Biologic tissue has the ability to repair itself after cyclic loading if the load is not too great and time is allowed before the cyclic loading is again applied.

We hypothesize that there is a disuse elastic range that is created from the patient going through decreased function following an injury. If you view this range as a decrease elastic range on the stress-strain curve, you will also notice that the plastic range would also slide toward and into the normal elastic range. It is feasible to theorize that when linear force stretching is accomplished, the disuse plastic range (if you will) is entered, and it is because we take the muscle into that range, permanent change is made. If we only took the muscle through its "disuse elastic range," we would use only that portion of the muscle (and those sacromeres) that were available in that range. To achieve full elastic range, that muscle must be moved through its allowable anatomical range, which in the case of a disuse elastic range would push that muscle into the disuse plastic range. By accomplishing this complete stretch, the muscle is allowed to return over time to its normal range and the tearing that would normally have occurred in the plastic range is avoided.[11]

## REFERENCES


1. Gray, H., *Anatomy,* Running Press, Philadelphia, 1974: 224, 1086–96.
2. Guyton, A.C., *Textbook of Medical Physiology,* 4th ed., WB Saunders Co., Philadelphia, London, Toronto, 1971: 113–16.
3. Gordon, A.M., Huxley, A.F., Julian, F.J., Tension development in highly stretched vertebrae muscle fibres, *J. Physio.* 1966A: 184: 143–69.
4. Gordon, R., Cornerstone Professional Education Inc., MUA course syllabus sponsored by the National College of Chiropractic, 5th ed., August 1998.
5. Gowers, W.R., Lumbago: Its lessons and analogues, *Br. Med. J.* 1904:1, 117–21.
6. Roy, S., Irvin, R., *Sports Medicine, Prevention, Evaluation, Management, and Rehabilitation,* Prentice-Hall, Englewood Cliffs, NJ, 1983: 125–28.
7. Alter, M., *The Science of Stretching,* 2nd ed., Human Kinetics Pub., Champaign, IL, 1988: 13–21, 23–31, 33–41.
8. Kisner, C., Colby, L.A., Stretching, from *Therapeutic Exercise Foundations and Techniques,* 2d ed., F.A. Davis, Philadelphia, 1990: 109–20.
9. Gordon, R., Cornerstone Professional Education Inc., MUA syllabus sponsored by the National University of Health Sciences, 5th ed., August 1998.
10. McKechnie, B., Manipulation under anesthesia; neurological effects of different modes of anesthesia, *Dynamic Chiropractic,* April 10, 1992: 14 and 25.
11. Ettema, G,, Huijing, P.A., Architecture and elastic properties of the series elastic element of muscle-tendon complex, from *Multiple Muscle Systems,* Biomechanics and Movement Organization. Springer-Velag, New York-Berlin-Heidelberg-London-Paris-Tokyo-Hong Kong, Jack Winters, ed., 1990: 57–68.
12. Gordon, R., Hickman, G., Gray, J., Proprioception as a prerequisite to SG cell response in inhibiting musculoskeletal pain using manipulation under anesthesia, *Dynamic Chiropractic,* May 3, 1999: 6-8, 43-45.
13. Guyton, A.C., *Textbook of Medical Physiology,* 4th ed., WB Saunders, Philadelphia, London, Toronto, 1971: 113–16.
14. Kotlke, F.J., Physical Medicine and Rehabilitation, WB Saunders, Philadelphia, 1982: 389–92.

15. Bond, M.R., Pain, its nature, analysis, and treatment; physiological mechanisms, Melzach and Wall, Eds., *Gate Control Theory,* Churchill Livingstone, 1979: 21–23.

16. Hill, D.K., Tension due to interaction between the sliding filaments in resting striated muscle. The effect of stimulation, *J. Physiol.* 1968: 199, 637–55.

# 5 Manipulative Energy

*Timothy S. Kersch*

## CONTENTS



## LOW- VS. HIGH-FORCE MUA

Energy is one of the most important concepts in the world of science. We think of energy in terms of foods we consume, electricity for the home, and fuel for automobiles. These ideas do not define energy. They just tell us fuel is needed to produce energy to do a job. Energy is the ability to produce action or effect and exists in many forms. Despite the many existing forms of energy, one constant principle remains: energy in any form transferred to another does not diminish the total amount — the total amount remains constant. This is the principle that makes the energy concept so useful. We will see that when one isolated system loses energy, then by the law of the conservation of energy,[1] the second system must gain an equal amount. This transformation of energy from one form to another is an essential part of the study of the science of manipulation.

In this chapter we look at how energy is passed from the Doctor to the patient. In doing so, we establish two unique systems of interest and evaluate each system independently. First, we look at the Doctor as a system of interest. We see how the Doctor's gravitational potential energy is turned into kinetic energy and propagated as an external force. Second, we look at the patient as a system that breaks the external forces as they are applied. We see how a complex series of events takes place in each of the two systems as they essentially push on each other. The distinction of the two systems is paramount in understanding the role of energy exchange. The distinction of the two systems will also help identify where the effects of anesthesia take place in MUA. We follow the energy, identifying where and when the manipulative treatment can be quantified. We evaluate and compare characteristics of a high-force manipulative treatment and a low-force manipulative treatment, so that an understanding of each can be obtained. The characteristics of each type of treatment will be identified using a "dynamic impression"[2] produced by measuring force over time. Thus, we can document velocity or do an acceleration analysis of the biomechanical energy exerted. As skilled providers of manipulative therapy, we must understand our clinical treatments. As clinicians, we must recognize that MUA extends our scope of clinical practice. A rudimentary understanding of the Doctor/Patient encounter is necessary to evaluate how the MUA procedure differs from other manipulative treatment options. This chapter provides a perspective that uses objective measurements to obtain a basic understanding of the forces passed from the Doctor to the patient. We identify how anesthesia changes the complex action/reaction sequence of events during a manipulative treatment.

## THE DOCTOR SYSTEM

Force is the intensity of power or impetus, produced by the actions of one system onto another.[3] We can assume from this that Newton's second law, $F = MA$ (force = mass $\times$ acceleration), appears to express properly the mechanics of the Doctor system and the clinician's energy exchange with the patient. It is erroneous to make this assumption.[4] To make this assumption, it would have to be assumed that the Doctor is a free-falling object in space with no external forces acting on him.[5] (See Figure 5.1.)

This simplified assumption is clearly not the case. An observation of an actual treatment in a clinical setting depicts a more realistic representation of the Doctor system[6] (Figure 5.2).

We can see in Figure 5.2 that there are forces acting on the Doctor system, which have to be taken into consideration. For the sake of simplicity, we will deal with the relevant forces acting on the Doctor system. Primarily there are three contact forces. The first two forces are the ground acting on the left and right foot of the Doctor, and the third contact force is from the patient to the Doctor. So mathematically, a more complex equation becomes necessary than Newton's second law. Such equations have been derived,[7] but the mathematics goes beyond the scope of this presentation. Regardless of mathematics, what Figure 5.2 shows us is that the Doctor is clearly not a free-falling object in space, and the adjustment is not an uncontrolled collision. In a realistic clinical situation, the Doctor experiences external forces. The Doctor uses these external forces to skillfully control his collision with the patient. While these conclusions might seem rudimentary to some, $F = MA$ is used inappropriately if used exclusively to represent a manipulative treatment. Newton's second law ($F = MA$), however, does apply to manipulation in a very important way. Mass and acceleration are the principal components when it comes to the finesse of adjusting. The mass of the Doctor stored as potential energy is put to work by the aid of the constant force of gravity on the doctor and allows him to create energy (Figure 5.3).

The amount of acceleration or the rate of change in the Doctor's downward direction is referred to as his acceleration. The gravitational potential energy transforms into kinetic energy in the Doctor system. The relative displacement of the Doctor dictates how much gravitational potential energy is converted to kinetic energy. This is important to the desired clinical outcome based on how much energy is needed for the treatment. The energy transferred from the Doctor (his mass and velocity) is considered kinetic energy.

Later in this chapter we will see acceleration again; this time it will play a different role. This role will be to contribute to the quickness of a high-force adjustment. At this point, I would like to address how the Doctor's acceleration plays a dual role in manipulation, first, as a source of energy (as gravitational potential energy is accelerated downward) and, second, by contributing to the treatment of velocity (quickness) in a high-force adjustment.

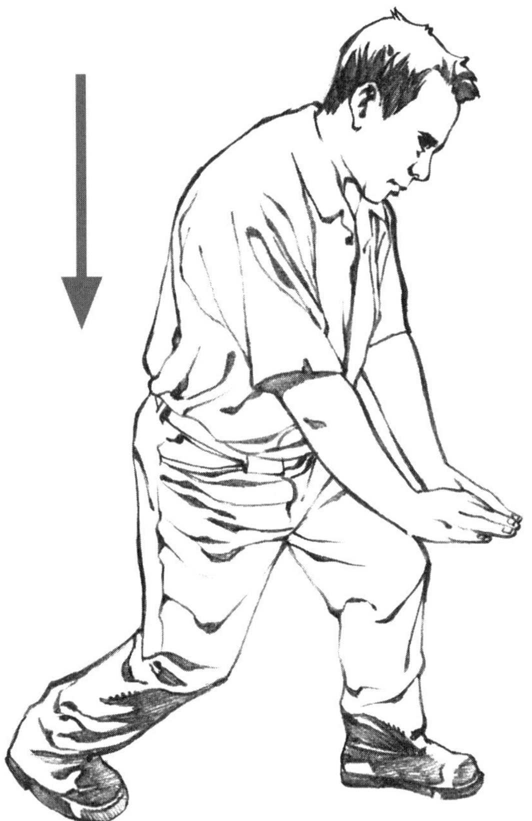


**FIGURE 5.1**

The Doctor system may be summarized as follows.

1. Gravitational potential energy is stored in the Doctor system.
2. As the Doctor moves his center of mass downward, the gravitational energy is transferred to energy stored in the Doctor. The energy is proportional to the distance the doctor has moved downward and the doctor's mass.
3. The energy stored in the doctor system is subject to external forces, including contact force in the hands and the force of the ground under each foot. These forces push back upon the doctor.
4. Energy initiated by the Doctor is transferred as kinetic energy to the patient.

## THE PATIENT SYSTEM

### PATIENT SYSTEM GRAPH

The patient (Figure 5.4) dissipates, or *brakes*, the incoming energy[8] or the adjustive force of the Doctor. As the Doctor controls his collision with the Patient, two distinct types of forces combine to act relative to the incoming energy. These are called *restoring* forces and *damping* forces. These

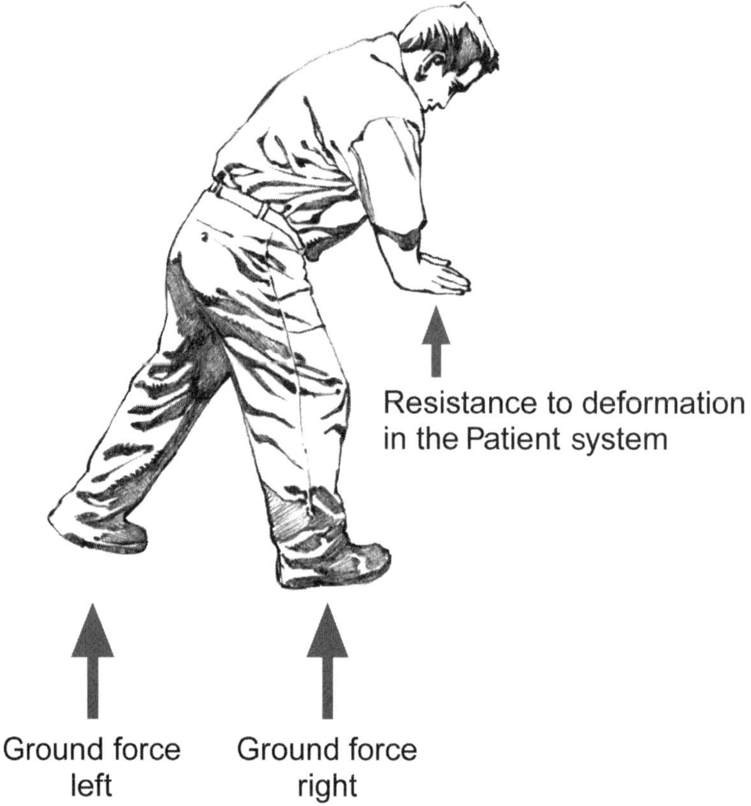



**FIGURE 5.2**

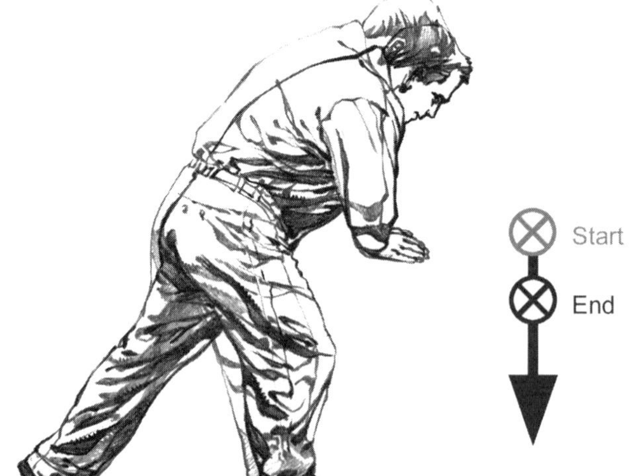



**FIGURE 5.3**

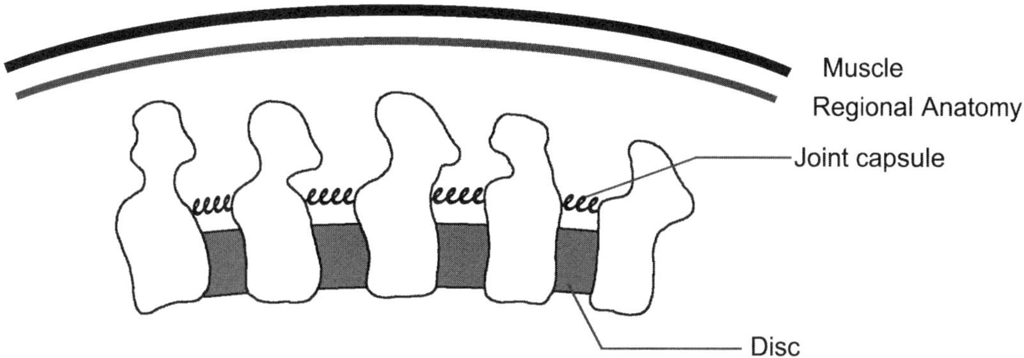



**FIGURE 5.4**

resistive forces contribute to the overall energy exchange by restricting and dissipating energy intended for the joint of interest in the patient. We will see later in our study of high- and low-force manipulation that the characteristics of the treatment and the rate of force application dictate what structures will be primarily responsible for braking the incoming energy.

## RESTORING FORCES

Restoring forces[9] are static forces that resist deformation and are best conceptualized as the Patient's stiffness. They are intrinsic forces that make the spine comparatively rigid and stable. This is vested primarily in the no-contractile properties of the spine.[10] The stiffness of the Patient dictates how much of the adjustment's energy can pass through this barrier (Figure 5.5).

Put another way, restoring forces are relative to the resistance to deformation (change in length and shape). The primary concept here is that the greater the stiffness of the patient, assuming the Doctor's rigidity remains the same, the greater the impact velocity. This is the impact velocity that

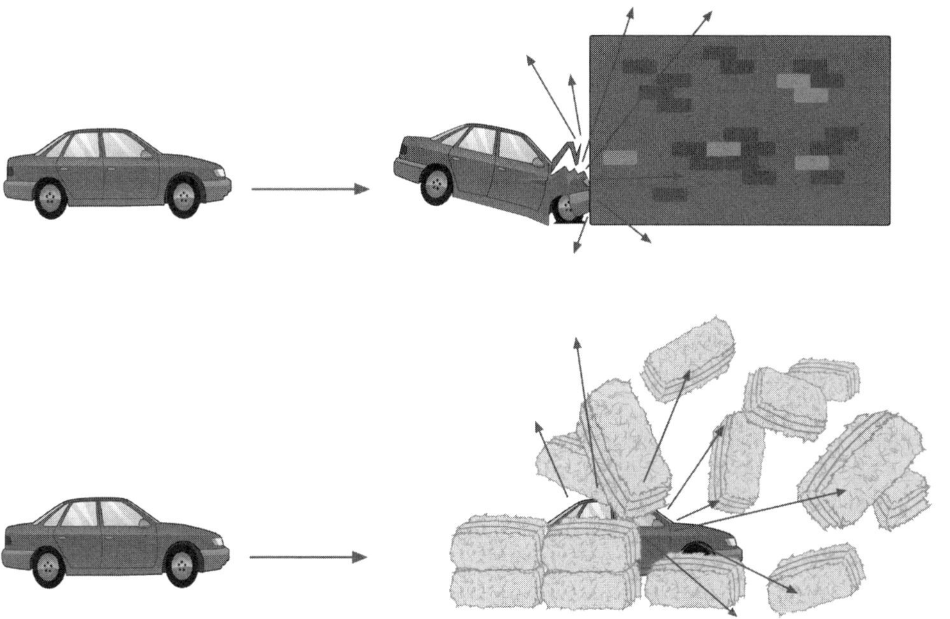

**FIGURE 5.5**

## <u>DAMPING FORCES:</u>  Dynamic Properties of the Patient

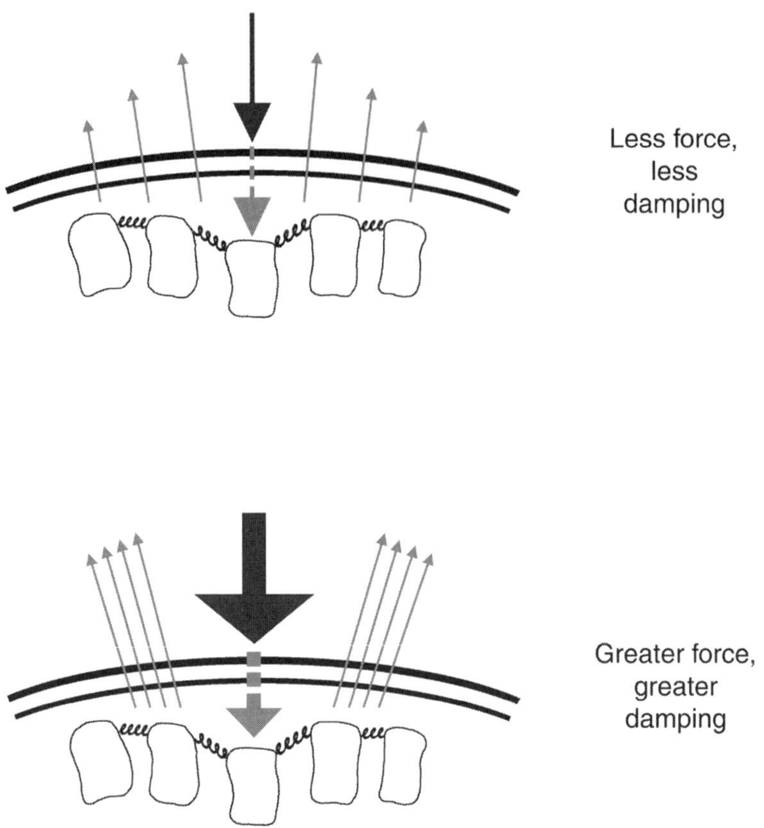


**FIGURE 5.6**

is experienced. Conversely, if a car hits bales of hay, there is less of a collision force because more energy can pass through the barrier.

### DAMPING FORCES

Damping forces act to resist motion and reduce the amplitude of the incoming energy.[11] Thus, the greater the velocity of motion, the greater the damping response by the body. Essentially, the presence of friction reduces the mechanical energy intended to the joint of interest and the motion is said to be *damped* as energy is lost to heat [12] (Figure 5.6).

Kinetic energy not lost to frictional damping is the measure of a system's elasticity.[13] The thickness and characteristics as well as tone of the soft tissue dictate its elasticity[14] (Figure 5.7).

Let's look, for example, at an elastic patient versus an inelastic patient. First, however, it is important to remember that, in a manipulative procedure, a large velocity produces large damping forces[15] as the patient's contractile structures react to resist motion.[16] The patient's damping resistance to deformation is relative to the characteristics of the incoming energy.[17] The more elastic the collision, the more energy remains to do the work in separating a joint.[18]

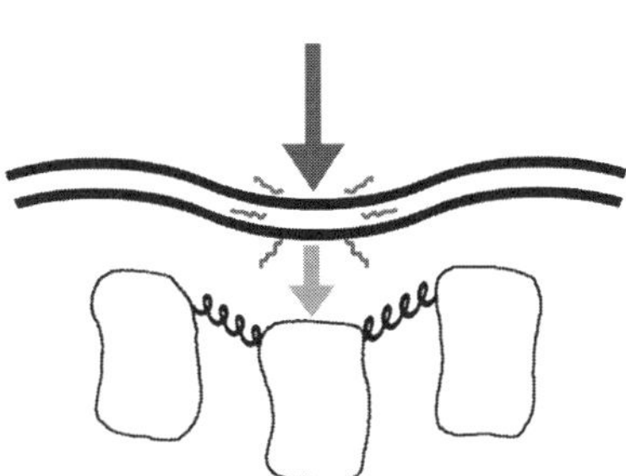


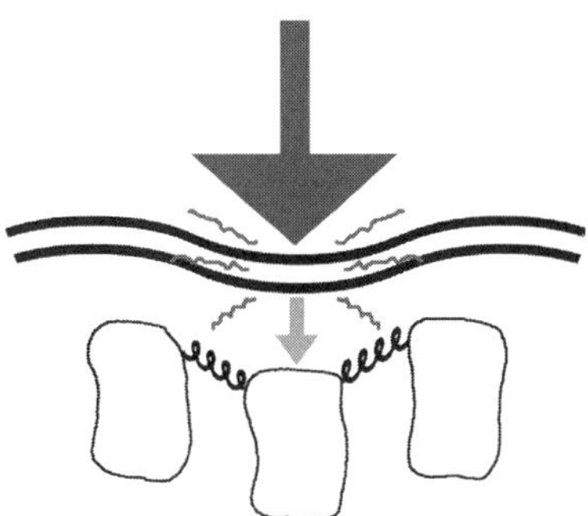


**FIGURE 5.7**

The combined mechanical resistance to deformation by both restoring or stiffness (which is a static property) and damping (which is a dynamic property) work together to absorb incoming energy.

It is important to clarify before leaving our discussion of the Patient system that connective tissues have both elastic and plastic qualities.[19] We are no longer discussing soft tissue braking incoming energy. Instead, these are characteristic behaviors of soft-tissue deformation in response to being loaded or stretched.

Elastic qualities include:

- Springlike connective tissue
- Elongates with a load
- Returns to normal length when load is removed

Plastic qualities include:

- Damping connective tissue
- Elongates with a load
- Changes shape when load is removed

We will see in our comparison of high- and low-force adjusting that the characteristics of soft tissue's elastic or plastic deformation[20] play a fundamental role in determining which manual therapy procedure will be most clinically effective in making the desired changes.

The Patient system may be summarized as follows:

1. The Patient system acquires the kinetic energy imparted by the Doctor.
2. The (static) restorative stiffness of an area restricts energy to the individual joints.

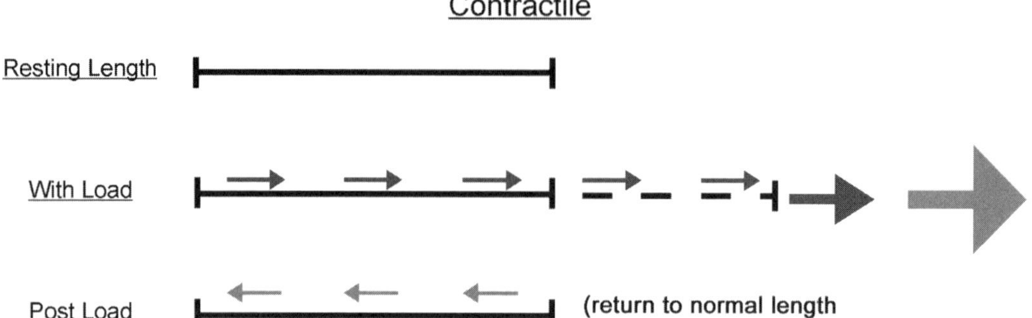



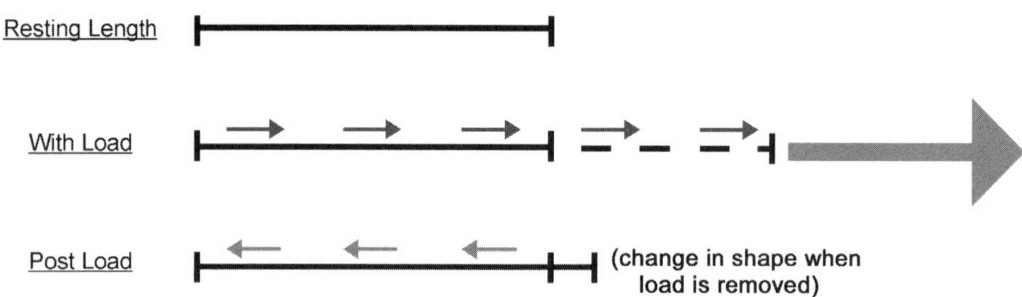



**FIGURE 5.8**

3. Secondary (dynamic) dampening forces also react to dissipate energy, reducing the amount that enters the individual joints.
4. Combined overall resistance to deformation by static and dynamic forces act to brake the incoming energy.


## A "DYNAMIC IMPRESSION"

The passing of energy created in one system and braked by the second, by nature, is complex. Yet, with this complexity recognized, chiropractors and osteopaths are producing what are considered successful manipulations repeatedly in their practices. The manipulative treatments and their unique characteristics have evolved to maximize clinical success.[21] The interplay of the doctor and the patient is a unique moment in time. It is at this moment we can measure energy and its relationship to time (Figure 5.9).

The analysis of objective information obtained can be used to evaluate the manipulative treatment. In the next section, we take a closer look at manipulative forces. We measure the forces the Doctor produces as well as quantify and evaluate those forces and their relative change as a treatment progresses from start to finish.

For simplicity, two types of normalized adjustments[22] will be evaluated: adjustments that are considered to be high force and those that are considered to be low force.

## The "Dynamic Impression"

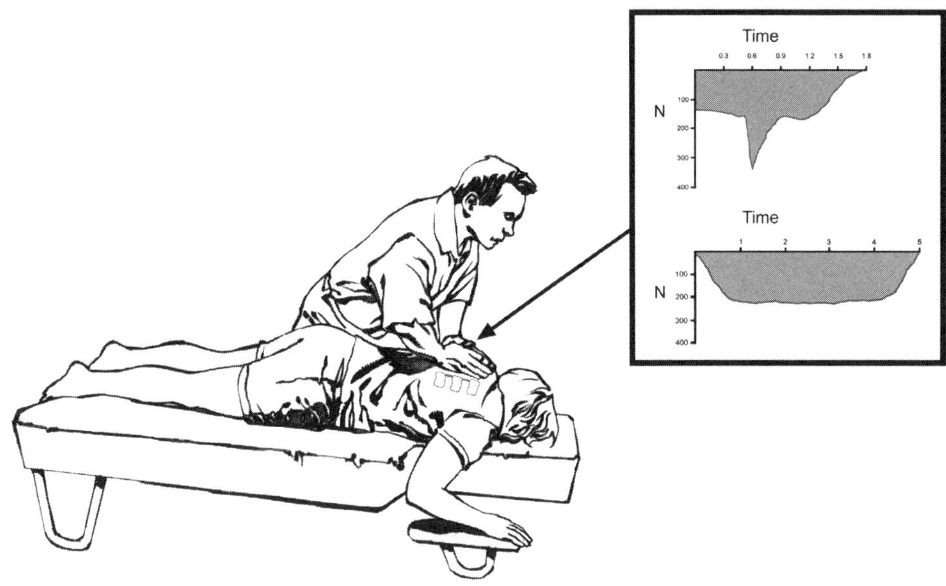


**FIGURE 5.9**

### HIGH-FORCE MANIPULATION

High-force manipulation is a primary tool used as a treatment for chronic problems of the spine. The goal in high-force procedures is to restore spinal joint biomechanics.[23] Quantifications of the high-force manipulation have long been established.[24] Force–time histograms can best express the relationship of how much force is being used and at what time in the treatment. A force–time profile lets us capture the "Dynamic Impression" of each spinal treatment. Thus, the visual representation can be used to objectively evaluate the actual treatment rendered by the Doctor (Graph 5.1).

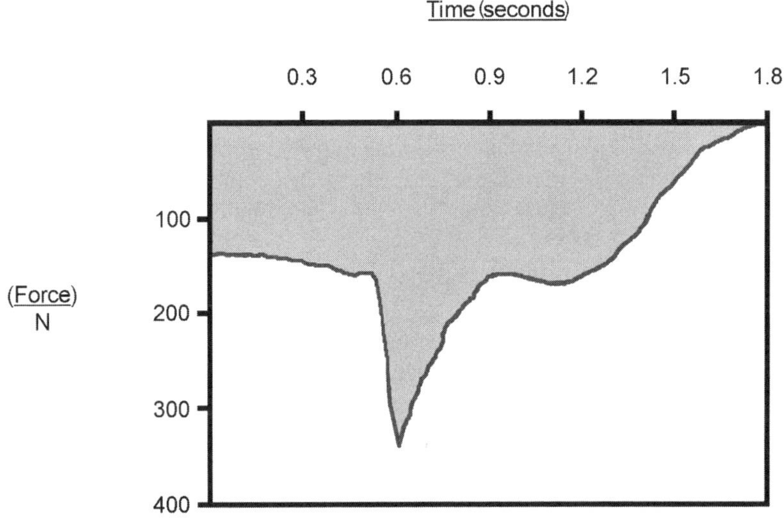


**GRAPH 5.1**  High-force spinal treatment.

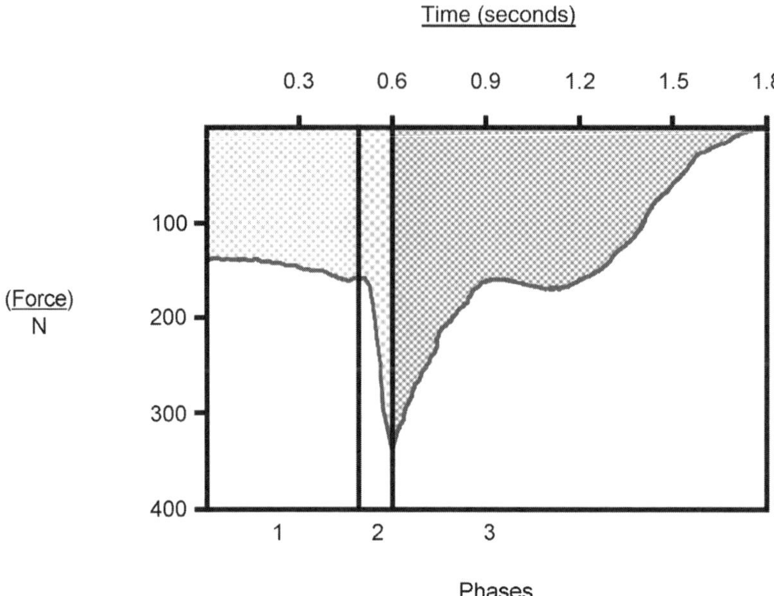


**GRAPH 5.2**   Three phases of a high-velocity manual procedure.

This continuum of applied force over time provides a scientific framework to evaluate each treatment. Note that high-force manipulation is characterized by a thrust of high speed for a short duration. The set on–off sequence produces a wavelike "dynamic impression" that is individual to each treatment. The unique variables of the kinetic energy passed from the Doctor to the patient can be evaluated. High-force manipulation is quick. In general, the treatment lasts around 0.7 sec once the preadjustive force is established.[25–27] A quick thrust or impulse of energy is moved into the patient. The acceleration phase lasts approximately 0.115 sec, average time.[28]

## MANIPULATION TIMELINE

Graph 5.2 shows the three phases of a high-velocity manual procedure. This timeline helps establish the behavior of the three phases of high-force treatment. We can see that the applied forces have different characteristics at different times during the treatment application.

The three phases of the dynamic thrust are preload, acceleration, and resolution.

The events of a high-force manipulation as they happen are shown as a timeline in Graph 5.3. *Phase 1* includes equilibrium, preload, and dip. *Phase 2* is comprised of initiation, acceleration, thrusting force, cavitation, and peak force (maximum amplitude). *Phase 3* is resolution/decline (return to equilibrium).

The various components of the different phases may be summarized in Graph 5.3 as follows.

1. **Equilibrium/start:** Contact with the patient is initiated.
A. **Preload phase:** A quasi-static load applied to the segment to be manipulated in the same direction as the intended loads of the manipulation. Its purpose is to reduce the elastic damping[29] of the spinal manipulative therapy force through compression of the soft tissues and movement of the joint through the available range of motion. It is hyphothesized that preload force may compress the soft tissue enough to cause it to behave in a predictable or at least a more predictable manner, but this also remains to be tested. It's a relatively constant force that can be applied for several seconds. The preload phase ends when a sudden increase in force is seen.

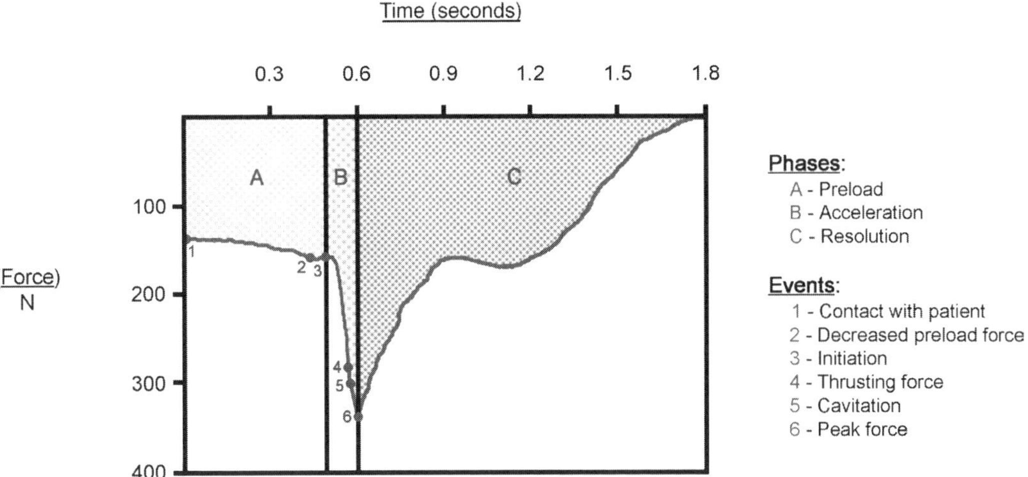



**GRAPH 5.3**  A timeline sequence.

2. **Dip:**[30] A short interval of decreasing preload force immediately before the dynamic impulse of spinal manipulative therapy. Its presence may vary and it is considered a negative attribute in manipulation. By easing up on the preload force, it is possible to lose the distraction and the benefits of preadjustive tension.

3. **Initiation:** Has no intrinsic principles of its own. It is a moment in time that marks the onset of the acceleration phase. It is general knowledge that the "best time to proceed" with a high-force adjustment is at the moment the patient relaxes. It is also well understood that the proper timing of the treatment to coincide with the patient's relaxation will optimize the manipulative procedure.[31]

B. **Acceleration phase:** The average slope of the thrust force onset. This slope can be used for acceleration analysis and may be divided into an upper and lower rate by dividing the rise time in half. Preliminary study suggested[32] that the two regions might have different behaviors.[33] The acceleration phase, which is the time frame from initiation to peak force, can be divided into two phases: the initial and the terminal phase. The time from the sudden increase in force to onset of the manipulation thrust to its peak development was 0.135 sec in a sample group from which this example is taken.[34] This is close to physiological reaction times. As a result, the duration of the thrust may be as important as the displacement in producing segment motion, but this has not been tested.

4. **Thrusting force:** The dynamic component of the total manipulative force. A rapid event, whose key component is speed. It is possible that this is the most important component in causing cavitation in high-force adjusting.[35] Force is a function of velocity and amplitude and can be categorized as either high or low. However, force is a continuum. The velocity and amplitude of the thrust should be chosen based on the intended outcome of the procedure. Controlled velocity and controlled amplitude are attributes of skilled manual therapy. When a sudden increase in force is seen, it is at this point that the thrust application begins.

5. **Cavitation:** Defined as the audible sound achieved by manipulation.[36] There is speculation that the state of tissue compliance prior to manipulation greatly influences the force required to achieve cavitation and may act as a predictor of the force required to

achieve cavitation. Cavitation is caused by an increase in joint volume and a corresponding decrease in fluid partial pressure, creating a gas bubble as intra-articular gases are
drawn out of solution. As a result, fluid rushes into the area of low-pressure volume,
collapsing the gas bubble, which releases energy that may be heard as a crack. Cavitation
has been related to a temporary increase in joint space and a concomitant increase in
active and passive range of motion of the cavitated joint.[37]

6. **Peak force:** The thrust application continues until a peak, or maximum, force is reached.
   At this time the joint of interest experiences its maximum amplitude. Amplitude is defined
   as the maximum distance that an object moves away from its equilibrium position.[38]

C. **Resolution phase/decline:** The decrease in force following the peak force is known as
   the resolution phase. This phase is considered to be post-adjustive and is characterized
   by the system's return to equilibrium.

## The Successful High-Force Manipulation

A successful high-force manipulation (see Graph 5.4) involves a thrust or impulse that moves the
joint beyond the elastic barrier into the paraphysiological space.[39] "More forceful procedures are
chosen when the intent is to break adhesions in the capsular fibers, restore normal tracking, reduce
capsular entrapment, stimulate articular nerve ending, or relieve mechanical blockage."[40] A successful manipulation is most often associated with a resulting cavitation or rapid gapping of the
joint. This audible crack is a result of creating sudden negative pressure within the joint space,
causing the liberation of synovial gases.

High-force manipulation employs brevity, which utilizes the principle of inertia.[41] Inertia is
sometimes referred to as Newton's first law, and it tells us that the tendency of an object is to
remain at rest until acted upon.[42] The sluggishness of the individual vertebrae keeps them in their
equilibrium position. In other words, the brief impulse of energy exploits inertia and, due to brevity,
facilitates joint isolation. This illustrates how the Doctor's quickness or the rapid acceleration of
energy into the patient is very important in the skill of manipulation. High speed coupled with
preadjusted tension, which has compressed the regional anatomy, leads to a single joint being
isolated.[43] By maximizing the manipulative energy into the desired joint, pushing it past the
paraphysiologic space, a successful adjustment has been achieved.

The brevity of the impulse isolates the individual vertebrae in a high-force adjustment. This
isolation of manipulative energy to one level with quickness is one of the primary "skills of joint
manipulation."

We can see from Graph 5.5 that the applied energy is very effective if we want to isolate the
intersegmental capsular fibers or restore proper tracking to an individual articulation. Understanding
of the structure and function of the posterior spinal joints is of primary importance[44] since high-force
manipulation is clinically directed at removal or reversible fixations in the posterior articulations.[45]

## Muscle Guarding Ineffectual

While the primary function of muscle is to produce movement, muscles can also effectively restrict
motion. The same contractile forces that produce movement can also oppose it.[46] The energy-
absorbing capabilities of skeletal muscle are no less important to the control of motion than its
energy-imparting function, both of which depend on muscle contracture.[47] It is well understood
that muscle spasms may increase muscle contracture. Dampening of energy is relative to the
incoming force and the muscle's response to that force. If the patient tenses to guard pain due to
involuntary muscle splinting, a large portion of the manipulated energy is dampened so as to be
insufficient to push the joint beyond the passive range of motion. This is considered to be an
unsuccessful manipulation because the paraphysiological space was not reached and joint separation
was not attained. (See Graph 5.6.)

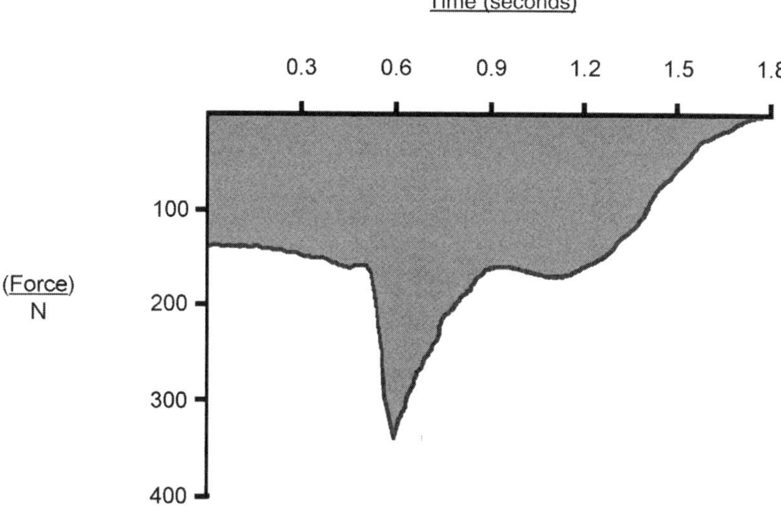



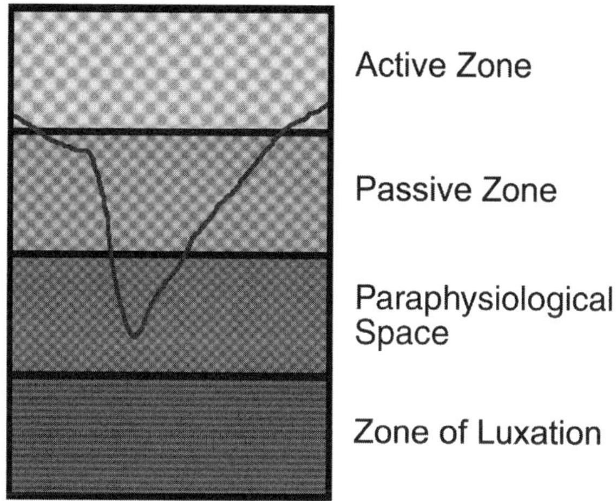



**GRAPH 5.4** A successful high-force manipulation.

## Low-Force Manipulation

Low-force manipulation is a unique type of clinical treatment. Low-force manipulation is a passive movement that tractions the joint to the end point of this elastic barrier.[48] Its unique characteristics make it the treatment of choice for some clinical situations. Let's look at the "Dynamic Impression" of a low-force spinal treatment.

We can see from Graph 5.7 that a low-force manipulation is uneventful. A tensile type of energy is passed from the doctor to the patient. Force application takes place for a longer duration and generally lasts from 3 to 5 sec. Overall, the low-force treatment is a quasi-static force for the treatment duration. It lacks the previously described phases; noticeably absent are the preload and

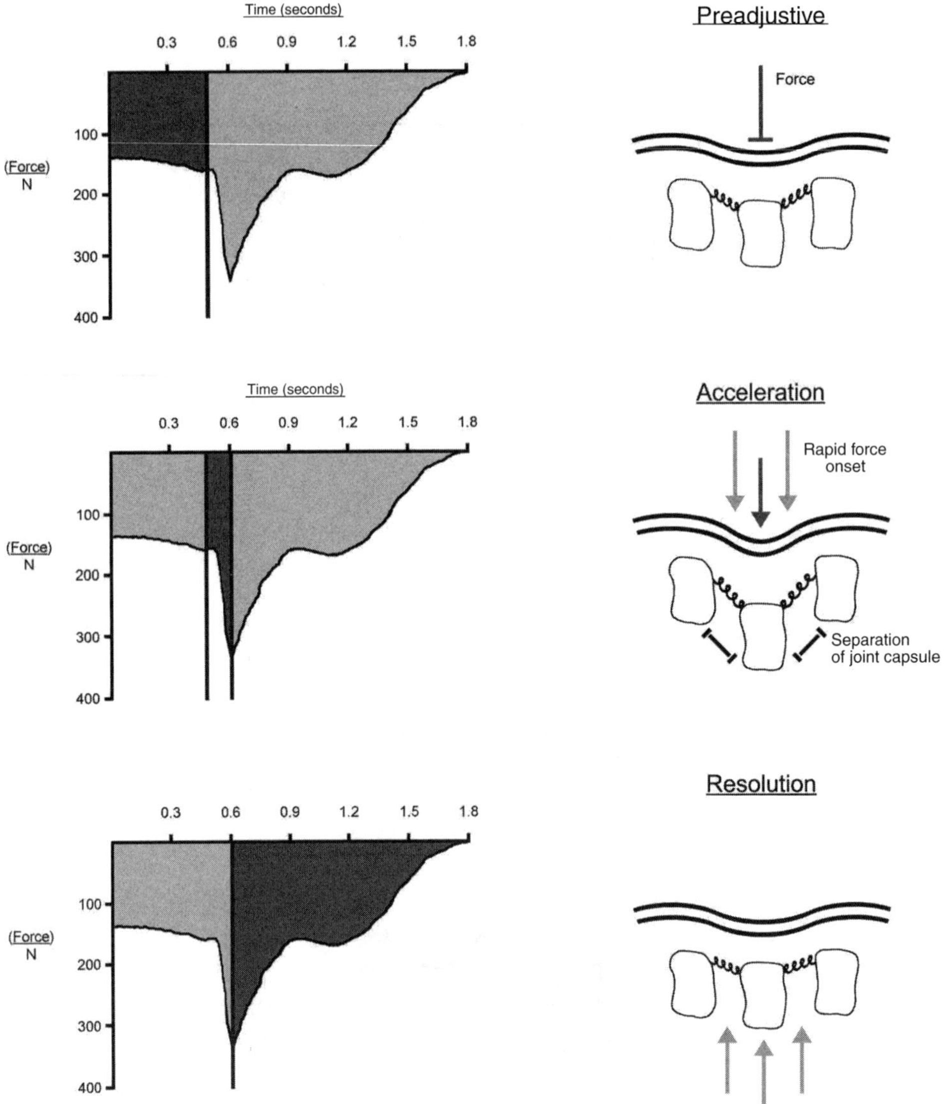



**GRAPH 5.5**   The phase function.

thrusting phases. This lack of variability in low-force treatment and its uneventful "dynamic impression" represent a purposely individual method of imparting energy into the patient.

As shown in Graph 5.8, the low-force procedure is often repeated. The repetition can be for a predetermined number of times or until the clinician feels that he has accomplished his goal. The low-force procedure is routinely done in succession, so the true application of energy would better be represented as shown in Graph 5.9.

By repetition of the procedure, the total energy of the treatment is equal to the cumulative work that was done to the joint of interest. What happens in the patient with a mobilization procedure? The slow, constant application of the energy allows continuous tensile forces within the physiological space. A mobilization procedure with its longer duration and constant application of force dictates what specific connective tissues work to brake the incoming energy in the Patient system. The slow, passive stretch affects the regional shortened soft tissues.[49] This is accomplished by using a constant force over a longer period. This results in a force application that is potent in creating

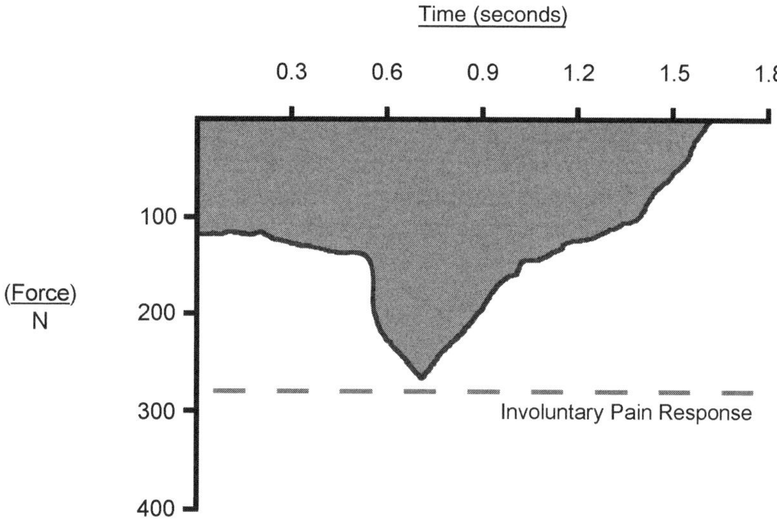


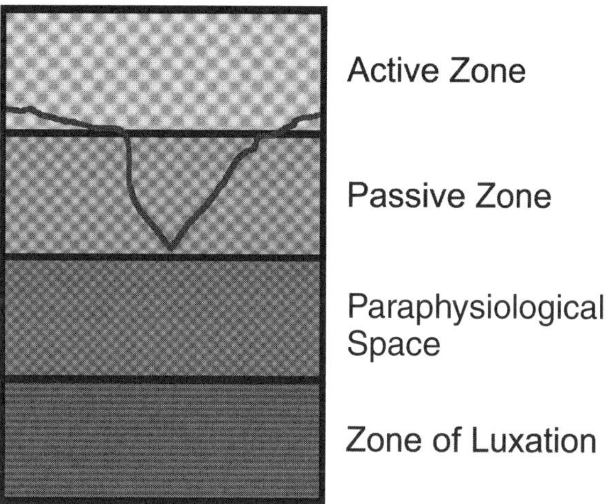


**GRAPH 5.6**  Ineffectual spinal treatment.

plastic deformation[50] in the globally shortened abnormal and thus more easily deforming soft tissue elements. The relative portion of plastic deformation versus nonpermanent elastic deformation favors plastic changes. This allows the restoration of the area's global range of motion. The low-force tissue stretching and its effects vary inversely with the time and force used. The loading of biological tissues produces a characteristic stress–strain curve,[51] as shown in Graph 5.10.

The elongation or deformation is measured in relationship to the applied load. After the initial slack in the ligament has been stretched, the ligamentous tissue quickly becomes stiffer. All connective tissue elements are effected by immobilization, each with its unique pattern of change.[52,53] When joints are immobilized, adhesions form between adjacent connective tissue structures.[54] Forced motion leads to a physical disruption of these adhesions, as well as a disruption

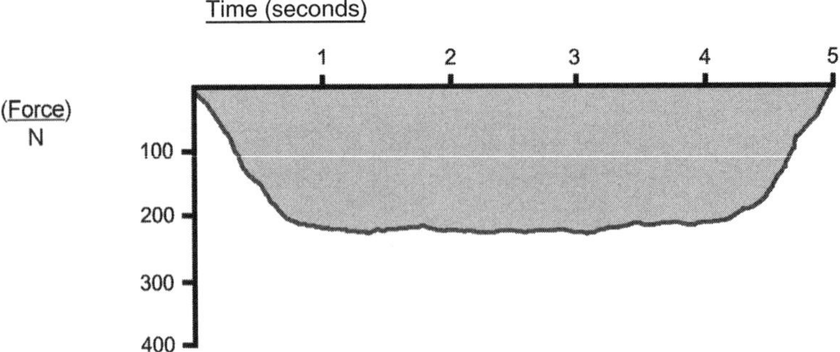



**GRAPH 5.7**   Low-force spinal treatment.

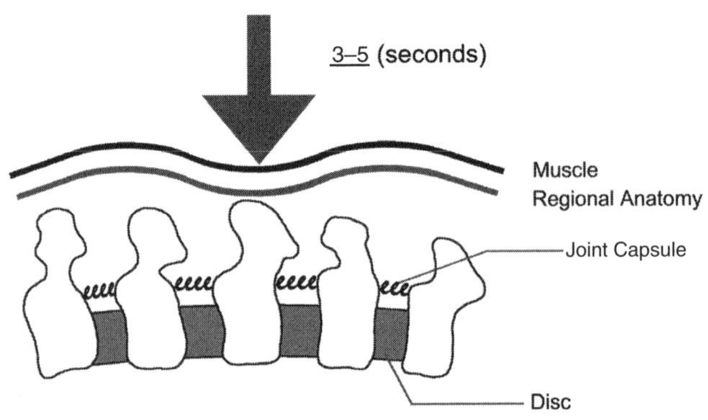



Low-Force Spinal Treatment

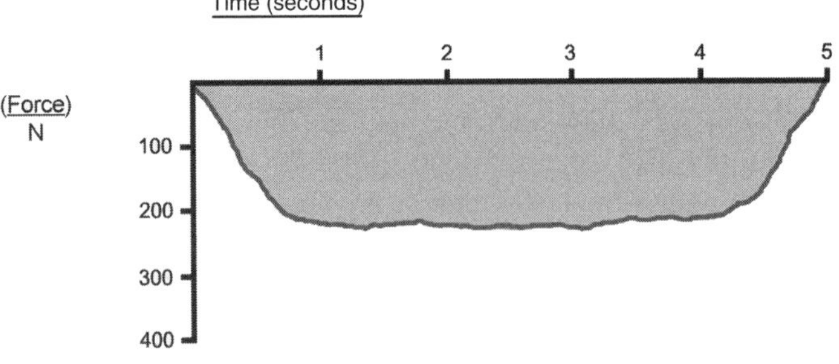



**GRAPH 5.8**   Low-force 3–5 sec/muscle regional anatomy.

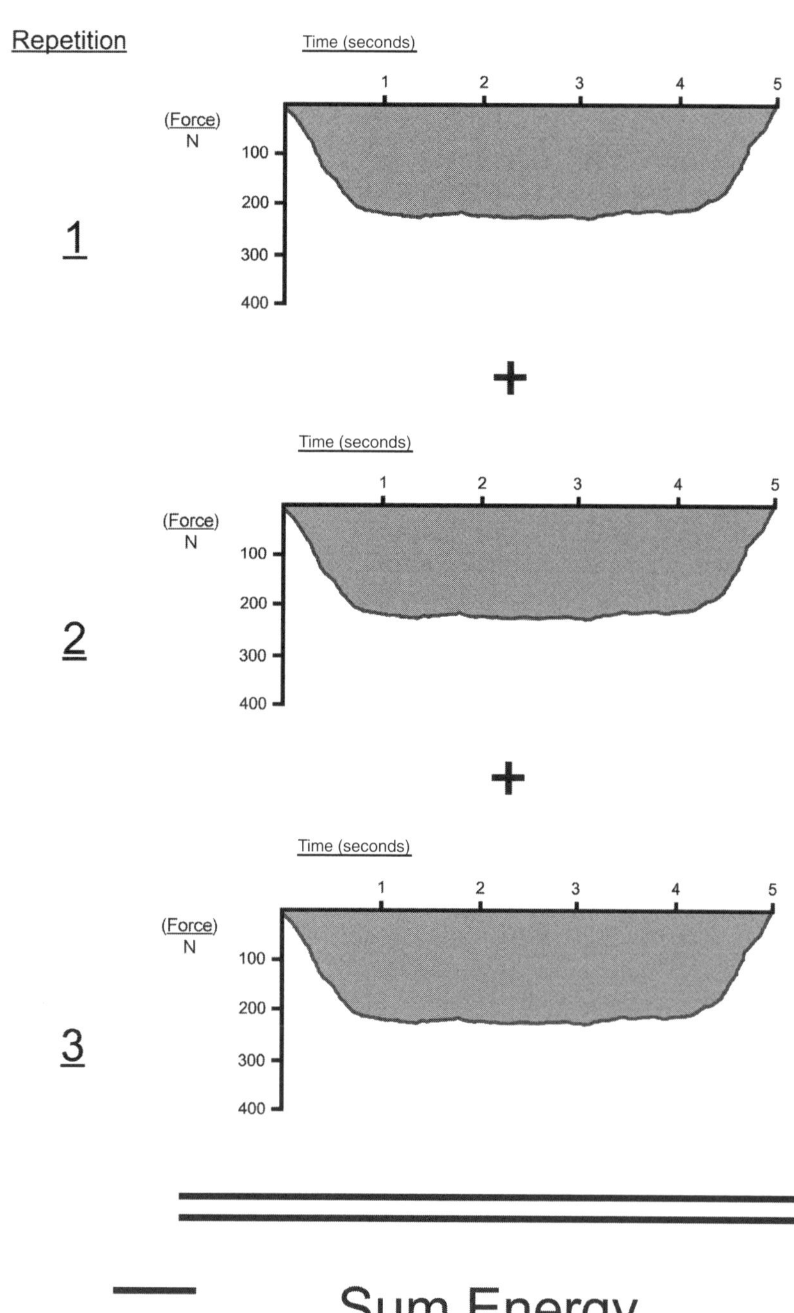



**GRAPH 5.9**  Sum energy/low force.

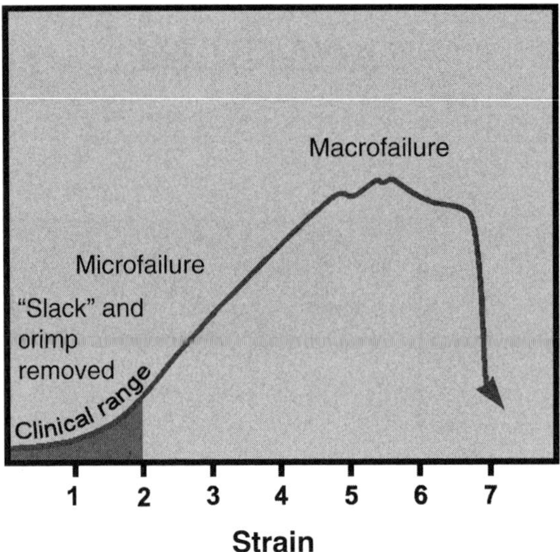



**GRAPH 5.10**  Stress–strain curve.

intermolecular cross-linkages. The further a structure is stretched beyond its slack phase, the more bonds that are broken and the greater the hysteresis.[55] According to Bogduk and Twomey,[70] the energy lost after prolonged or repetitive loading is called hysteresis.[56]

This stress–strain curve illustrates hysteresis (see Graph 5.11). After repeat loading, tissue creep will occur. This is resulting from the gradual rearrangement of collagen fibers, proteopolycans, and water in the tissues being stressed.[57] Essentially, when the external forces are removed, the structures regain shape at a different rate than it was deformed. Any difference in the initial and final shape is called a "set."[58] The set or difference in the initial and final length of the tissues stretched is the work done by the energy of the low-force adjustment. The gains accomplished in the hysteresis set are what help in the restoration of an area's global range of motion.[59]

## HIGH FORCE VS. LOW FORCE

What is the role of each treatment? Some general rules would be

**Low force:** If the intention of the procedure is to stretch ligaments, a low-amplitude, long-duration procedure is indicated. This helps restore the global range of motion to an area.[60]

**High force:** If the intention is to affect a joint that is mistracking, a high-force procedure is indicated.[61] This could be due to, but not limited to, capsular fibers, specifically, fibers that do not align along the normal lines of stress in that joint and limit or alter the joint's tracking.

The type of manual therapy used determines whether the elastic or plastic properties of the soft tissue are affected.[62] A high-force manipulative treatment and its characteristic high force results in elastic deformation.[63] A low-force manipulative treatment over a long period results in plastic deformation.[64] It should be noted that force is a continuum and the relative ratio of plastic and elastic deformation can vary widely depending on how and under what conditions the therapy is applied.[65] Due to the duration of the adjustment, there are different total amounts of energy characteristics to each treatment. Let's evaluate the "area" referring to the region under the force time curve. The total work done by a varying force is equal to the "area" under the force displacement curves. (See Graph 5.12.)

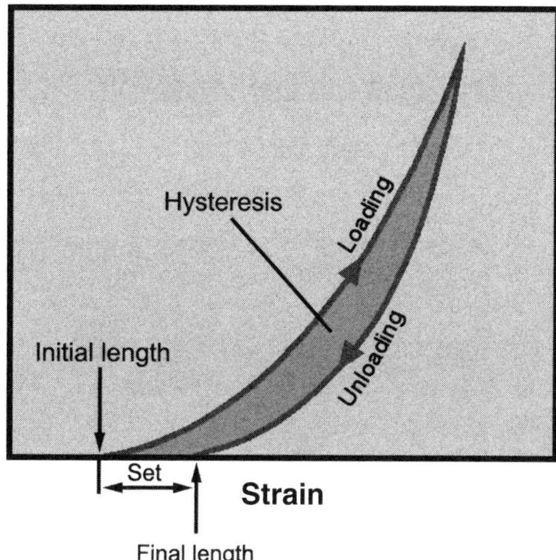


**GRAPH 5.11**   Rehab of spine: hysteresis.

This obvious difference in the amount of total energy produced by each treatment should be noted by the clinician. Clearly each treatment type is unique and can accomplish different effects on the patient.

## DOSE–RESPONSE

We see that in comparing high-force and low-force manipulative treatments, the energy passed on to the patient can be highly variable. The identification of this principle can help determine what spinal adjustments are more effective than others.[66] A scientific database could help document and measure individual spinal adjustments with the pursuit of more effective patient adjustments and clinical outcomes. Similar clinical outcomes can benefit from previous manipulative trials. The data can be used by the clinician to develop a more effective and accurate manual therapy procedure plan. Other treatment methods such as medications are commonly prescribed in a dose–response relationship. Could a manipulative prescription someday direct treatment?

Sample of dose recommendation for manipulative therapy is

* Appropriate manual procedures
* Frequency of treatments necessary for change to occur
* Duration – how long is it necessary for treatment to proceed?

Further understanding of how manipulative therapy achieves its clinical therapeutic benefits would be beneficial for the manipulative profession. But most important, such an understanding will aid the patient by maximizing the effectiveness of manual procedures. Manipulation will benefit from increased utilization as treatment outcomes document clinical success.

## SAFETY

Any adjustment with too great of an amplitude threatens the joint from overdistention past the limit of anatomical integrity. Again, amplitude is defined as the maximum disturbance as an object moves away from its equilibrium point. Graph 5.13 shows Sandoz zones.

## ENERGY PRODUCED

### High Force = Spinal Treatment

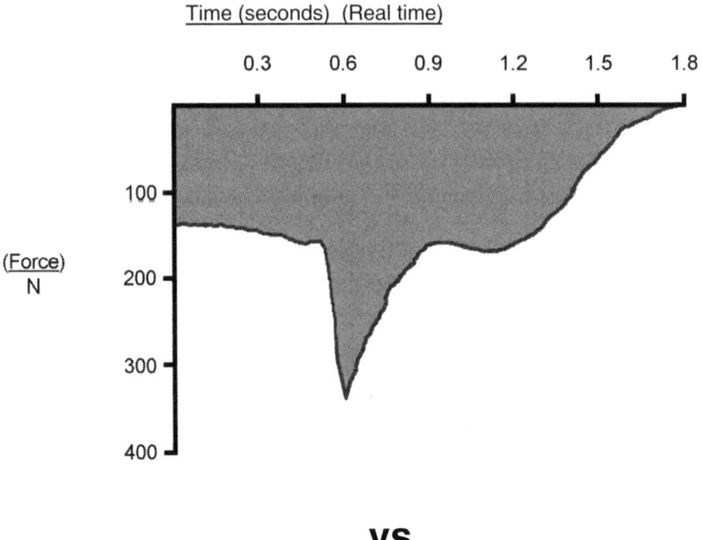


## VS.

### Low Force = Spinal Treatment

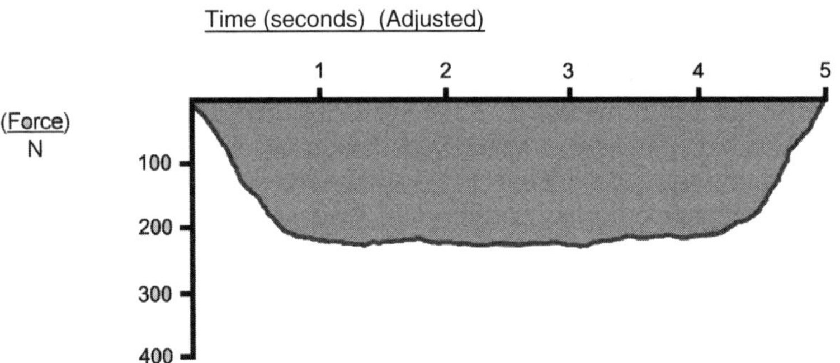


**GRAPH 5.12**   Low-force vs. high-force energy produced.

Controlling the depth of a high-force adjustment is an important psychomotor skill.[67] The clinician should have a clear understanding by this point that amplitude is not an independent characteristic. It takes the generation of a inordinately large velocity or an extremely long duration to produce sufficient energy for overdistraction of the joint, causing joint injury. Graph 5.14 shows HF (max amp) LF (max amp).

## THE MUA PROCEDURE

The manipulative portion of the MUA procedure is a combination of 70% stretch and 30% articular manipulation.[68] Both high-force and low-force manipulations are used in the MUA protocol. The purpose of anesthesia is to reduce muscular tension which translates into a decreased overall patient

## ANATOMICAL INTEGRITY

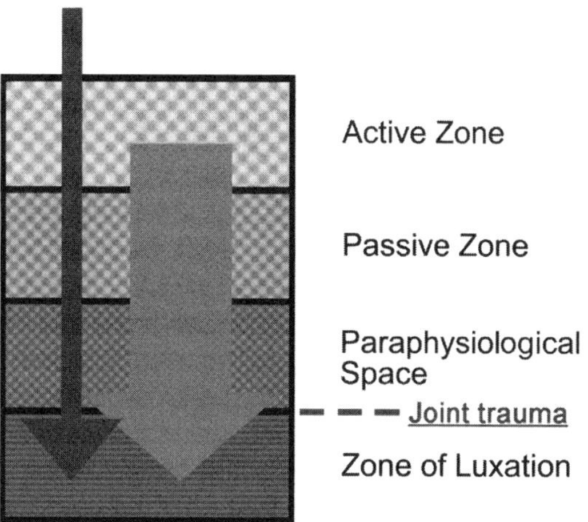


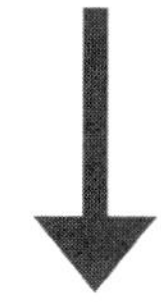

**GRAPH 5.13**

resistance to deformation. This is accomplished mostly by decreasing the secondary contractile damping forces surrounding the area. Decreasing the dynamic attenuation of the energy results in a decreased resistance to deformation. This in turn allows more energy to reach the intended joint.

This example (Graph 5.15) has been simplified to convey a concept — that by reducing the secondary damping forces in the patient, more of the energy enters the individual joint. This graph should allow the clinician the ability to conceptualize how equal external forces cause different relative displacements in patients with and without anesthesia.

Our rudimentary understanding or how manipulative energy is passed from one system to anther is sufficient to understand that by changing the Patient system, we have a different type of manipulative treatment. This fact should not be overlooked! With MUA, a far greater amount of tissue compliance can always be obtained than in the regular office setting.

According to Gordon,[68] "The biochemical activity of the anesthetic causes the brief interruption of afferent response to joint, joint capsule, and surrounding muscular reaction by the mechanore-

## AMPLITUDE

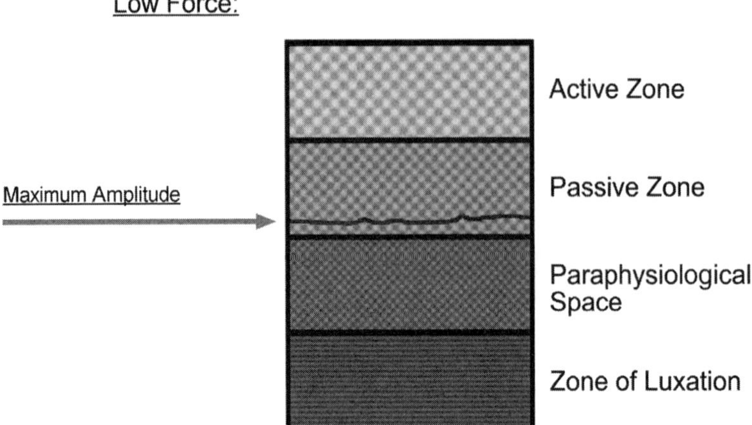


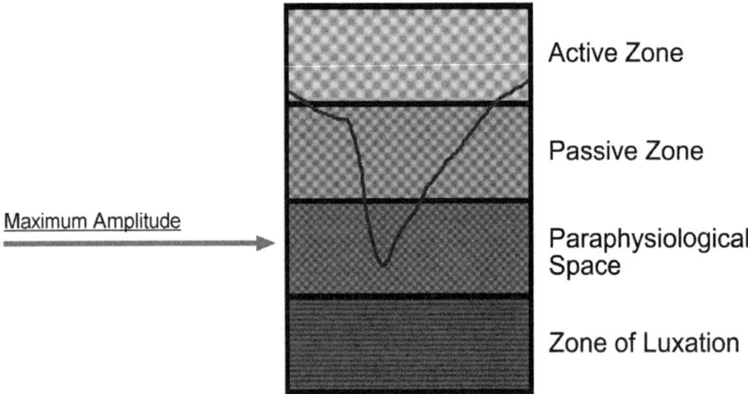


**GRAPH 5.14**  HF (max amp) LF (max amp).

ceptors so that these areas are able to be moved without the immediate afferent response of protective muscle splinting that would normally occur with the manipulation if anesthesia were not used."[69]

## FROM ART TO SCIENCE

Technology has helped quantify the manipulative art. As manipulation moves to a modern era, the basic building blocks of a manipulative science have been set in place. The foundation of understanding and quantification has been hard. Art became science and, as such, could be measured, reproduced, and controlled. We have witnessed this throughout history — the stars guiding the early explorers on the open sea or uncharted land in a quest for knowledge and rewards. Today, science and technology have advanced to the point where anyone can purchase an inexpensive global positioning satellite unit and, with accuracy beyond the imagination, know their position anywhere on the planet. Likewise, with the advance of science and technology gained from

# RELATIVE DISPLACEMENT

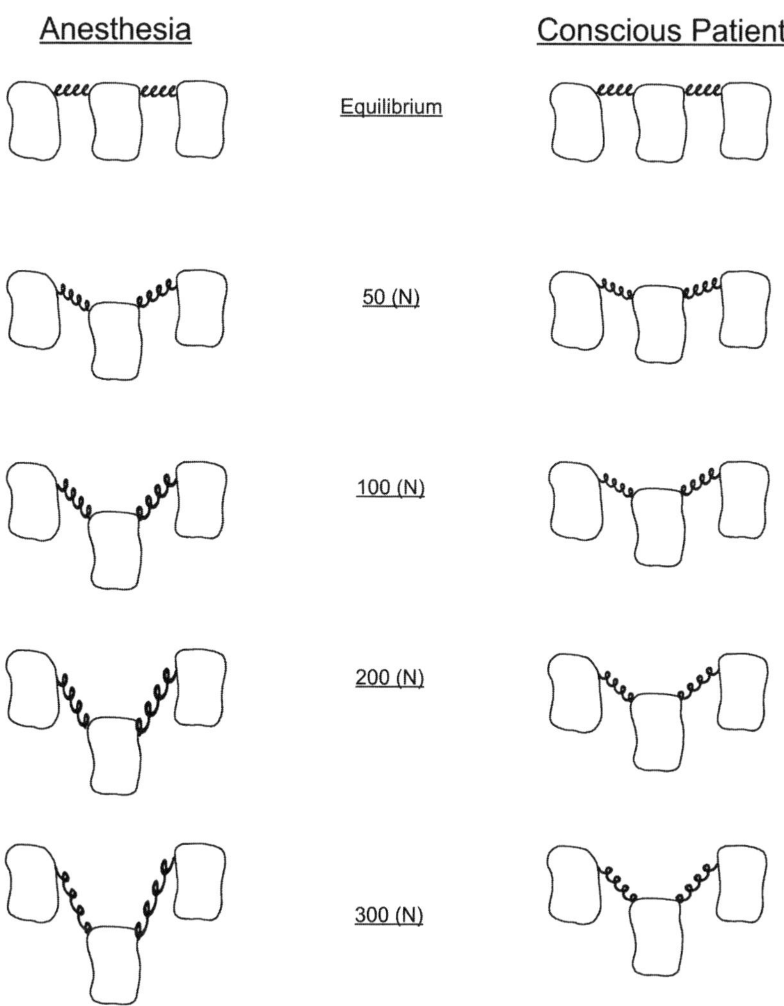


**GRAPH 5.15**   Relative displacement.

understanding or quantification the "Gift of Art" will no longer be a trial-and-error process. Skill and clinical accuracy gained through clinical advances and manipulative repetition will be enhanced. Both the positive and negative attributes of manipulation will be universally established, and once again, science and technology will remove any guesswork and help establish guidelines based on scientific evidence. The energy of the manipulative treatment to the patient will have a better chance of clinical success due to the honing and forward advancing of the positive characteristics of manipulation therapy. The goal would be to have a target energy or force with each treatment as determined by a dose–response relationship. Negative or unneeded aspects of manipulation that have entered the modern era via specific technique systems or outdated thinking could be eliminated. We could, in a sense, make manipulation or manipulation therapy more effective. This predictability could have a profound impact, including, but not limited to, a safer and more potent manipulative treatment.

To predict at this point the future of manipulation therapy is a risky proposition. What is the optimum force in the adjustment, what is the optimum amplitude of the adjustment, and what is the ideal speed of the adjustment? If the answers to these questions were known, it would simplify greatly the teaching of chiropractic/osteopathic techniques, but these are not easy questions to answer. With manual adjusting, it is almost impossible for the adjuster to control all of these factors in a consistent, reliable, and reproducible manner that lends itself to clinical studies. We are sure to encounter more challenges as the evolution of manipulation takes place. While the eventual destination of manipulation is a more positive and predictable outcome for the patient, the precise criteria have yet to be established. The tools of exploration have been developed. These tools, though rudimentary at this time, have added insight and are paramount in the first stages of scientific quantification and the progression of the manipulative art. "Our facts must be correct. Our theories need not be if they help us to discover important new facts."[2]

## REFERENCES


1. Serway, R., Foughn, J. 1992. *College Physics*, 3rd ed. Orlando, FL: Saunders Publishing, 118.
2. Kersch, T.S. 2003. Personal papers. Vista, CA.
3. Serway, R., and Foughn, J. *College Physics*, 80.
4. Haas, M. 1990. The physics of spinal manipulation. Part I. The myth of f = ma. *J. Manipulative Physiol. Ther.*, 13: 204–6.
5. Ibid.
6. Herzog, W. 1992. The physics of spinal manipulation. *J. Manipulative Physiol. Ther.*, 15: 402–6.
7. Ibid., graph 11.
8. Haas M. 1990. The physics of spinal manipulation. Part IV. A Theoretical consideration of the physician impact force and energy requirements needed to produce synovial joint cavitation. *J. Manipulative Physiol. Ther.* 13: 378–83.
9. Ibid.
10. Gatterman, M. 1990. *Chiropractic Management of Spine Related Disorders*, Baltimore, MD: Williams and Wilkins, 28.
11. Haas, M. 1990. The physics of spinal manipulation. Part II. A theoretical consideration of the adjustive force. *J. Manipulative Physical. Ther.* 13: 253-57.
12. Ibid.
13. Ibid.
14. Kersch, T.S. Personal papers.
15. Herzog, W. The physics of spinal manipulation, 402–6.
16. Gatterman, *Chiropractic Management of Spine Related Disorders,* 43.
17. Herzog, W. The physics of spinal manipulation, 402–6.
18. Haas, M. 1990. The physics of spinal manipulation, Part IV, 378–83.
19. Bergmann, T., Peterson, D., Lawrence, D. 1993. *Chiropractic Technique Principles and Procedures*. New York: Churchill Livingstone, 32–37.
20. Ibid.
21. Kersch, T.S. Personal papers.
22. Ibid.
23. Herzog, W., Conway, P.J., Zhang, Y., Hasler, E., Ladly, K. 1993. Forces exerted during spinal manipulative therapy. *Spine* 18: 1206–12.
24. Kersch, T.S. Personal papers.
25. Kersch, T.S. 1999. Knowsis Corporate Material, Operation Guidelines. Vista, CA.
26. Herzog, W., Conway, P.J., Zhang, Y., Hasler, E.M., Ladly, K. 1991. Forces exerted during spinal manipulative treatments of the thorasic spine. Proceedings of the International Conference of Spinal Manipulation.
27. Herzog, W. et al., Forces exerted during spinal manipulative therapy, *Spine*, 1206–12.
28. Kersch, T.S. Knowsis Corporate Material.
29. Cohen, E., Triano, J., McGregor, M., Papakyriakou, M. 1995. Biomechanical performance of spinal manipulation therapy by newly trained vs. practicing providers. *J. Manipulative Physiol. Ther.* 18: 347–52.

30. Ibid.
31. Gatterman, M. 1995. *Foundations of Chiropractic Subluxation*. St. Louis: Mosby Publishing, 101.
32. Cohen, E. et al., 347–52.
33. Kersch, T.S. Knowsis Corporate Material.
34. Ibid.
35. Haas, M. 1990. The physics of spinal manipulation. Part III. Characteristics of adjusting that facilitate joint distraction. *J. Manipulative Physiol. Ther.* 13: 305–8.
36. Bergmann T., Peterson D., Lawrence D., *Chiropractic Technique Principles and Procedures*, New York, Churchill Livingstone, 1993, p. 140–41.
37. Bergmann et al., *Chiropractic Technique Principles and Procedures*, 140–41.
38. Serway and Foughn, *College Physics*, 423.
39. Gatterman, M. *Chiropractic Management of Spine Related Disorders*, 50.
40. Gatterman, M. *Foundations of Chiropractic Subluxation*, 97.
41. Haas, The physics of spinal manipulation, Part III, 305–8.
42. Serway and Foughn, *College Physics*, 78.
43. Haas, The physics of spinal manipulation, Part III, 305–8.
44. Gatterman, M. *Chiropractic Management of Spine Related Disorders*, 48.
45. Gatterman, M. *Foundations of Chiropractic Subluxation*, 101.
46. Gatterman, M. *Chiropractic Management of Spine Related Disorders*, 43.
47. Liebenson, C. 1996. *Rehabilitation of the Spine*. Media, PA: Williams and Wilkins, 17–19.
48. Gatterman, M. *Foundations of Chiropractic Subluxation*, 92.
49. Ibid., 97–98.
50. Ibid., 101.
51. Liebenson, C. *Rehabilitation of the Spine*, 16–17.
52. Jackson, R. 1978. *The Cervical Syndrome*. Springfield, IL: Charles C Thomas.
53. Akeson, W.H., Amiel, D., La Violette, D. 1967. The connective tissue response to immobility. *Clin. Orthop.* 51: 183–98.
54 Gatterman, M. *Foundations of Chiropractic Subluxation*, 158.
55. Liebenson, C. *Rehabilitation of the Spine*, 16.
56. Ibid.
57. Gatterman, M. Foundations of Chiropractic Subluxatio, 158–59.
58. Liebenson, C. *Rehabilitation of the Spine*, 17.
59. Ibid.
60. Gatterman, M. *Foundations of Chiropractic Subluxation*, 101.
61. Ibid.
62. Ibid., 99.
63. Bergmann, T. et al., *Chiropractic Technique Principles and Procedures*, 34.
64. Ibid.
65. Liebenson, C. *Rehabilitation of the Spine,* 16–18.
66. Grostic, J. 1998. The adjusting instrument as a research tool. *Chiro. Research J.*, 1(2): 47–55.
67. Kersch, Knowsis Corporate Material.
68. Gordon, R. 2001. An evaluation of the experimental and investigational status and clinical validity of manipulation of patients under anesthesia. *J. Manipulative Physiol. Ther.* 24: 603–10.
69. Ibid.
70. Bogduk,N., Twomey, Lt: Clinical Anatomy of the Lumbar Spine. 2nd ed. Melbourne, Churchill Livingstone, 1991.

# 6 Indications and Contraindications for MUA

*Robert C. Gordon*

## CONTENTS



The "chronic patient," as the term pertains to the MUA patient, is a patient who has developed patterns of pain or restriction of movement over a prolonged period of time and who returns regularly for similar problems that are located in similar areas of the body.

The definition of "acute," as it pertains to the MUA patient, is based on severity. When a patient who has undergone a reasonable period of conservative chiropractic/manual therapy care remains pain expressive and symptomatically unchanged, or has an exacerbation of a recurrent problem, they may express an acute episode, but the condition has had a history of care. (Acute trauma or immediate injury is contraindicated with the MUA procedure in most instances.) A reasonable period of conservative care is 4–6 weeks.[1,2,3]

Deviation from this protocol is left to the discretion of the treating practitioner based on objective documentation of necessity. An example of this would be intractable pain and muscle splinting with little or no relief that interferes with activities of daily living, such as sleep, where no therapy, including pharmacologic intervention, is relieving the pain.

Indications for MUA with regard to objective and subjective clinical observations are as follows:

1. Neuromusculoskeletal conditions where manipulation and adjustment have had incomplete results but where manipulation is the treatment of choice.
2. Neuromusculoskeletal conditions that fall within the parameters for manipulation, but are so painful that narcotics and other analgesics have had little if any benefit and that may have been causing unwanted side effects.
3. The chronic patient who has reached maximum medical improvement (MMI) but who continues to have exacerbations that require therapeutic intervention to maintain the level of physical impairment.

4. Patients who have been treated for 2–8 weeks but who continue to have a pain threshold that does not allow manipulation or adjustments when this is the therapy of choice. (The decision early on in conservative care would be based on the pain interfering with sleep and normal daily functional activities.)
5. Patients who cannot control voluntary contracture or muscle splinting during manipulation or adjusting, and where treatment is being delayed or prolonged. In these cases, MUA would greatly reduce the patient's treatment period.
6. Patients who are candidates for manipulative and adjustive therapy in the office, but the extent of the injury has caused ineffective results and prolonged care because greater movement to the involved joint is necessary to produce expected clinical results.
7. Patients who are considered disc surgery patients but who fall within the parameters of MUA, which may be an alternative or interim step and may be useful as either a therapeutic or a diagnostic tool in determining the prognosis of this patient's care.
8. The patients who are candidates for manipulative or adjustive therapy but, due to restrictive adhesions causing articular fixation, are responding only minimally to conservative clinical care.

Simply because the patient did not respond to conservative care is not a reason to use the MUA procedure. The patient needs to fall within the parameters of varying indications for MUA. Those indications for MUA that have been shown to be most responsive include but are not necessarily limited to:

- Unresponsive pain, which interferes with the function of daily life and sleep patterns but which falls within the parameters for manipulation treatment
- Unresponsive to manipulation and adjustment when these are the therapies of choice
- Unresponsive muscle contracture, which is preventing normal daily activities and function
- Bulging, protruded, prolapsed, or herniated discs without free fragment
- Failed back surgery
- Restricted motion, which causes pain and apprehension from the patient, but manipulation is the therapy of choice
- Frozen or fixed articulations from adhesion formation
- Compression syndromes with or without radiculopathies caused from adhesion formation but not associated with osteophytic entrapment
- Post-traumatic syndromes from acceleration/deceleration or deceleration/acceleration types of injuries that result in painful exacerbations of chronic fixations
- Chronic recurrent neuromusculoskeletal dysfunction syndromes that result in regular periodic treatment series that are always exacerbations of the same condition
- Neuromusculoskeletal conditions that are not surgical candidates but that have reached MMI, especially with occupational injuries

## INDICATIONS

The following conditions have been found to respond well to manipulation under anesthesia. You will notice that one particular condition might involve more than one set of etiological symptoms as listed here:

1. Nerve entrapment
   Radicular — toward or close to spinal nerve root (i.e., facet syndrome); peripheral — causing blockage; away from the spinal cord (i.e., piriformis muscle contracture around sciatic nerve)

2. Chronic myofascitis
   Peripheral; muscular, fibrotic adhesion formation (i.e., chronic muscle splinting or contracture)
3. Chronic fibrositis
   Can be muscular or articular; related to fibrotic adhesion buildup (i.e., facet joint encapsulation or encapsulitis with chronic restriction of joint motion)
4. Traumatically induced restricted motion could be peripheral or radicular; may encompass all of the above entities; a differential diagnosis (d.d.) would be to rule out disc involvement (i.e., torticollis; spontaneous disc herniation)
5. Chronic muscle contracture
   Peripheral in nature; away from the spinal cord; could be related to vertebral misalignment; a different diagnosis (d.d.) would be to rule out muscle disease or muscle involved tumor (i.e., chronic muscle shortening from severe biomechanical postural change or congenital shortening of extremity, short leg syndrome, pelvic tilt, or rotation occipital shifting)
6. Acute muscle spasm associated with subluxation
   Can be peripheral or involve radicular if subluxation closes off IVF; encompasses many of the previously listed entities (i.e., chronic rib head subluxation causing dorsal paravertebral muscle spasm and intercostal neuralgia; subluxation of C6-C7-T1, causing chronic upper trapezius spasm; combination of both)
7. Chronic productive arthritis, such as spondylosis; spondylarthritis, or spondylarthrosis. Can be multiple joints or articulations (i.e., degenerative osteoarthritis causing multiple fibrotic adhesive sites)
8. Lumbarization associated with chronic acute (relating to MUA acute) pain
   Peripheral in nature; causing muscle splinting; fibrotic adhesions; chronic spasm
9. Sacralization associated with chronic/acute (relating to MUA acute) pain
   Peripheral; can cause chronic muscle splinting, contracture, spasm; fibrotic adhesion formation (i.e., relating to degenerative changes)
10. Chronic disc changes associated with fibrotic adhesions from degenerative changes
11. Disc bulge; can be peripheral or radicular pain, but usually associated with radicular (having to do with nerve root). May be chronic or acute (i.e., spontaneous disc herniation from traumatic entity).

The following is a list of spinal dysfunction conditions that have been shown to respond well to the MUA procedure. Note that this is only a partial list of conditions to be used as an example; they are not the only conditions that have responded to MUA.

## CERVICAL SPINE

Cervicalbrachial syndrome
Torticollis
Cervicogenic headache
Cluster headaches
Migraine headaches
Cervical facet syndrome
Cervical articular dyskinesia
Cervical discogenic spondylosis
Cervical disc herniation (contained within the annulus, with medical intervention)
Myofascitis of the trapezius and occipital muscular band
Acceleration/deceleration and deceleration/acceleration injuries (chronic)
Segmental dysfunction of the cervical spinal area(s)
TMJ and fibromyalgia

## Thoracic Spine

Mainly myofascial problems related to segmental joint dysfunction and rib head articular
   dyskinesia
Medial scapular border myofascitis
Thoracic scoliosis and concomitant articular dyskinesia

## Lumbar Spine

Discogenic spondylosis
Lumbar radiculopathy
Lumbopelvic articular dyskinesia
Lumbar facet syndrome
Dics herniation (contained with no fragmentation)
Myofascitis secondary to discogenic involvement
Lumbar segmental dysfunction
Chronic myofascial paravertebral muscle spasm
SI dysfunction with secondary myofascitis
Hip/pelvic rotation secondary to segmental dysfunction (or in conjunction with lumbar
   scoliosis)

The contraindications for MUA must be differentiated from more common symptoms that
might not indicate severity unless investigated further diagnostically. Those conditions that would
be contraindicated to manipulation under anesthesia are

- Any form of malignancy
- Metastatic bone disease
- Tuberculosis (TB) of the bone
- Acute fractures
- Direct manipulation of old compression fractures
- Acute inflammatory arthritis
- Acute inflammatory gout
- Uncontrolled diabetic neuropathy
- Syphilitic articular or periarticular lesions
- Gonorrheal spinal arthritis
- Osteoporosis, advanced as indicated diagnostically
- Evidence of cord or caudal compression by tumor
- Widespread staph or strep infection
- Infectious bone disease
- Sign of, or symptom of, aneurysm

The algorithm for determining indications and contraindications for MUA is

1. Identify primary site of patient discomfort.
2. Identify onset of symptoms (i.e., immediate, progressive).
3. Identify related past history and social history.
4. Identify pertinent physical characteristics (i.e., age, weight, skin color, growths on
   body, etc.).
5. Identify related symptoms from review of systems (i.e., discal articular, muscular, systemic, metastatic, etc.).

6. Identify orthopedic tests that reproduce patient's discomforts (use phrase "reproduce patient discomfort" rather than positive or negative in your H&P report).
7. Identify neurological tests that classify patient symptoms into these categories: upper motor involvement; lower motor involvement; peripheral; radicular (nerve entrapment, nerve root, respectively); sensory deprivation; motor deprivation.
8. Identify primary postural abnormalities that relate to the patient symptoms (i.e., patient gait; antalgia; scoliosis; short legs; pelvic rotation, etc.)
9. Identify primary site of palpatory tenderness that increases patient symptomatology and follows a dermatomal pattern.
10. Identify any laboratory tests that support patient's primary symptoms.
11. Identify diagnostic tests that support patient's primary symptoms.
12. Identify working diagnosis from differential diagnosis using findings from this algorithm.

In the following we show some sample uses of the algorithm for indications/contraindications.

## NERVE ENTRAPMENT

Lumbar motion unit L4-L5.
Acute recurrent exacerbation.
Patient has had recurrent back pain; last time 4 months ago.
Patient has problems extending backward but can bend forward to relieve symptoms; no urinary or bowel dysfunction.
Patient has no symptoms when doing Braggards; SLR (straight leg raising) causes muscle pull in low back bilaterally; trunk rotation and lateral bending cause discomfort.
Patient has deep tendon reflexes of 2+ and brisk bilateral lower extremities; Babinski is normal.
Patient has trouble moving around when sleeping at night; has trouble moving doing work as a secretary, especially turning from one location to another when typing, etc.
Patient has tenderness, muscle spasm, and rigidity over paraspinal muscles in lumbar spine.
Lab tests indicate normal findings except for slight increase in alkaline phosphates.
X-rays show early osteoarthritis; joint facet articular spaces are moderately thinned in neutral position and are jammed together in extension.
Patient has localized pain; pain on extension, lateral bending and rotation; has no radicular pain and no radiation of extremity pain, tenderness, tingling or numbness.

### Diagnosis

Nerve entrapment in lumbar facet articulation; facet syndrome with chronic fibrotic adhesions.

## ACUTE GOUTY ARTHRITIS

Patient (a 44-year-old male) has lumbar pain at the level of L5-S1 and constant pain in the right foot and first three toes when walking. Also has pain in the foot awakening the patient early in the morning.
Patient has had the pain come on gradually over the past 4 months, but the pain has lately been acute, especially in the foot.
Patient has been told that he has arthritis of the lower spine, and has had back pain and periodic right foot pain about a year or so ago that seemed to go away. The foot pain never seems to go away completely.
The patient has some small nodules on his elbows; the patient has soreness in the foot when he wears his right shoe, and there may be some slight reddening. The patient has trouble controlling his weight and is obese.

Patient has full range of motion in the lumbar spine. Has some tension when bending forward.
  SLR is only tight and causes discomfort from stretch; Braggards reproduces foot pain,
  especially when pulling on the great toe. Patrick-Fabere is only painful from tight ligaments. Ely's and Yeoman's do not reproduce the patient's low back pain.
Patient has deep tendon reflexes of 2+ and brisk in the lower extremities; Babinsky was
  normal, but the great toe did not respond in a normal full dorsum extension.
The patient limps a lot, favoring the right lower extremity, and puts weight on left leg when
  he rises from a chair.
The patient only has mild to moderate muscle spasm in the lower paravertebral muscles
  bilaterally and has a slight piriformis spasm in the left sciatic notch area.
The lab tests were run for purposes of investigating patient's response about arthritis, and
  also, due to patient's age, a gout profile was requested.
The lab tests showed increase in alkaline phosphates, serum uric acid, and urine uric acid,
  which were specifically related to the patient's symptoms. There was also an increase in
  white blood cell (WBC) count and a decrease in hemoglobin.
The x-rays show moderate arthritis of the osseous structures of the lumbar spine in this
  patient. Disc space is somewhat thinned; articular space is fair without any specific
  pathology. An x-ray of the feet bilaterally shows the right foot with acute monarticular
  arthritis in the first metatarsophalangeal joint and early arthritis of the same joint on the left.

## Differential Diagnosis

Fibromyositis of the lower paralumbar muscles and acute gouty arthritis. In this case, because of
the inflammatory results of the lab tests, plus the x-ray findings, I would suspect more of an
inflammatory condition going on than would be considered safe for MUA. This would be a
contraindicated case and would be monitored for improvement of the low back pain so that with
medication and conservative care, the MUA procedure might be indicated at a future time.

## DISC PROTRUSION (AS INDICATED ON MRI)

The patient indicates lower back pain with pain that goes down his left leg and extends
  down into the middle three toes.
The patient had the pain come on suddenly after lifting a cinderblock while working at a
  construction site.
The patient has had low back problems on three occasions over the past 10 years, but never
  this bad, and never had pain down into the leg.
The patient does not report any bowel or bladder dysfunction. The patient has pain when
  he strains at the stool but is able to move his bowels. The patient has to climb up his
  thighs to get to a standing position, and then has trouble fully straightening out.
The patient states he can't sleep and is in severe pain when turning to the left, or bending
  to the left side.
The patient has several orthopedic tests that reproduce his pain. Laseque's on the left to 20;
  double leg raising with more pain when lowering the legs; Kemps test on the left side;
  Braggard's test on the left causes moderate discomfort in the low back; and flexing the
  foot also reproduces the pain.
The patient has lower extremity patellar reflexes on the right of 2+ and brisk and 1+ on the
  left; and has an Achilles reflex of 2+ and sluggish on the right and 1+ on the left. Babinsky
  is normal, as are Oppenheim, Chaddocks, and Gordon's.
The patient has an antalgic posture leaning to the right side. The patient also has trouble
  standing or sitting for any length of time. The patient has to limp when he walks, but does
  not have foot drop in either foot.

The patient has severe paraspinal muscle spasms from the middle to lower lumbar spine. The patient has muscle tension in the upper gluteal muscle on the right and has muscle contracture of the tensor fascia lata on the left side.

The patient also has tenderness in the middle calf of the left lower extremity and point tenderness in the sciatic notch on the left and directly over the L5 supraspinous ligament on the left.

Laboratory tests came back within normal limits in this case.

The patient had x-rays of the lumbar spine taken to include anterior/posterior (AP), lateral, and oblique views, flexion/extension and lateral bending bilaterally. There was moderate thinning of the L5-S1 disc space. There was a right lateral scoliosis of the lumbar spine and a drop on the pelvis on the right with compensatory anterior rotation of the vertebrae and pelvis. Since the patient has pain into the leg an MRI is requested and shows bulging discs at L4-L5 and L5-S1, with more bulging present at L4-L5. The bulge is 3–4 mm, and there is slight thecal indentation but no cord compression.

## Differential Diagnosis

Disc herniation, bulge, protrusion, or space occupying lesion, causing the pain in the back and the paresthesias down the leg. Since the MRI shows a moderate bulge, this case would be indicated for MUA following the recommended 4–6 weeks of conservative chiropractic care in the office. This is based on what improvement had taken place in the conservative program and the progress taking place in the office setting.

## REFERENCES

1. Capps, S., Texas College of Chiropractic, syllabus: Manipulation under anesthesia; postgraduate course of study, 1992.
2. Gordon, R., with contribution from Furno, P., Cornerstone Professional Education, MUA syllabus currently sponsored by the National University of Health Sciences, 5th ed., August 1998.
3. The National Academy of MUA Physicians Standards and Protocols, 1995, St. Louis chapter.

# 7 MUA Principles and Practices

*Robert C. Gordon*

## CONTENTS



Today manual therapy techniques have been refined to a point where specific maneuvers can be accomplished to reestablish much of the integrity of the joint involved and accommodate physiological and biomechanical reintegration of the elements of the articulations involved.

The purpose of using the technique of manipulation under anesthesia (MUA) is to provide adjustments of the spinal motion units and muscular stretching in an atmosphere where there is a slowdown of the normal response to muscle splinting and contracture, and loss of patient apprehension to the maneuver. It is also used because the patients having the procedure completed are more responsive to this form of technique, it is less invasive, they lose less time from work, and the program is considerably more cost-effective than long, drawn-out conservative therapy programs and potential surgical intervention.

"Manipulative treatment of the spinal region is the art, science and practice of the nonoperative restoration of the function of bones, joints, muscles, tendons and ligaments."[1] The overall objective of manipulation under anesthesia is to relieve the patient's pain and disability with a minimum amount of expense to the patient, and loss of time from work and other activities in an environment of relaxation.

MUA is used in both acute and chronic conditions. In the acute case, the procedure is used when severe spasms with accompanying pain, prevent the use of joint mobilization, and corrective physical or pharmacological interventions. Here the use of MUA has been found to greatly improve the flexibility in the joints, and considerably reduce the patient's pain.[2–5] In the chronic case, the use of MUA alters fibrotic adhesions that have accumulated around the involved joint from disuse and, as has been discussed, will greatly increase the mobility of a hypomobile joint.[4–8]

The general indications for the use of MUA are primarily conditions in which manipulation is the therapy of choice but the patient only responds minimally without the use of anesthesia.[2,4,5,7,9] In these instances the patients have plateaued from the conservative regime but are still manipulative/adjustive candidates. They are responsive to manipulative/adjustive techniques, but it is not possible to complete the entire process either because of muscle splinting, patient apprehension, or a combination of many factors that make the office environment unproductive.

Manipulation or adjustment under anesthesia combines the concept of mobilization of soft tissue with the specific adjustment of an articulation whether in the spine or the extremities. It is essentially a team or multidisciplinary approach and involves the certified manual therapy practitioner as the primary provider, a first assistant certified manual therapist, the anesthesiologist as a close partner, and, in many cases, advice from knowledgeable neurologists or orthopedic surgeons who work closely with the team to help determine the patient's risk or nonrisk for the procedure. All work is in harmony to develop the procedure that will ultimately improve the patient's condition, and all the team players are essential for success.

But why use anesthesia for manipulation of the spinal motion unit? The answer lies in the physiology of anesthesia, in this case monitored anesthesia care (MAC). The postural tone of the muscles is relaxed using this type of anesthesia. The muscle function of joint stabilization and the muscle splinting action of the muscles of the joint structure are delayed. Under anesthesia, especially using light sedation, there remains only ligamentus and tendonous action and articular changes to limit motion. This enables the MUA provider to put an articulation through its normal range of motion, reduce the restrictive adhesions, and mobilize the involved vertebral motion unit.[2,7]

## MUA PRINCIPLES AND PRACTICE

Standard of care is a huge concern in the scientific community. A procedure that has a standard of care has direction and validity. MUA is slowly becoming accepted in more manual therapy circles as having not only validity but also real potential as an alternative to prolonged conservative care or potential surgical intervention with properly selected cases. The selection of proper cases for MUA intervention must be aligned with proper historical selection criteria. The selection of proper cases for the MUA procedure is a part of the standard-of-care issue. Most facilities where MUA is performed are interested in the types of cases that will be performed, and they are looking for guidelines as to how the cases for MUA are selected by the practitioner performing this procedure.

Several years ago most practitioners who used MUA had no guidance as to which patients were the best candidates and which were better treated in other forms using other modalities. In 1995 the National Academy of MUA Physicians was formed to address these concerns and focused on conceiving standards and protocols for standards of care and parameters for patient selection, facility responsibilities, nursing standards, anesthesiology considerations, and considerations for patient processing through the MUA program. The following standards and protocols have been established as evolutionary and will stay stable until other studies indicate that additional information is needed to improve these concepts as more information becomes known about the MUA procedure. (These are provided with permission from the National Academy of MUA Physicians.)

### STANDARDS AND PROTOCOLS

(Reprinted with permission from the National Academy of MUA Physicians, Manchester, Missouri.)

### Clinical Justification

- The patient has responded favorably to conservative, noninvasive chiropractic and medical treatments, but continues to experience intractable pain and/or biomechanical dysfunction.
- Sufficient care has been rendered prior to recommending MUA (standard is 2–6 weeks).
- Manipulative procedures have been utilized in the clinical setting during the 2–6-week period prior to recommending MUA.
- The patient's level of reproduced pain interferes with lifestyle (sleep, daily functional activities, work habits, etc.).

- When medical pain management parameters for immediate acute care protocols are met, and if it is recommended by the medical pain management specialist, the MUA procedure can be used in conjunction with medical pain management for treatment of acute pain.
- Diagnosed conditions must fall within the recognized categories of conditions responsive to MUA. The following disorders are classified as acceptable conditions for utilization of manipulation under anesthesia:
  - Patients whereby manipulation of the spine or other articulations is the treatment of choice; however, the patient's pain threshold inhibits the effectiveness of conservative manipulation.
  - Patients whereby manipulation of the spine or other articulations is the treatment of choice; however, due to the involuntary contraction of the supporting tissues (splinting mechanisms), patient treatment is delayed or may be prolonged.
  - Patients whereby manipulation of the spine or other articulations is the treatment of choice; however, due to the extent of the injury mechanism, conservative manipulation has been minimally effective in 2–6 weeks of care and a greater degree of movement of the affected joint(s) is needed.
  - Patients whereby manipulation of the spine or other articulations is the treatment of choice; however, due to the chronicity of the problem and/or the fibrous tissue adhesions present, conservative manipulation is incomplete.
  - When the patient is considered for spinal disc surgery, MUA is an alternative and/or an interim treatment and may be used as a therapeutic and/or diagnostic tool in the overall consideration of the patient's condition.

## Diagnosis

### Establishing Medical Necessity

Every condition treated must be diagnosed and justified by clinical documentation in order to establish medical necessity. Documentation of the patient's progress and the patient's response to treatment are combined to confirm the working diagnosis. Those diagnoses that are most responsive to MUA include, but are not limited to, the following:

- Sclerotogenous pain from the medial branch of the dorsal rami
- Cervical, thoracic, and lumbar myofascial pain syndromes
- Intervertebral disc syndromes without fragment, sequestration, or significant osseous encroachment with or without radiculopathy
- Cervical brachial pain syndrome associated with torticollis
- Chronic recurrent headaches
- Failed back surgeries that do not involve hypermobile motion units and have been responsive to clinical therapeutic trials of manipulation
- Adhesive capsulitis relative to articular motion of the appendicular skeleton
- Paravertebral muscle contraction related to functional biomechanical dysfunction syndromes (vertebral subluxation syndrome)

## Frequency and Follow-Up

### Guidelines for Determining the Necessity and Frequency of MUA

The National Academy of MUA Physicians recommends the following considerations when determining the necessity and frequency of manipulation under anesthesia:

- The patient's progress and response to previous conservative care
- Consideration of functional lifestyle

- The patient's psychological acceptance of the MUA procedure, and the psychosomatic response to overcoming chronic pain and discomfort
- Prevention of additional gross deterioration
- Prevention of possible surgical intervention

*Guidelines for Determining the Necessity and Frequency of MUA*

- Chronicity
- Length of current treatment and patient progress
- Patient age
- Number of previous injuries to the same area
- Level of intractable pain considering standard 2–6-week protocol parameter
- Patient tolerance of previous treatment and procedures
- Muscle contraction level (beyond splinting)
- Response to previous MUAs based on objective clinical documentation and protocols for determining patient progress
- Fibrous adhesion from failed back surgery or prior injury

*Protocols for Determining the Frequency of the MUA Procedure*

- Single spinal MUA is most often recommended when the patient is of a younger age, and when the injury to the area is of the first order (first injury to area).
- Single spinal MUA is most often recommended when conservative care has been rendered for a sufficient time (2–6 weeks) and the patient's lifestyle and daily activities are interrupted in such a fashion as to warrant immediate relief.
- If the patient is treated for intractable pain with a single MUA procedure and responds with 80% resolution, the necessity for future MUAs is reduced.
- Serial MUA is recommended when the patient's condition is chronically present and when conservative care as described in the Academy standards and protocols has been rendered.
- Serial MUA is recommended when the injury is recurrent in nature and fibrotic tissue and articulator fixation prevents a single MUA from being effective.

*Protocols for Performing Serial MUAs*

- If the patient regains 80% or more of normal biomechanical function during the first procedure and retains at least 80% of functional improvement during post-MUA evaluation, then serial MUA is usually unnecessary if post-MUA therapy and rehabilitation is performed.
- If the patient regains 50%–70% or less of normal biomechanical function during the first procedure and retains only 50%–70% of improvement during post-MUA evaluations, a second MUA is recommended.
- If the patient continues to improve with the second MUA, but does not achieve at least an 80% improvement in function, then a third MUA is recommended and has been found to be of significant benefit.
- If the patient has not achieved an 80% increase in function, then a fourth or fifth MUA is recommended. This number of MUAs is rare especially when the procedure is completed in consecutive series. Some procedures have been repeated at a later date, and the patients have improved more rapidly than when the MUA was originally performed.

- If the patient shows a 10%–15% improvement during the first MUA and continues to show a 10%–15% functional improvement during post-MUA evaluations, it is recommended that additional evaluation be completed to establish the appropriateness of additional MUAs.
- Since most patients gain between 50 and 75% improvement during the first day of a serial MUA treatment plan, a small improvement in function may indicate more extensive involvement. This is important since MUA has been found to be both therapeutic and diagnostic by surgeons in establishing objective evidence for surgical intervention.

Parameters for determining MUA progress may include but are not limited to

- Subjective changes
  - Patient's pain index, visual analogue scale, faces of pain
  - Patient's ability to engage in active range of motion
  - Patient's change in daily routine activities
  - Patient's change in job performance
  - Patient's change in sleep patterns
  - Patient's dietary change
- Objective changes
  - Change in measurable muscle mass
  - Change in muscle contractibility
  - Change in EMG and/or nerve conduction studies
  - Change in muscle strength
  - Change in controlled measurable passive ROM
  - Change in radiological studies (x-rays, CT, MRI)

*General Post-MUA Therapy*

- Therapy following first MUA
  - Lay patient in side posture on table.
  - Heat area for 5 minutes.
  - Repeat MUA stretching.
  - Set interferential on acute settings with ice for 15 minutes.
  - Patient rest at home (not in bed).
- Therapy following second MUA
  - Same as first day
  - No manipulation
  - May add proprioceptive neuromuscular facilitation (PNF) exercises during stretching if tolerated
- Therapy following last MUA
  - Same protocol as above with PNF
  - Perform same manipulation as during MUA procedure
- Week following last MUA
  - May put the patient in prone position if tolerated same as above with PNF and manipulation
  - Patient may use heat at home if indicated (usually after day 7)
  - Treat patient daily
- Next two weeks
  - Perform full protocol (stretching, PNF, manipulation)
  - Treat patient two times per week for two weeks
  - Begin home rehabilitation exercises — two to three times per week

Start prerehabilitation (i.e., theraban exercise mild resistive stretching)

- Next four weeks
  - Perform full protocol (stretching, PNF, manipulation)
  - Patient treated once per week for four weeks
  - Active progressive resistive strength/stabilization exercises, supervised/unsupervised —two to three times per week (advanced rehabilitation before discharge)

## Safety

The Academy documents the need for certified MUA physicians as first assistants. The Academy recognizes two important factors regarding MUA and the certified first assistant.

### Patient Safety

Manipulation under anesthesia is performed using the anesthesia technique determined by the anesthesiologist to be appropriate for the patient. MUA is performed with the patient in a semi-conscious state. The primary doctor and the first assistant move the patient in specific ranges of motion to accomplish the procedure. In this capacity, the patient depends on the primary doctor and first assistant to protect the patient from bodily injury. Since the patient is responsive only to painful stimuli and does not have the ability to respond to proprioceptive input, both the primary physician and the first assistant are key to a safe and successful procedure.

The first assistant is responsible for patient stability, patient movement, patient observation, and completing portions of the procedure should the primary physician need assistance or be unable to perform the procedure. Because there are several instances during the procedure when the primary doctor has to move the patient, stabilizing and working with the patient would be unsafe without assistance from another certified physician.

### Doctor Safety

Manipulation under anesthesia is a very physically demanding therapeutic procedure. Since the patient is in a semiconscious state, the doctor has the added responsibility of ensuring that the patient's extremities and torso do not fall from the treating surface. The doctor must also be able to move the patient without the assistance of patient response.

The first assistant is responsible for helping the primary doctor move the patient through the prescribed ranges of motion. The first assistant is present to ensure that all movements are accomplished without injury to the patient or to the primary doctor performing the procedure. As a result of the added weight of the patient in a semiconscious state, there is a high risk of injury to the doctor and the patient if only one doctor were to attempt the complex moves necessary for the MUA procedure. A certified first assistant physician is the only safe way to perform this procedure.

In the cervical spine, the first assistant must secure the patient's shoulders to obtain the necessary traction for this part of the procedure. In the thoracic spine, the first assistant turns the patient and applies proper traction for the adjustment. In the lumbosacral area, the first assistant coordinates movements with the primary doctor, assists with the actual procedure, and can complete the MUA procedure if necessary.

A certified MUA physician carries the appropriate malpractice insurance to perform MUA. Since noncertified assistants may not carry malpractice coverage for MUA, utilization of ancillary staff to assist with the MUA procedure places the entire team at risk.

### Facilities

All MUA procedures should be performed in the highest quality facility available and within the parameters of state regulations. The Academy recommends performing MUA in hospitals, ambulatory surgery centers, or other specialty centers that meet the American Society of Anesthesiology standards, and adhere to Academy standards of care.

## ROLE OF THE MEDICAL SPECIALIST IN MUA*

MUA is analogous to a tool in the toolbox of a professional craftsman. There may be occasion where the use of more than one tool may be similarly indicated. In these instances, a thought process must occur so as to prioritize the use of these tools. Ultimately, the choice will be made based on training, experience, and an awareness of prevailing information on the subject.

Only when a definitive diagnosis has been rendered can medical decision making occur. While the provision of MUA falls most routinely within the disciplines of chiropractic and osteopathy, it may be appropriate to consider the timing of medical and surgical specialty referral, to assist in the confirmatory diagnosis of a prospective MUA patient. The collaborative assistance of an orthopedist, neurologist, neurosurgeon, anesthesiologist, physiatrist, and others represents a "built-in" second opinion by specialists who routinely treat pain patients within their respective practices. These providers are not only familiar with the history taking and physical examination of patients with spinal pain, but are also able to consider the relative necessity of additional diagnostic studies, so as to assist in the determination of whether MUA is "the right tool at the right time."

Often a medical or surgical specialist will see patients who have already completed and possibly failed various therapies, to include the simple passage of time and medication as well as physical and/or manipulative therapies performed in an office setting. There are instances where the patient has failed conservative care by a chiropractor or osteopath not familiar with MUA or not certified in it. However, the medical specialist, once becoming familiar with the criteria necessary for a patient to be considered an MUA candidate, would be in a position to refer that patient to an MUA provider, for a confirmatory opinion. In documenting this referral, the specialist will opine as to the potential use of MUA, as it compares with other treatment options that the specialist has considered. In this fashion, the utility of MUA may be undertaken in patients whose pain problem has been considered by more than one discipline, enhancing access to MUA as a treatment option.

Specialists are able to evaluate a spinal pain patient in considering the utility of MUA as it compares to alternative or concomitant treatments such as trigger point injections, diagnostic and therapeutic spinal injection, or surgery, some or all of these treatments being available through that particular specialist.

A specialist who is familiar with the indications for MUA can evaluate a patient and determine what treatment options exist, working in a collaborative fashion with the MUA provider, so as to prioritize those options. This collaborative approach enhances patient care, improves interprovider communication and education, and optimizes patient outcome and satisfaction.

## REFERENCES


1. Capps, S., Texas College of Chiropractic, syllabus: Manipulation under anesthesia; postgraduate course of study, 1992.
2. Gordon, R., Cornerstone Professional Education, MUA course syllabus sponsored by the National University of Health Sciences, 5th ed., August 1998.
3. Gordon, R., Justifying MUA within the standard chiropractic scope of practice, *FCA J.*, November/December, 16–19, 1995.
4. Melzach, R., Wall, P.D., Pain mechanisms: A new theory, *Science* 150: 971, 1965.
5. Morgan, D.L., Separation of active and passive components of short-range stiffness of muscle, *Am. J. Physiol.*, 232: C45–C49, 1977.
6. Cailliet, R., *Neck and Arm Pain*, 5th printing, F.A. Davis Co., Philadelphia, January 1972.


---

* Robert Mathews and Matt Miller contributed this section.

     


7. Gordon, A.M., Huxley, A.F., Julian, F.J., Tension development in highly stretched vertebrae muscle fibres, *J. Physiol.* 184:143–169, 1966A.
8. Gray, H., *Anatomy, Descriptive and Surgical*, Running Press, Philadelphia, 224, 1086–96, 1966.
9. Sherman, S., Which treatment to recommend: Hot or cold, *Pharmacology* 20 (8): 46–49, 1980 [clinical justification for the use of MUA].

# 8 Support for MUA: Evidence-Based Research and Literature Review

*Robert C. Gordon*

## CONTENTS



Many authors have documented the results obtained by using the fibrosus release procedure with manipulation under anesthesia (MUA) since the late 1930s.[1,2,3] Although much of the reference to this procedure is somewhat anecdotal,[4] a significant number of authors over the years have documented remarkable outcomes when properly selected patients have undergone this procedure.

This chapter addresses specifically documented research, current referenced literature, trends in understanding how the MUA procedure is being performed today, and the need for further study into how this procedure fits into the field of pain management from a very practical standpoint.

Because MUA has been given a CPT code for reimbursement in the Current Procedural Terminology (which is published by the American Medical Association), it has to have undergone scrutiny from a clinical standpoint. The following statement is made in that publication: "inclusion of a descriptor and its associated 5-digit identifying code number in CPT is generally based on the procedure being consistent with contemporary medical practice and being performed by many physicians in clinical practice in multiple locations."[5]

The CPT code book is used by insurance carriers as a guide in establishing those procedures that have been used within the parameters and given a code number that represents reasonable and customary reimbursement parameters. Procedures that are experimental and have not been found to be safe and effective for use with the patient population are not given a code and fall within an "unlisted code" parameter such as 20999 "by report."[5,6] Manipulation of the spine requiring anesthesia has met the requirements for inclusion in the CPT code book of reimbursable procedures because over time it has been practiced by clinicians of varying specialties throughout the U.S. who commonly achieve the same or similar results by applying the same or similar techniques.[5]

In a letter from the director of CPT Editorial Research and Development of the American Medical Association dated April 6, 2004, it was determined that CPT code 22505 falls within the Category I types of codes for reimbursement: "In developing CPT code 22505—*Manipulation of the spine requiring anesthesia, any region,* CPT code 23700—*Manipulation under anesthesia, shoulder joint, including application of fixation apparatus (dislocation excluded),* and CPT code 27275—*Manipulation, hip joint, requiring general anesthesia* as with all new and revised CPT codes, the CPT Advisory Committees and the CPT Editorial panel require that:

- The service/procedure has received approval from the Food and Drug Administration (FDA) for the specific use of the device or drugs
- The suggested procedure/service is a distinct service performed by many physicians/practitioners across the U.S.
- The suggested service/procedure is neither a fragmentation of an existing procedure/service nor currently reportable by one or more existing codes
- The suggested service/procedure is not requested as a means to report extraordinary circumstances related to the performance of a procedure/service already having a specific code."

This chapter will address why this procedure has been given a code for reimbursement, and how the clinical papers published in support for MUA, although they may be anecdotal in theory, have laid the groundwork for the research that is presently being conducted in the field of manipulation under anesthesia. This falls within the parameters for all procedures that have gone through this same process as mainstream medicine has adopted new procedures continually throughout history. Today this process is referred to as evidence-based medicine and is being reintroduced to help to continue to develop good procedures that show significant change in patient outcome assessment, as does the MUA procedure.

Literature reviews indicate that a considerable body of material has been written on the subject of MUA, including references in manual therapy texts.[7] It is important to mention some of the more prominent writers who have supported the use of MUA over the years. Their comments about MUA directly relate to the historical safety and effectiveness of this procedure and support the findings that are being documented now and that will be observed and documented in the future. MUA continues to be successful today based on past reference to its use, continued adherence to standards and protocols, and advances in manual therapy techniques.

Harold Clybourne was one of the earliest writers in the U.S. (in 1948) to write an article about his clinical findings after using manipulation while the patient was under general anesthesia. He states that "I have had the opportunity to use manipulation under anesthesia on a sufficiently large number of cases to realize its scope and limitation."[8] Siehl and Bradford both wrote articles about MUA in the early journals of the American Osteopathic Association, but in one of the articles[9] they refer to a study from Piersol's International Medical Clinic, in which 200 MUA procedures were performed with a 94%–97% recovery from nonspecific low back pain. What makes that significant today, however, is that this is a study that was conducted in the UK and referred to by Siehl in his clinical paper regarding MUA. The results that were obtained (94%–97% recovery) are still being achieved with this procedure today with properly selected cases. The significance of this cannot be overlooked as anecdotal if the procedures today are less forceful, use anesthetics that are certainly more patient friendly, and are more conducive to protecting the body's natural reflexes. Historical reference to MUA included the use of general anesthesia, intubation, loss of reflex and end range, and unspecified procedural formats that today have been changed dramatically.

Today with the more advanced types of anesthesia, the anesthesiologist works as a team member to provide a specific level of semi-consciousness that allows the manual therapist to perform the desired stretches and manipulation techniques within protective barriers to help the patient recover from the condition that has not responded in the past to conservative therapy but that has been responsive minimally to the manual therapy techniques.

In 1963 Siehl wrote, "A conservative regime which includes manipulative treatment of the lower lumbar intervertebral disc syndrome under anesthesia eventuates in a significantly high percentage of satisfactory results to warrant its use as an essential part of conservative therapy."[10] He acknowledged this by a presentation of an 11-year study of 723 cases of MUA at the annual meeting of the Osteopathic Academy of Orthopedics in Bal Harbour, Florida, October 31, 1962.

Even in 1963 we were seeing dramatic changes occurring with the MUA procedures, yet the research that was completed did not eventuate into the types of outcome studies that we are looking for today. That does not mean that MUA was not achieving significant results. Reporting clinical documentation and key case studies were the more prevalent forms of reporting patient outcomes at that time. Call it anecdotal or experimental, or inconclusive, or any other adjective you want to assign to delay the inevitable use of this procedure in mainstream pain management, but it still does not change the fact that MUA is achieving remarkable results. Today we are getting the same results that were being achieved back when Siehl was completing his studies. The end results are better now than in the past, however, because today we are using techniques that are far more sophisticated with medications that are far more responsive to our needs than Siehl had access to in the mid- to late 1960s.

As we move forward historically, Krumhansl and Nowacek, in their book, *Modern Manual Therapy*,[11] make the following comment regarding the efficacy of using MUA: "The importance of fascial lengthening, tendon stretching and ligamentous mobilization are as important as the realignment of joints. Patients with long-standing, intense pain resulting from motor vehicle accidents, industrial accidents and falls gradually compensate. Eventually even "normal" joints of the spine and proximal extremities become involved. Most frequently there develops a zigzag pattern of muscle tightness and locked facets, either in individual segments or in groups. Manipulation under anesthesia is a final step in a long sequence of medical and physical treatments for patients who have endured prolonged and intractable pain and who have not responded to the more conventional methods of treatment. It is neither new nor revolutionary. Orthopedic surgeons in the United Kingdom have practiced it for many years. Osteopaths in the United States have relied on its efficacy. A few American orthopedists have incorporated this approach into their treatment regimes."[11]

References like this have been around for many years. Manipulation with the patient under a medication to induce more relaxation for fixated joints is not a new concept. For years orthopedists have used this form of therapy for frozen shoulders and fixated joints of the knee when surgery would only further deposit more scar tissue in an area that already had joint fixation from adhesion formation. The concept of using monitored anesthesia care (MAC) to accomplish this same end result is only about 12 to 15 years old and was brought into mainstream manual therapy healthcare delivery primarily by the chiropractic profession. The practitioners in the chiropractic profession (initially, Francis, Capps, Beckett, Ciccarillo, Gordon, Mills, and Morovati) were interested in the early osteopathic approach to MUA and wanted to see the more specific adjustive techniques that are performed in the chiropractic profession brought over into the field of MUA. As more and more was learned about positive outcomes, more manual therapists and chiropractic physicians became interested in adapting their techniques to the techniques in the past.

Beckett and Francis[12] reported on a controlled study on MUA completed by Chrisman et al.[13] that included 39 patients, all of whom had low back pain, sciatica, and positive findings on at least one sciatic nerve stretch test, with at least one reflex, motor, or sensory deficit finding. By using guidelines from an earlier study by Mensor,[14] it was found that 27 of the 39 patients had positive myelograms for disc herniation. The average duration of the symptoms was 6 years, with a range of 10 days to 25 years. For their last attack of back pain, these patients had received conservative management including heat, analgesics, muscle relaxants, bracing, flexion exercises, and rest. (Reference is not made to the amount of previous manual therapy provided by an osteopath or a chiropractor prior to having MUA, as is our protocol today.) These patients then received MUA.

A similar group of 22 patients received conservative management with no MUA. Chrisman et al.[13] reported that "the effects of MUA were frequently dramatic and more than half of the patients reported their sciatic symptoms lessened within 24 hours." According to Mensor's criteria,[14] Chrisman et al.[13] reported that 21 of the MUA patients had excellent or good outcomes at 5 to 10 months follow-up, 4 patients had fair outcomes, and 14 patients had unsatisfactory results. Overall, they reported that 51% of the patients with an unequivocal picture of ruptured intervertebral disc unrelieved by conservative care had good or excellent results after MUA. The 22 patients who did not have MUA did poorly, and 16 eventually required surgery. The findings of Chrisman et al. were consistent with the findings of Mensor in an earlier study.[13,14]

Their findings are also consistent with clinical reasoning that if a procedure has a record of positive patient outcomes and includes similar techniques and procedures from earlier studies, it is hard to argue against its effectiveness, safety, and reliability. Even though the techniques used were not as refined as they are today, the results from all of the clinical data that has been gathered over the past 70 years still point to the fact that MUA is a reliable form of therapy that has historically caused dramatic improvement in populations of patients with neuromusculoskeletal conditions of the spine and proximal extremities when other more conservative types of therapies have failed and the patients do not have categorical indications for surgery, such as bowel and bladder dysfunction with a true ruptured/fragmented lumbar disc.

More recently, Kohlbeck and Haldeman published a technical assessment paper on Medicated Assisted Spinal Manipulation in the journal *Spine* (2002), in which they completed a literature search. They also presented an abstract at the World Federation of Chiropractic in Orlando, Florida, in May 2003. The purpose of the review "was to provide a review of the literature and present a description of current clinical practice methods for the application of the different techniques of medication assisted spinal manipulation therapy followed by a discussion of the current clinical support and the published indications, contraindications and the complications for each procedure."[4] Their conclusions were "that medication assisted spinal manipulation therapies have a relatively long history of clinical use although the evidence for the effectiveness of the protocols remain largely anecdotal there is sufficient theoretical basis and positive results from case series to warrant further controlled trials on these techniques."[15]

We certainly agree with this statement and continue to focus today on increasing our awareness of patient outcomes by instituting several studies where local sites that practice MUA can measure patient response to MUA using both pre- and post-standards of measurement from acceptable measuring devices as well as comparison studies of conservative care with no MUA involved. By employing these standards of measurement and then publishing the results in a timely fashion, we will not only be able to relate our findings to those who have published in the past, but we will also be able to direct our vision for this procedure for the future. MUA has not had a chance to prove its reliability as have other techniques and continues today to be scrutinized by people who have incomplete information about how this procedure is done. I hope that in the next few years you will see more than just anecdotal opinions based on clinical outcome papers. What I envision are good controlled studies that once and for all will eliminate the backwash of insecure unintelligent propaganda that has surrounded this procedure for so long. The results that we get when we perform this procedure on cases such as fibromyalgia simply cannot be swept under a carpet because someone does not understand the procedure. This text is a testament to the legitimacy of this procedure and the diligence of many practitioners who have kept the clinical light burning for so many years. It is, after all, the patients who enjoy the benefits of that diligence.

Chapter 6 has a partial list of diagnoses that have responded well to MUA. Referring to this chapter will give you an understanding of the types of patient conditions selected for the MUA procedure and will also support the efficacy of continued need for research as we learn more about the responses to the MUA procedure.

## PROTOCOLS FOR DETERMINING PATIENT PROGRESS PRIOR TO AND FOLLOWING THE MUA PROCEDURE

### SUBJECTIVE CHANGE

- Patient visual analog scale (patient pain analysis)
- Patient's ability to engage in active range of motion
- Patient's change in daily routine activities
- Patient's change in job performance
- Patient's sleep habit changes and patterns
- Patient's dietary change

### OBJECTIVE CHANGE

- Change in measurable muscle mass
- Change in muscle contractibility
- Change in EMG, nerve conduction studies
- Change in muscle strength
- Change in controlled measurable passive range of motion (ROM)
- Change in radiological studies (x-rays, CTs, MRIs).

### HYPOTHESIS FOR PARAMETERS IN DETERMINING NUMBER OF MUAS REQUIRED FOR COMPLETION OF DESIRED THERAPEUTIC RESULT

- Chronicity
- Length of current therapy program and progress as determined by progress protocols
- Patient age
- Numbers of previous injuries to same area (past history)
- Level of intractable pain given 4–8 weeks protocol parameter
- Patient acceptance
- Muscle contracture level (beyond splinting)
- Consideration of social life (interference with normal lifestyle)
- Consideration of prolonged care with little hope of much improvement
- Possible surgical intervention if procedure isn't complete (meaning one might still make patient a surgical candidate — two or three might alleviate the problem completely)
- Adhesion buildup from failed back surgery — rely on progress protocol clinically

### PARAMETERS FOR SELECTION OF THE NUMBER OF MUAS

As with any treatment technique, determining the exact number of treatments is like trying to look into a crystal ball and being right with what you see.

The amount or number of treatments required to get the desired results is more accurately determined if we place numerical or response indices with patient reaction to the procedure and then factor in the parameters that have already been established in the protocols and standards in determining numbers of MUAs required (chronicity, age, etc.).

The spinal MUA procedure is a procedure that has seen transition and historical evolution. Today with the advancement in mobilization, manipulation, and adjustive techniques, which are being used extensively and exclusively within the chiropractic/osteopathic professions, the MUA technique has taken on significant importance in the care of many neuromusculoskeletal conditions. In the past these patients and conditions were not responding to care and were not surgical candidates, so the patient was simply left to "live with the discomfort." These new parameters for determining the number of MUAs comes from the outcome assessments of a 60-case study, from clinical trials of some 6,000 cases completed over the past two to four years, and current studies being completed.

The following are recommended considerations when determining the need for MUA and the addition of serial MUA to the treatment protocol:

- Patient response and progress to rendered conservative care
- Patient's response to the ability to function with everyday activities given the current care being rendered
- The patient's psychological acceptance of the MUA technique, and the psychosomatic response to overcoming chronic pain and discomfort given the length of time the patient has been away from the workload environment
- Prevention of further gross deterioration if the MUA procedure was performed given the amount of time the patient has been under conservative and/or surgical care
- Prevention of or the diagnosing of specific parameters for surgical intervention
- Correction of failed surgical intervention

In comparing clinical reaction to MUA that has been observed with the studies that are currently being completed, the following parameters for continuing with the plan for single or serial MUA have been recommended:

- Single-spinal MUA is most often performed when the patient is of a younger age, and when the injury to the area is of the first order (determined to be the first injury to the involved area.)
- Single-spinal MUA is most often performed when the injury is of the first order and the care being rendered has had sufficient time (protocols determined 2 to 4 weeks) of conservative care and where the patient's lifestyle and daily activities are being interrupted in such a fashion as to warrant immediate relief. (Medical intervention and evaluation is recommended.) Note: It is generally agreed that if the patient is treated for the intractable type of pain with a single MUA procedure and responds well, the necessity for future MUAs is greatly reduced.
- Serial MUA (more than one MUA) is recommended when conservative care has been completed and when the condition is chronically present, when the injury is recurrent in nature, and when it is determined that fibrotic tissue and articular fixation prevents a single MUA from ever being effective. The following parameters should be a guide to continuing with the serial MUA treatment plan, or discontinuing the procedure for further evaluation:
    - If the patient gains 80% or better of the normal biomechanical function back during the procedure and continues to show at least an 80% functional improvement during post-MUA evaluation on the same day as the MUA, then the serial series has been found to be unnecessary as long as the proper follow-up post-MUA therapy and rehabilitation is performed.
    - If the patient has less than 50%–70% improvement in desired function during the MUA procedure and continues to show only a 50%–70% improvement during post-MUA evaluations, the second MUA is recommended and found to be of great benefit.
    - If the patient continues to improve with the second MUA, but does not achieve at least an 80% improvement in function during the MUA and in the post-MUA evaluation, then the third MUA has been found to be of significant benefit. Note: At this time most patients have responded very well to the 3-day procedure. However, if the patient has still not achieved an 80% increase in function, then a fourth or fifth MUA

has been clinically documented. (This number of MUAs is rare however, especially when done all in a row. Some cases have been repeated at a later date, and have shown to improve at a faster rate than when the MUA was originally performed.)

- If the patient only shows a 10%–15% improvement during the first MUA and continues to only show a 10%–15% functional improvement during post-MUA evaluations, then it is recommended that further evaluation be completed on that patient to determine if the MUA procedure is the treatment of choice.

Since most patients gain between 50% and 75% improvement during the first day of a serial MUA treatment plan, a small improvement in function may indicate more extensive involvement than what was determined in the initial treatment plan. The importance of this is that MUA has been found to be both therapeutic and diagnostic and has been used by both neurosurgeons and orthopaedic surgeons in deciding objectively that surgical intervention is the right choice since the conservative therapeutic regime of office therapy and MUA were performed with little significant change in the patient's condition.

(The preceding information was taken from a 60-case study that took place at Newport News General Hospital, completed in 1993 by Burt Rubin, DC, DABCO, and Robert C. Gordon, DC.)

## INTRODUCTION OF MUA TO PATIENT

There are several ways to introduce MUA to your patients. The following describes two ways that I have found to be beneficial.

The first approach is casual and takes place in a relaxed atmosphere while you are adjusting your patient. This is usually your comfort zone and the patient is placed in a position where he or she is less likely to argue about treatment. As you are trying to get your patient to adjust, casually comment that you have a new procedure available that would make it easier for the patient to be adjusted. Add that the patient would respond to this new procedure at least twice as fast as he or she would respond normally.

Then again, in a casual manner talk about the MUA procedure with the enthusiasm that you have developed by using it with your other patients.

As the patient becomes more interested, have the patient come into the consultation room and give him or her a brochure about the procedure, and then have the individual discuss the procedure on the next visit. Remember, this is the casual approach, so there is no pressure to try and sell the whole procedure. Let patients absorb the brochure and then answer questions the next visit. You might also like to invite the spouse to come in on the visit to discuss the procedure if you notice a significant interest. I use the term "sell" only as an information word. We are not trying to sell used cars here; we are presenting information about a procedure that we know other patients have responded well to and we feel strongly will help this patient as well.

The second approach is more formal and works better for those patients whom you feel may have immediate hesitation. During her regular office visit, you tell Mrs. Jones that on her next visit you want to see her in consultation. You go to the front desk with her and tell your receptionist you want extra time with Mrs. Jones on her next visit. You also explain that it is important for her spouse to come in with her. Impress upon Mrs. Jones that you really need to have this consultation and that it is important that you spend time with her discussing her case. The approach with this patient is to present a concise appraisal of what the problem is, what you have been doing, what has been accomplished and what will occur if the treatment continues on the same course. Of course, you have followed the protocols for establishing the selection of this patient for the MUA procedure, so your report of findings in this case is to emphasize to the patient the logical necessity for having MUA. This then becomes a more educational environment initially than the other approach, which will give them the most confidence to (1) have the procedure done and (2) have you perform the procedure.

It is a good idea when doing either of these reports to present anesthesia in a direct way, but emphasizing that other similar procedures, such as colonoscopies, are done every day with similar anesthesia approaches (refer to this procedure as IV sedation or twilight sedation). The patient needs to understand the risks of anesthesia, but does not need to be frightened by the word "anesthesia."

If the patient has anesthesia concerns, refer the patient to the anesthesiologist.

## OBTAINING PATIENT ACCEPTANCE FOR MUA

The patients who are candidates for MUA are those who are minimally improving with manipulation and who have exhausted other forms of conservative care but for whom manipulation is the therapy of choice. In most cases patients who are facing the following options may want to consider MUA as an alternative to prolonging their current conservative care:

- Possible future surgical intervention
- Chronic exacerbation of the same condition
- Severe muscle contracture that is unresponsive to conservative care, drug therapy, or any other alternative and that is affecting the patient's lifestyle
- Intractable pain that is unresponsive to medicinal intervention and is ruled a nonsurgical or possible surgical case

Most cases that will respond favorably to MUA fall into one or more of these categories.

If the patient has been given the prescribed protocol of 4–8 weeks of conservative care, has been referred for diagnostic evaluation, has been seen for evaluation by various specialties and is still not responding, the alternative that should be considered is manipulation under anesthesia.

Considerations to be discussed with your patients might be as follows:

- They have been to many types of doctors with only minimal results.
- They have been treated for ___ weeks with no appreciable difference in their condition.
- Chiropractic/osteopathic certified MUA physicians offer alternatives to prolonged care, drug therapy (which is only temporary), and surgery.
- If the condition they have doesn't begin to change and the fibrous tissue continues to become more and more dense around the injury, even MUA may not work.
- The MUA procedure may save them from possibly or probably having surgery.
- An anesthesia is used (IV sedation, monitored anesthesia care MAC), but the level of anesthesia is minimal compared to having to undergo a surgical procedure using general anesthesia, even if multiple days or serial MUA is performed.

## DEVELOPING A RAPPORT FOR AUTHORIZATION

The certified MUA physician who intends to perform MUA must be conscious of three major factors when making his or her decision:

1. Does the patient need the procedure and have all conservative measures been exhausted?
2. Has the patient accepted your recommendation and is he or she educated to accept the need for the procedure?
3. Have you taken the time to prepare your case for authorization?

(Refer to the section "A Case for MUA" in Chapter 16.) The following section is specifically written to give you some guidelines to follow to help facilitate insurance authorization.

When dealing with insurance adjustors, it is best not to approach them with an intimidating attitude. Adjustors are usually prompted to try and be relatively fair within established company financial parameters. If you are to get authorization, you must help them see that you fall into that parameter and that there is clinical justification for the MUA procedure in the future of their claimant, your patient's, treatment. If you can show the relevance of performing this procedure, in order to help their claimant return to a more normal life style that will reduce or terminate the current care being rendered, you have a better chance of receiving approval for the procedure rather than denial.

There are several key elements in establishing that "comfort zone" for the insurance adjustor:

1. Be honest. If there is litigation at some future time, you need reliable, honest records to establish your credibility and that of your treatment(s).
2. Do not change your diagnosis to match your treatment at the time. Your diagnosis may vary as you move into the MUA arena, but if you did not have a diagnosis for the cervical spine before MUA, don't try and do work in the cervical spine when doing MUA.
3. Always provide a clinically justifiable diagnosis for each area of the spine or extremities.
4. Establish the need for MUA by the clinical history and the probable clinical deterioration or extended care without the procedure.
5. Explain that MUA has been listed with its own diagnostic code (22505) for a number of years and is established as a viable alternative form of treatment.
6. Give a clear and concise reason for wanting to do MUA, and back your decision with objective diagnostic evaluation.

## REFERENCES


1. Gordon, R., An evaluation of the experimental and investigational status and clinical validity of manipulation of patients under anesthesia: A contemporary opinion, *J. Manip. Physiol. Ther.*, October: 603–11, 2002.
2. Gordon, R., Manipulation under anesthesia: an anthology of past, present, and future use, in Weiner, R., Ed., *Pain Management: A Practical Guide for Clinicians*, 6th ed., Boca Raton, FL: CRC Press, 2002, 701–14.
3. Palmieri, N., Chronic low back pain: A study of the effects of manipulation under anesthesia, *J. Manip. Physiol. Ther.*, 2001.
4. Kohlbeck, F. and Haldeman, S., Technical assessment: Medication assisted spinal manipulation, *J. North American Spine Society*, 2002.
5. *Current Procedural Terminology: CPT/American Medical Association*, 4th ed. Chicago: AMA, 2004. p. ix.
6. California Industrial Medical Council, ad hoc committee for MUA consensus, 2003.
7. Krumhausl, B.R. and Nowacek, C.F., Manipulation under anesthesia, in Grieve, G.P., Ed., *Modern Manual Therapy of the Vertebral Column,* Edinburgh: Churchill Livingstone, 1986, pp. 777–786.
8. Clybourne, H.E., Manipulation of the low back region under anesthesia, *J. Am. Osteopathic Assoc.* September 1948: 10–11.
9. Siehl, D. and Bradford, W.C., Manipulation for low back pain, *J. Am. Osteopathic Assoc.* 32: 239–42, 1952.
10. Siehl, D., Manipulation of the spine under general anesthesia, *J. Am. Osteopathic Assoc.* 62: 35–39, 1963.
11. Krumhansl and Nowacek, Manipulation under anesthesia.
12. Beckett, R.H. and Francis, R., Spinal manipulation under anesthesia, in *Advances in Chiropractic*, St. Louis: Mosby, 1994, pp. 325–40.
13. Chrisman, O.D., Mittnacht, A., Snook, G.A., A study of the results following rotatory manipulation in the lumbar intervertebral disc syndrome, *J. Bone Joint Surg.*, 46: 517–24, 1964.

14. Mensor, M.C., Nonoperative treatment, including manipulation for lumbar intervertebral disc syndrome, *J. Bone Joint Surg.* (AM) 5: 925–36, 1955.
15. Kohlbeck, F., Haldeman, S., Hurwitz, E., Dagenais, S., Medication-assisted manipulation for low back pain, World Federation of Chiropractic 7th Biennial Congress, Orlando, FL, May 1–3, 2003.

# 9 Evaluation of the MUA Patient

*Robert C. Gordon*

## CONTENTS



The typical chiropractic/osteopathic patient who is a candidate for the MUA program has been receiving care anywhere from 4 weeks to 4 months (on average) or has been evaluated for "intractable" pain in a 2-week period. The patient has undergone regular adjustive techniques that have had only minimal results.

To be a candidate for MUA, specific procedures should be followed in a sequential format. The necessary forms are a history and physical, pre-operative diagnosis report, operative report for each day, and a discharge summary report with followings. Samples of these reports can be found in Chapter 17.

## THE IMPORTANCE OF THE HISTORY AND PHYSICAL

The patient must have received a conservative regime of manipulative therapy prior to being considered for the MUA procedure. This is an advanced form of manipulative therapy, and it would obviously not be advised to place a patient into an advanced manual therapy program who had never experienced office-based manipulation.

A systemic evaluation and a neuromusculoskeletal evaluation need to be completed on the patient.

It is important to note here that, if a patient is referred for MUA and has not undergone manipulative therapy, the same standard of care applies. Evaluate the patient to see if manipulative therapy was the therapy of choice, and then proceed with a reasonable amount of time in a conservative office-based manipulative therapy program.

If the patient has received manipulative therapy and is referred for MUA, evaluate the patient for selection criteria.

It has been very encouraging to see the trend for referrals that has taken place in the past 2–3 years. Referrals for MUA have come from allopathic, chiropractic, and osteopathic sources who see the benefits of the MUA technique.

What needs to happen is to secure a better understanding from the health-care community as to when the patient should be referred for MUA, and then what the criteria is for that patient to then become a candidate for MUA. That understanding needs to include the necessity for consideration of the amount of manipulative therapy that the patient has undergone, and the response to that manipulation. This is the primary reason why a history and physical has to be completed on every new MUA candidate. This holds true for referrals as well as for those selected from the practitioner's patient base.

The history and physical is considered one of the most important phases of a patient health-care program. "Common errors at this level of the differential process arise when insufficient data are available as a result of careless interview or examination techniques."[1] Proper acquisition of the data from the initial patient interview and a review of the significant positive findings from examinations develop the pattern for the differential diagnosis and ultimately the proper treatment program. Part of the history and physical should always be a systems analysis and an assignment of systems placement. An example is placing emphasis on weakness in all extremities or bilateral paresthesias, which might suggest spinal stenosis or could indicate an encroaching tumor. The emphasis by the patient of constipation or vertigo are not necessarily specific for cause, and when taking a history and applying the significant examination findings to the patient symptoms, ranking the findings in accordance to specificity helps to rule out secondary discomfort nonspecific to the primary diagnosis.

## EXAMINATION AND TESTING STRATEGY

The examination of the MUA candidate should always include an orthopedic, neurological, and chiropractic/osteopathic spinal analysis, as well as routine vital signs and specific testing of symptom-oriented patient discomfort.

"Appropriate test selection, whether lab, imaging, or physiological (i.e., electrocardiography, electrodiagnostic testing) is necessary for diagnostic orientation, patient safety, and cost effectiveness. Battery 'shotgun' or routine testing is to be avoided."[2] The MUA patient is not to be considered as a "special case" but rather as a comprehensive continuation of care from the conservative office care to a more advanced/intensive form of manipulative therapy.

Some of the testing that is routinely done in the office setting will carry over into the MUA program, but an EMG, nerve conduction studies, MRIs, or CTs is important to consider if symptoms warrant this type of testing. It is not an "overcautious" doctor who takes the initiative to use diagnostic tools that are available to him to feel comfortable that the MUA procedure will significantly help the patient. It is important to understand that coming as close to proving your concerns for why the patient has the symptoms, and what the MUA is going to accomplish, is as important as doing the procedure.

However, "the physician is now faced with the decision of whether to proceed directly with treatment or employ testing procedures to eliminate further the differential diagnostic considerations. The outcome of this decision will be determined by the level of certainty or confidence operating over the differential, the presence of conditions capable of inflicting significant morbidity or mortality, and the cost effectiveness of further testing."[2]

## RESPONSIBILITIES FOR THE CERTIFIED MUA PRACTITIONER IN RECORDING A COMPLETE PATIENT CHART

The patient's chart must include a concise record of the patient's history of symptoms, a record of onset and social history, a comprehensive physical examination, diagnostic testing (if required),

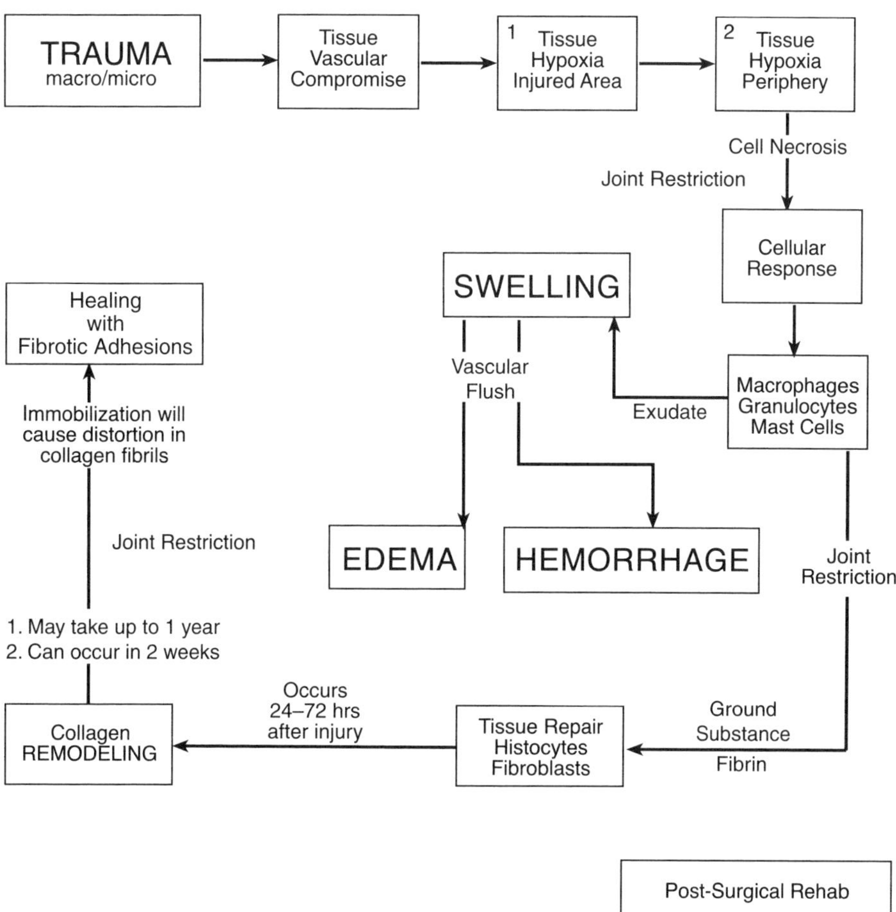


**FIGURE 9.1** The inflammatory cycle.

diagnostic impression from a breakdown of the differential diagnosis, and a working plan of action that has as its cortex the ability to be flexible to the patient's response to treatment.

## HISTORY

The purpose of a history is to record all the pertinent information that the patient relates regarding the primary and secondary symptoms that brought the patient to you. In most instances, it is necessary to ask specific and open-ended questions about the patient's feelings, both physical and mental, since the coordination of both physical and mental entities control the patient's perception of discomfort or what the patient will describe as pain.

A good history should include the following information:

1. **Primary patient complaint:** What exactly does the patient feel and where is the discomfort principally located? Is there more than one location? Is the sensation the patient feels descriptive or nondescriptive (i.e., pain in my back and burning pain down my leg? What are the sensation descriptors? Tingling; numbness; burning; achiness; surgery, pain at night; constant; intermittent, etc.?)
2. **Onset of the patient's primary complaint:** A description of the onset of the patient's primary symptoms is important in ruling out other entities with similar symptoms, and whether the problem is acute traumatic, acute recurrent, or chronic.

3. **Past history:** Has the patient had these same or similar symptoms in the past, and have these symptoms been treated by other physicians? What was the previous diagnosis and what was the outcome? It is good here to list all previous care for the patient's current symptoms.

4. **Social history:** What familial history relates to the patient's symptoms? What kind of physical activities is the patient engaged in (i.e., exercise program, etc.)? What kind of home life does the patient have? Is the patient depressed? Does the patient want to return to work? How much does the patient smoke and drink? Does the patient use drugs?

5. **Personal profile:** The profile should contain age, marital status, number of children, and the spouse's occupation (which may directly relate to how symptoms appeared if wife or husband do same or similar work, etc.). This would also be an area of the history to inquire about how the patient is able to handle the stress in his or her life. Sleeping habits would fall into this category.

6. **Specifics as described by the patient:** This is a section of the history in which I let the patient personally describe the sensation he or she is experiencing, point with fingers to the exact location, and tell what makes the symptoms better and what makes them worse. This portion of the history can be redundant, but also may bring out small facts that could lead to significant findings. Here we must be specific. (Use the P2 QRST format described later in this chapter, under "Guidelines for creating an H&P.")

7. **Work habits:** Be very specific about the patient's job description here. You are the type of provider that industry needs to listen to these days. The leading cause of employee absenteeism in industry today is repetitive motion and overexertion injuries, and we see that type of patient in our practices all the time. When you return these patients to the worksite after they have undergone MUA, which you will easily do with this procedure, you need to have a solid foundation on which to base the changes you recommend for continued improvement. As a side note, if you are looking to get involved in the industrial field, employers need to know the benefits of the MUA procedure for injured employees with a history of chronic back and neck pain. The results have been long lasting and exceptionally rapid, and have shown significant changes in productivity for the industrial field primarily in manual lifting injuries and manufacturing injuries involving the low back.

## The Physical Examination

If the history is taken carefully, the practitioner should have a fairly good idea of what is causing the primary discomfort, or at least the most likely areas in which to concentrate his or her effort.

The physical examination should contain an examination of systems related to the symptoms, but should also be a review of systems with the patient.

Vital signs are always a good way to begin, and will many times dictate the flow of the entire exam as the patient initially feels that the whole body is being examined. The examination should be based on a systems review to rule out additional, or related, problems and should be comprehensive with an emphasis on the patient's complaint or a neuromusculoskeletal problem. Additional testing that is paramount to discerning a differential diagnosis of neuromusculoskeletal etiologies are

- An orthopedic examination, to include those factors specifically related to the area of primary patient discomfort. At this time, doing several orthopedic tests that are not specific to the primary area of discomfort is a waste of time, and might cause undue stress on the patient. Be concise, and establish a pinpoint location, if possible.
- The neurological tests should rule out upper motor and sensory dysfunction. They should also rule out peripheral from radicular, or cord discomfort:

Simplified:
Peripheral — involving components away from the intervertebral foramen (IVF).
Radicular — relating to a nerve root source, affecting the elements of the cord, up to and including the IVF.
**Note:** The phrase "reproduces patient discomfort" rather than "positive" or "negative" should be used as more descriptive terminology in both orthopedic testing and neurological testing.

- The postural analysis should include observation of the patient's gait, stance, pelvic level, scoliosis, if any, normal or abnormal postural curvatures. Included here would be an examination of motion palpation, etc.

The muscular movement, skin, and outer body observation should be a part of this examination. (Refer to Chapter 2, which describes predisposing factors.)

## RADIOGRAPHIC CONCERNS WITH MUA

Yochum, Rowe, Kettner, and Guebert[2,3,4] have all stated that a better concept in radiology is to discover the primary problem using all the hands-on skills and experience at your disposal, and then using differential diagnostic skills to decide whether to x-ray.

If radiological studies are indicated, the optimum views should be taken and reviewed. In most instances, anterior/posterior (AP) and lateral views are basic, but oblique views are also very helpful in diagnosing joint space occlusion. Also, with MUA lateral bending and flexion/extension studies are good diagnostic studies.[3,4]

A report of the x-ray findings should always be a part of the patient's chart, and should accompany the patient when referrals are made for further consultation.

The standard for diagnosis in most neuromusculoskeletal conditions is plain film radiographs to rule out more complicated osseous concerns. With MUA it is imperative that plain films and in many cases MRIs and CT scans be a part of the diagnostic work-up. The standard of care would suggest that if the patient has been undergoing care for several months and still has similar symptoms such as radiculopathy a follow-up MRI would be indicated. Since we are talking about radiological concerns in this section, we will only briefly mention that with radiculopathy another diagnostic concern would be to recommend electrodiagnostic studies to confirm MRI findings.

X-rays must be foremost in the mind of practitioners who practice mobilization/manipulation. X-rays add the blueprint for providing information on how the patient is progressing at the time the MUA is being performed, and they provide quality comparison outcomes when compared to past x-rays that may have been taken in the patient's progress.

In many cases since previous x-rays and MRIs have been taken the MUA practitioner needs to determine the time frame for additional films or follow-up MRIs. If a patient has not been x-rayed in the past 6 months and is experiencing similar problems that are requiring continued care, we recommend that additional films and another MRI be ordered, especially if the patient is experiencing radicular components as part of their continued symptomatology.

It is not advocated that an MRI is required in every case that undergoes MUA. Modifications that may be made so that even though a disc is protruded, for instance, with the proper idea of the position of the disc, the certified MUA practitioner can take the basic technique and modify it, so that the surrounding areas can be treated but the disc is put under very little, if any, distraction or compression because of the medications and the procedures that we use today with MUA. We would not be able to determine this change in technique without a full understanding of what the disc was doing, disc anatomy, and biomechanical factors that might affect the treatment using MUA as the technique of choice. The following is considered to be one of the more recent guidelines for interpreting the clinical progression of the disc while reading an MRI.

## RADIOLOGICAL NOMENCLATURE AND CLASSIFICATION OF LUMBAR DISC PATHOLOGY

Since it is estimated that 70% of the MUA procedures performed involve the lumbar spine with the potential for discogenic involvement, I felt it necessary to mention the newest information concerning standard terminology that is being recognized to describe disc pathology.

The following nomenclature has been endorsed by the American Academy of Orthpaedic Surgeons; American Academy of Physical Medicine and Rehabilitation; American College of Radiology; American Society of Neuroradiology; American Society of Spine Radiology; Joint Section on Disorders of the Spine and Peripheral Nerves of the American Association of Neurological Surgeons and Congress of Neurological Surgeons; European Society of Neuroradiology; North American Spine Society; and Physiatrics Association of Spine, Sports and Occupational Rehabilitation.

Through the efforts of the North American Spine Society, these standards have been proposed and used to help clarify disc pathology. "Though the NASS 1995 effort has been the most comprehensive (endorsement) to date, it remains deficient in clarifying some controversial topics, lacking in its treatment of some issues, and does not provide recommendations for standardization of classification of reporting. To address the remaining needs, and in hopes of securing endorsement sufficient to result in universal standardization, joint task forces were formed by NASS, the American Society of Neuroradiology (ASNR), and the American Society of Spine Radiology (ASSR)."[5] The nomenclature listed here is the product of those task forces and is the most commonly used terminology used in standard format.

The general classifications of disc lesions are

Normal (excluding aging changes)
Congenital/developmental variant
Degenerative/traumatic lesion
Anular tear
Herniation
    Protrusion/extrusion
    Intravertebral
Degeneration
    Spondylosis deformans
    Intervertebral osteochondrosis
Inflammation/Infection
Neoplasia
Morphologic variant of unknown significance

### Clarification of Nomenclature

**Normal disc** is referring to disc material, including the nucleus, within the confines of the annulus within the apophysis and means that the disc is fully and normally developed and free of any changes of disease, trauma, or aging. Some people are clinically "normal" even though they have morphologically abnormal discs (e.g., minor bulges of annuli, marginal vertebral body osteophytes, etc.).

**Annular tear/fissures** is used to refer to localized radial, concentric, or horizontal disruption of the annulus without associated displacement of disc material beyond the limits of the intervertebral disc space. There is general agreement about the various forms of loss of integrity of the annulus; however, some authors have recommended that such lesions be termed "fissures" rather than "tears," primarily for fear that the word "tear" could be misconstrued as implying a traumatic etiology. It is unwise to recommend contrary to ingrained common usage but wise to reiterate the caveat that the term "annular tear" does not imply traumatic etiology. In the case where a single, traumatic event is clearly the source of loss of integrity of a formally normal annulus, such as with documentation and findings of violent distraction injury, the term "rupture" of the annulus is appropriate, but use of the term "rupture" as synonymous with commonly observed tears or fissures is contraindicated.[5]

**Disc degeneration/traumatic** changes includes all processes, including aging of degeneration of the disc, and does not compel the observer to differentiate the pathologic from the normal consequences of aging. It does allow the observer to report distinction with appropriate data with a degree of confidence. The two degenerative processes involving the intervertebral disc that have previously been described by Schmorl and Junghanns[6] are classified as "spondylosis deformans," which affects essentially the annulus fibrosus and adjacent apophysis, and "intervertebral osteochondrosis," which affects mainly the nucleus pulposus and the vertebral body end plates, but also includes extensive fissuring of the annulus fibrosus, which may be followed by atrophy.[5]

**Herniated disc** material must be displaced from its normal location and not simply represented as acquired growth beyond the edges of the apophysis. Displacement, therefore, can only occur in association with disruption of the normal annulus or, as in the case of the intervertebral herniation (Schmorl's node), a break in the vertebral body end plate. For general purposes the term herniation is a broader term that can encompass various permutations of displaced disc material beyond the intervertebral disc space. Herniated disc, herniated nucleus pulposus, ruptured disc, prolapsed disc (used nonspecifically), protruded disc (used nonspecifically), and bulging disc (used nonspecifically) have all been used in the literature in various ways to denote imprecisely defined displacement of disc material beyond the interspace. Generally the term herniation needs to lend delineation to a specific anatomical consideration that would include disc material beyond the apophysis.

The term **bulge** refers to an apparent generalized extension of disc tissue beyond the edges of the apophysis. Such bulging occurs in greater than 50% of the circumference of the disc and extends a relatively short distance, usually less than 3 mm, beyond the edges of the apophysis. "Bulge" describes a morphologic characteristic of various possible causes. Bulging is sometimes a normal variant, resulting from degenerative changes, vertebral body remodeling, or ligamentous laxity in response to loading or angular motion, and can be an illusion from volume averaging (particularly with CT axial images).

A disc is **protruded** if the greatest distance, in any plane, between the edges of the disc material beyond the disc space is less than the distance between the edges of the base of the same plane. Protrusions may be "focal" or "broad based." The distinction between focal and broad based is arbitrarily set at 25% of the circumference of the disc. Protrusions with a base less than 25% (90 degrees) of the circumference of the disc are "focal." If the disc material is herniated so that the protrusion encompasses 25%–50% of the circumference of the disc, it is considered "broad-based protrusion."

A disc is **extruded** when any one distance between the edges of the disc material beyond the disc space is greater than the distance between the edges of the base measured in the same plane or when no continuity exists between the disc material beyond the disc space and that within the disc space. Extruded disc material that has no continuity with the disc of origin may be further characterized as "sequestered." Disc material that is displaced away from the site of extrusion, regardless of continuity, may be called "migrated," a term that is useful for interpretation of imaging studies because it is often impossible from images to know if continuity exists.[5]

Herniated disc material can be **contained** or **uncontained**. The test of containment is whether the displaced disc tissue is wholly held within the confines of the annulus. Strictly speaking, containment refers to the integrity of the outer annulus covering the disc herniation. The technical limitations of currently available noninvasive modalities (CT or MRI) usually preclude the distinction of a contained from an uncontained disc herniation. Note: In chiropractic we refer to this phenomenon as the disc being either "intra-annular" or "extra-annular" to help us distinguished the disposition of the disc material.

A **free fragment** is synonymous with a "sequestered fragment" and not the same as "uncontained," as the latter refers only to the integrity of the outer annulus and has no inference as to the continuity of the displaced disc material with the parent disc. A fragment should be considered "free" or "sequestered" only if there is no remaining continuity of disc material between it and the disc of origin.[5]

The term **migrated** disc or fragment refers to displacement of disc material away from the opening in the annulus through which the material has extruded.[5]

The previous material is taken from the "Nomenclature and Classification of Lumbar Disc Pathology"[5] produced by the *American Journal of Neuroradiology*, updated in 2003 and available for review on the Internet. The material was condensed from its original version for practical purposes for this chapter to help the reader evaluate discogenic involvement in the process of evaluation of a candidate for MUA who might have discogenic changes that must be addressed prior to moving the patient into the MUA arena. By using standard terminology when referring to the pathology that is representative of a particular disc involvement, we as practitioners will be able to describe in universal fashion the symptomatology, the description of anatomical dysfunction, the potential causation for patient discomfort, and the potential treatment method that might be appropriate for a particular patient based on the patient's pain complaint. This nomenclature has been needed for many years to help move health-care providers together, and more specifically manual therapists together, in their description of exactly what the patient is suffering from in hopes of increasing more productive outcomes with the various modalities that are used for treatment. In this case we use this nomenclature to provide guidance in the field of MUA to indicate in a descriptive manner the necessity as either contraindicative or indicative of this modality as a productive form of treatment in the case of discogenic pain.

## DIAGNOSTIC IMPRESSION

The diagnostic impression should include a complete summary and both a primary and secondary diagnosis of the patient's problems. The initial diagnosis is recorded as a working diagnosis since the problem the patient comes in for may change as treatment continues. The patient will ultimately level out and the diagnosis will become more permanent until maximum medical improvement (MMI) is achieved.

The practitioner will be responsible for documenting an entry diagnosis into the MUA program and a discharge diagnosis, which may or may not be the same.[7,8,9]

# GUIDELINE FOR CREATING AN H&P*

(To be written in narrative form)

**Patient's Full Name**                              Date of Examination
**Attending Physician**
**Patient Vitals**
**History**
**Chief Complaint**
**Present Complaint**
**Location** (use P2 QRST format for each area)
    P – Palliative (what makes discomfort better)
    P – Provocative (what makes discomfort worse)
    Q – Quality (aching, sharp, burning, numbness)
    R – Radiation (location, where pain goes) –)
    S – Severity scale 1–4 (mild, moderate, severe)
    T – Temporal – (rare 10%, occasional 25%, intermittent 50%, frequent 75%, constant
        100%)
**History of present illness** – concise, with all treatment the patient has received, including
    the duration, type, and patient's response.
**Past medical history** – all past accidents, falls, other injuries; surgeries; illnesses; past
    history of present chief complaint.
**Social history** – work type and duties, smoking habits, drinking habits, recreational drugs, etc.
**Allergies**
**Medications** – all prescription and OTC presently taking (this also includes all vitamins
    and herbs or natural remedies the patient is taking)
**Review of systems** – all current medical conditions. Include names of doctors being seen
    presently. Include a current pre-anesthesia consult if under care for cardiac, respiratory,
    kidney, or other condition that may be adverse for anesthesia use.
**Physical Examination**
    **General** – Well developed, well nourished, alert, acute, distress, gait, posture, antalgic, etc.
    **Cervical** – Spinal tenderness, paraspinal muscle tenderness spasm, trigger points, ROM,
        Ortho tests, etc.
    **Thoracic** – Spinal tenderness, paraspinal muscle tenderness spasm, trigger points, nota-
        ble articular dysfunction (rib head subluxation).
    **Lumbar** – Spinal tenderness, paraspinal muscle tenderness spasm, trigger points, ROM,
        Ortho. tests, etc.
    **Extra spinal** – (i.e., hip, shoulder, knee, wrist, ankle, etc.).
    **Neurological** – DTRs, sensory, motor testing, EMGs, etc.
    **Radiographic imaging** – Reports attached, or interpretation of all films, MRIs, CTs, etc.
    **Clinical impression** – Record your diagnosis verbally which will coincide with your OP
        report. Do not use insurance dx code numbers.
    **Recommendations** – State your rationale for MUA and whether single or multiple pro-
        cedures will be rendered and why.

**Rationale Example:** The patient has chronic recurrent headaches which manifest in the
    occipital area with radiation to the forehead. Review of systems is unremarkable for
    systemic pathology. Imaging studies in the form of plain film x-rays reveal hypomobility
    of the C4–5 motion units and static movement at C5 6. The patient continues to suffer

---

* B.H. Rubin contributed to this section.

from chronic paravertebral muscle contracture in the cervical and mid to upper thoracic spinal areas from C2 to T9. A working diagnosis of torticollis with secondary cervico-thoracic myofascial radiculitis has been used and the patient has undergone three months of noninvasive conservative care to include physical therapy and specific chiropractic manipulation with minimal articular motion. The patient is also under a regime of medical care to include both pain management and muscle relaxants with little improvement. To date this patient has responded only minimally to his therapy program. This patient falls within the standard acceptable forms of conditions that have responded favorably to MUA as documented in other cases and referenced case studies throughout the country. I am recommending MUA as an alternative to chronic prolonged conservative care or possible future surgical intervention. The patient will receive a series of two MUAs in accordance with chronicity and patient response to previous therapy. This follows protocols as established by the National Academy of MUA Physicians (NAMUAP).

## SAMPLES OF HISTORY AND PHYSICAL

### Case 1

*History*

Chief Complaint – Neck pain, headache, and low back pain. Mrs. S. is a 36-year-old female of Caucasian descent. She stated that she exercises occasionally. She drinks alcohol occasionally and also smokes tobacco (1 pack per day.) She is currently employed as a nurse. She is 5 foot 1 and weighs 190 pounds. Her resting pulse was 72 bpm. The left brachial blood pressure was 136/92. Today, Mrs. S. described having frequent moderate right upper neck symptoms which were dull in character. She states that her neck catches when she turns to the right. She further reported having right occipital pain. She describes that it feels like a stick in her right upper neck. She was also experiencing intermittent moderate diffuse right upper back symptoms of an achy and dull nature. She further reported having mid-line lower back pain that seems to come and go since the auto accident. She also states that she has some intermittent right ear pain that she has noticed since the accident. The symptoms were first noticed after an automobile accident. She was the driver of her vehicle and was wearing her seatbelt. She stated that the other vehicle failed to stop and struck the right front quarter panel of her vehicle. She reports that this caused her to be thrown into the driver's side door. She does have a past history of neck and lower back pain but she says not to this extent. She states that in the past usually a couple of adjustments will fix the problem. She states that since the accident after she is treated she will feel better for a while but her symptoms gradually return. She also related that a couple of weeks ago she thought for a few days that she was over it but her symptoms have returned. Her diagnostic workup for this condition has included plain lumbar and cervical x-rays. Treatment has consisted of physiotherapy (interferential electrical muscle stimulation), progressive resistance exercises of the cervical spine, ice/heat, traction and spinal manipulation. She is using a cervical pillow and lordotic cervical traction at home. She denies having any known drug allergies. She is currently taking Prozac. She states that her family physician prescribed this to her about one month ago and she states this is helping her get through some mild depression. I asked if she feels her symptoms and/or the accident are related to the depression and she said she did not think so. She said that she was on Prozac a few years ago for a while when she was going through a divorce. She also takes ibuprofen occasionally for the pain. Neck Disability Index (NDI) is graded at 22%, which is considered by the questionnaire to be a mild disability. The review of systems was unremarkable.

*Physical Exam*

On palpitation, moderate spasm and tenderness was noticed in the superior trapezius on the right and to a lesser degree on the left, moderate tenderness was found in the levator scapulae and superior trapezius bilaterally. On further digital palpitation, mild tenderness was found in the sacroiliac region bilaterally and tenderness was found in the lumbo-sacral region. Active trigger points were found in the superior trapezius on the right. On active testing in the cervical region, extension was painful, right lateral flexion was mildly restricted by pain, and right rotation was mildly restricted by pain. All other active cervical ranges of motion were unrestricted. All active thoraco-lumbar ranges of motion were mildly restricted. The head was positioned slightly anterior when viewed from the side. There was no antalgia present. All heart sounds were normal to auscultation. The lungs were normal to auscultation and percussion. Routine examination of the eyes, ears, nose and oral cavity was unremarkable. She is somewhat obese. All of the standard upper extremity muscle strengths were graded 5/5. All of the standard lower muscle strengths were grade 2/2. Dermatomes were found to be unremarkable with the use of pinwheel. Cervical compression was found to be negative. Cervical distraction decreased the neck pain. Shoulder depression was found to be positive bilaterally for the neck pain. George's test was found to be negative during the standard procedure. Seated straight leg raise was negative bilaterally to 90 degrees. Kemp's test was found to be negative bilaterally. Routine x-rays of the cervical and lumbar spinal areas were taken. On spinal evaluation, moderate joint dysfunctions were noted at the right occiput, C1, C5, T2, T3, L5, and the right sacroiliac joint.

*Clinical Impression*

The primary diagnosis is cervicocranial syndrome with associated myofascitis. The secondary diagnosis is lumbar somatic dysfunction, which is complicated by L5 Grade 1 Spondylolisthesis.

*Recommendations*

I have spoken with the patient and her husband in detail with regard to other options of treatment for her condition. We spoke in depth about MUA, manipulation under anesthesia. I have given her written research information and a video to watch in regard to the MUA procedure. I feel that due to her plateaued response to her recent care she would be an excellent candidate for the procedure. She has failed to gain prolonged relief of her symptoms with the recent care given.

I feel that MUA is a viable alternative to continued prolonged conservative care. Given the chronicity of her condition, I believe that a series of three MUA procedures will be needed to achieve the expected gain. This follows protocols as established by the National Academy of MUA Physicians.

Sincerely,

**Case 2**

*History*

Chief Complaint — Ms. Y described her neck pain as follows. She stated that it felt like she had to hold her head up with her hands. She described a deep soreness to the neck and upper trapezius area, which got to be a throbbing type of pain occasionally. She stated that this was just about daily. She further stated that her neck pain worsened as the day progressed and this was consistent seven days a week. Her neck pain was aggravated by prolonged sitting, which was required in her duties as an administrative secretary. At the time of presentation she reported no numbness or tingling into the upper extremities, but she did report some immediately following the motor vehicle accident. The pain was mostly on the left side of her neck and into her shoulders; however there was also persistent pain on the right side of her neck. Ms. Y described her headaches initially as starting at the base of her skull and in the neck and it would radiate forward to behind the eyes in a C-type pattern on each side of her head. These were very severe at least a few times per month and lasted from three to four days. She had severe nausea accompanying these headaches and also vomiting on a regular basis. On her initial presentation the headaches had returned full blown and were worsening once again and even waking her through the night occasionally. Her low back pain was initially described as an irritating kind of pain where she could not sit down. It had eased up a little bit over the few days prior to her initial visit, but it had overall been a very persistent problem. She also noticed some constipation relative to increases in back pain. There was a sharp component to the low back pain with certain movements, but by and large this was a dull achy soreness.

### History of Present Illness

Following a traffic accident, the patient did not go to the hospital. On her way home the patient started feeling neck pain and started feeling a severe headache coming on. The pain got worse through the night and her low back started hurting quite badly. She did not go to work the next day and she thought "she was going to die because of the low back and neck pain." At that time she called her family physician, Dr. R, who scheduled her right away. He diagnosed her condition after having examined her as a cervical strain. He prescribed for her exercises, stretching, ibuprofen, and Norflex. These treatments did not seem to help Ms. Y very much, although Dr. R did monitor her weekly for three to four weeks at which time due to lack of progress, he referred her to Dr. H. Dr. H performed x-rays, which revealed no broken bones, and he diagnosed her as having a soft tissue injury. Ms. Y reports that Dr. H gave her a book of stretches and exercises and referred her to a physical therapy program. Ms. Y was given physical therapy for three to four months. Her physical therapy treatments involved heat, muscle stimulation, ultrasound, home ice, in-office exercises, and some home exercises. She was released after this period of time.

### Past Medical History

Prior medical history involved a motor vehicle accident in which she was rear-ended. She was a passenger in that vehicle. She did sustain some facial cuts and stitches due to the fact that she was not wearing a seatbelt and struck an object in the vehicle. She also reported previous accidents where her car was barely hit in the front end. No injuries were sustained in that accident. All of these injuries had been resolved and she had no similar complaints prior to this most recent motor vehicle accident. All other past medical history was unremarkable.

### Social History

Patient is nonsmoking and light drinker. Patient reports no use of recreational drugs. Patient is an administrative secretary, which requires prolonged periods of sitting and typing, which aggravate her neck pain. Social activities of daily living include Nordictrack, line dancing, some light weight lifting at the YMCA, and playing tennis.

### Allergies

Patient states no known allergies.

### Medications

Ibuprofen.

### Review of Symptoms

Patient was referred by Dr. H for present condition. Patient reports no other current medical conditions.

### Physical Exam

General – On initial physical exam, Ms. Y presented as a well-developed, well-nourished alert 38-year-old Caucasian female with good blood pressure of 102/62. She weighed 125 lbs. and is 5'6" tall.

Cervical – Numerous myofascial trigger points were found in the paravertebral musculature. Specific areas of tenderness and dysfunction were noted as well. There was an exquisite amount of tenderness found over the greater and lesser occipital nerves bilaterally. Ranges in motion were markedly diminished due to pain and muscle spasms. Foraminal compression test were found to be positive bilaterally as well as a positive left Spurling's test, which reproduced the patient's discomfort.

Thoracic – Digital palpation revealed myofascial trigger points and multiple vertebral misalignments.

Lumbar – Noted decrease in all ranges of motion with paraspinal muscular spasms. A positive right Yeoman's test with localized pain to the sacroiliac joint and slightly positive left Yeoman's also localizing to the left sacroiliac region indicating bilateral SI lesions. Lumbar joint dysfunction was identified.

Neurological – Examination at this time was essentially unremarkable and this included scans of cranial nerve function, posterior column function, cerebellar function, deep tendon reflexes in the upper and lower extremities, and sensitivity to the pinwheel and dermatomal ranges in the upper and lower extremities.

Radiographic imaging – A-P and lateral full spine radiographs were taken. X-ray revealed decreased cervical curve with vertebral rotational disc relationships in cervical, thoracic, and lumbar spine. Pelvic distortion was noted. No osseous interruptions or gross pathologies were identified as visualized.

Clinical impressions – My impression is that the patient was suffering from occipital neuralgia secondary to the most recent motor vehicle accident; chronic myofascitis secondary to chronic cervical sprain/strain which occurred as a result of the most recent motor vehicle accident; chronic lumbar myofascitis and dysfunction as a sequel to her lumbar sprain/strain which was resultant from the accident, sacroilititis and fibromyositis both secondary to the motor vehicle accident.

Recommendations – My initial recommendations were that the patient undergo spinal manipulative therapy with passive modalities with the possibility of needing to progress treatment to manipulation under anesthesia due to the chronicity of her condition at the time of initial presentation. Patient is recommended at this time for three MUA procedures.

*Rationale Example*

The patient has chronic recurrent headaches which manifest in the occipital area with radiation behind the eyes. Review of systems is unremarkable for systemic pathology. Imaging studies in the form of plain film x-ray reveal decreased cervical curve with multiple rotational disrelationships of the cervical thoracic and lumbar spines. A working diagnosis of chronic myofascitis secondary to chronic recurrent cervical sprain/strain, chronic lumbar myofascitis and dysfunction, sacroilitis, and fibromyositis bilaterally. After undergoing 18 months of conservative chiropractic care, including electro-muscle stimulation and specific adjusting with minimal articular motion, pharmacological intervention, and pain management, the patient's treatment has plateaued and she has slowed her recovery, making minimal progress toward returning to normal activities. Therefore, I am recommending MUA as an alternative to chronic prolonged conservative care or possible future surgical intervention. The patient will receive a series of three MUAs. This follows protocols as established by the National Academy of MUA Physicians.

## REFERENCES


1. Clybourne, H.E., Manipulation of the low back region under anesthesia, *J. Am. Osteopathic Assoc.* September 1948, 10–11.
2. Kettner, N.W., Guebert, G.M., Yochum, T.R., Intervertebral disc derangement: the magnetic resonance imaging perspective, *Applied Diagnostic Imaging*, May/June 1989, vol. 1, no. 3, 17–25.
3. Kettner, N.W., Guebert, G.M., Yochum, T.R., The radiology of segmental instability, *Applied Diagnostic Imaging,* September/October 1989, vol. 1, no. 5, 37-48.
4. Yochum, T. and Rowe, L.J., *Essentials of Skeletal Radiology,* Williams & Wilkins, Baltimore, vols. 1 and 2, 1987, 253–7.
5. "Nomenclature & classification of lumbar disc pathology," update 2003, presented by American Society of Neuroradiology, American Society of Spine Radiology and North American Spine Society; copyright 2001 Lippincott, Williams & Wilkins; http://www.asnr.org/spine_nomenclature/discussion. asp.
6. Schmorl, G., Junghanns, H., *The Human Spine in Health and Disease*, 2nd American ed., trans. E.F. Besemann, New York: Grune and Stratton, 1971, 141–48, 186–98.

7.  Capps, S., Texas College of Chiropractic, syllabus: Manipulation under anesthesia, postgraduate course of study, 1992.
8.  Gordon, R., with contribution from Furno, P., Cornerstone Professional Education, MUA syllabus currently sponsored by the National University of Health Sciences, 5th ed., August 1998.
9.  Greenman, P.E., Manipulation with the patient under anesthesia, *J. Am. Osteopathic Assoc.* September 1992, vol. 92, no. 9, 1159–70.

# 10 Anesthesia

*Anthony Rogers and Robert C. Gordon*

## CONTENTS



# Introduction

*Robert C. Gordon*

Manipulation under anesthesia (MUA) is not a procedure to be used on every patient who comes through your door. Manipulation under anesthesia, if followed with proper protocols, is an excellent technique to add to the therapeutic regime that a doctor of chiropractic/osteopathy has to use in the restoration of a patient's health.

Three very important principles must be followed if MUA is to be successful:

1. Careful selection of the cases
2. Careful and cautious application of the techniques

3. A careful, well-planned post-MUA program that will continue to help prevent the redevelopment of the adhesions.[1,2]

Manipulation under anesthesia should be used in very specific conditions. A differential diagnosis is required to establish which condition is most beneficial. (See Figure 10.1.)

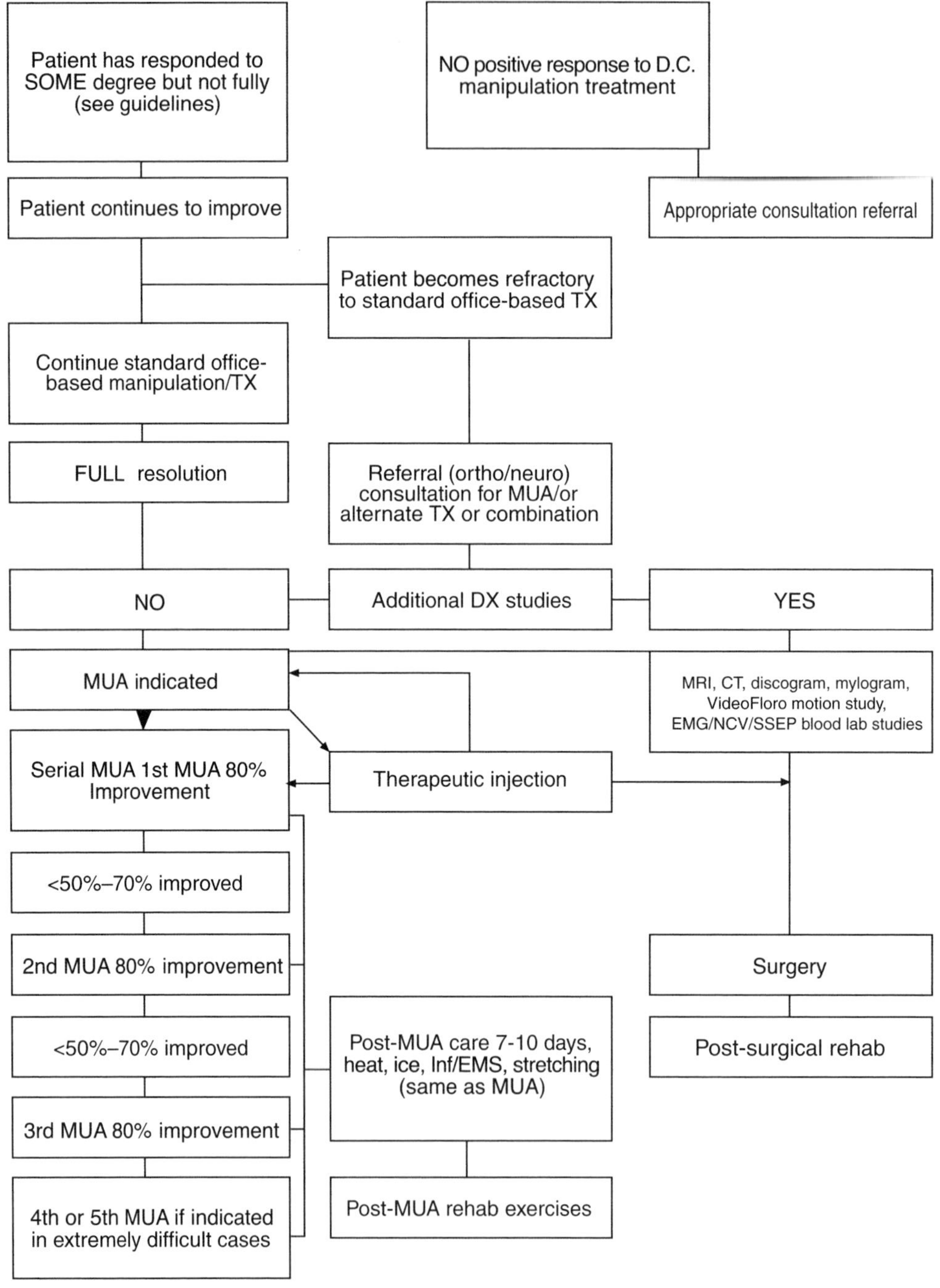


**FIGURE 10.1** Differential diagnosis for evaluating a patient for MUA.

## SCIENTIFIC VALIDITY FOR MUA

### WHY SHOULD WE USE MUA?

- Extended or prolonged conservative care is not working.
- The patient may be a borderline surgical candidate and MUA could be a deciding procedure.
- MUA has now proven to return patients to the work site faster with more productivity than other forms of advanced treatment programs.
- The rate of recurrence of injury has been found to be very low in MUA patients.
- The MUA procedure is considerably more cost effective than prolonged conservative care, disability income coverage for undetermined periods, or surgical intervention (when found to be questionable).

### WHAT MAKES MUA THE PROCEDURE OF CHOICE OVER OTHER TREATMENTS?

- Results are more rapid.
- Patients respond well.
- Treatment programs are fairly regimented and prescribed by protocol. (If unresponsive in the prescribed period, patients are placed into more intensive programs with clinical justification.)
- Results are long lasting with low percentage of reoccurrence.
- Patients who have been away from the work site for long periods of time are returning with renewed productivity.

### WHAT MAKES MUA DIFFERENT FROM CONSERVATIVE THERAPY?

- Twilight sedation places patient in a position to be responsive to therapy, but nonapprehensive to treatment.
- Mobilization, manipulation, and adjustments are completed without resistance.
- Proprioceptive change occurs. (Body's perception of movement/biomechanics changes.)
- Fibrotic adhesions are altered better and are remodeled for more productive movement and body function.

# Anesthesia Component in MUA

*Anthony Rogers*

Anesthesia is defined by *Stedman's Medical Dictionary* as "a state characterized by loss of sensation, the result of pharmacological depression of nerve function or of neurological disease" and by *Webster's Dictionary* as "a loss of sensation with or without loss of consciousness."

Anesthesia falls under several categories. These categories are defined by the type of anesthesia used, the level of consciousness, or a combination of both. There is general anesthesia, regional (local) anesthesia, monitored anesthesia care, and conscious sedation.

General anesthesia is a drug-induced loss of consciousness during which patients are not arousable. The components of general anesthesia consist of amnesia, analgesia, lack of movement, and control of sympathetic nervous system responses that are evoked by noxious stimulation. Additionally there is a loss of protective reflexes, including the loss of the ability to independently maintain a patent airway, and there is a loss of ability to respond purposefully to verbal commands or tactile stimulation. This is achieved by the use of a combination of drugs that may include inhaled and/or injected anesthetics with or without muscle relaxants. These drugs are selected on the basis of a specific goal (i.e., to control pain, blood pressure, heart rate, muscle relaxation, etc.).

Anesthesia with general anesthetics occurs in four stages, which may or may not be observable because they can occur very rapidly:

Stage One — Analgesia. The patient experiences analgesia or a loss of pain sensation but remains conscious and can carry on a conversation.

Stage Two — Excitement. The patient may experience delirium or become violent. Blood pressure rises and becomes irregular and breathing rate increases. This stage is typically bypassed by administering a barbiturate, such as sodium pentothal or propofol, before the anesthesia.

Stage Three — Surgical anesthesia. During this stage, the skeletal muscles relax, and the patient's breathing becomes regular. Eye movements slow, then stop, and surgery can begin.

Stage Four — Medullary paralysis. This stage occurs if the respiratory centers of the brain that control breathing and other vital functions (medulla) cease to function. Death can result if the patient cannot be revived quickly.

General anesthetics may be gases or volatile liquids that evaporate and are inhaled along with oxygen. Other drugs can function as anesthetics and are typically given intravenously. The level of anesthesia produced by inhalational anesthetics can be titrated rapidly, if necessary, by adjusting the concentration of the anesthetic in the oxygen that is inhaled by the patient. The degree of anesthesia produced by an intravenously injected anesthetic is fixed and cannot be changed as rapidly.

## INHALATIONAL ANESTHETICS

Halothane (fluothane) is potent and can be easy to overdose. This drug causes unconsciousness but little pain relief, so it is often used concomitantly with other agents to control pain. Very rarely, it can be toxic to the liver in adults. It also has a pleasant odor, and it is often the anesthetic of choice for use with children.

Enflurane (ethrane) has a more rapid onset of anesthesia and a faster recovery than halothane. This anesthetic is not recommended in patients with kidney failure.

Isoflurane (forane) is not toxic to the liver but can induce heart rhythm abnormalities.

Sevoflurane (sevorane, ultane) is an excellent induction agent, provides rapid emergence, and allows excellent anesthetic depth control.

Suprane (desflurane) has a pungent odor and is less likely to be used for inhalation induction than halothane or sevoflurane. It allows for rapid emergence and excellent anesthetic depth control.

Nitrous oxide (laughing gas) is used with other drugs, such as thiopental, to produce surgical anesthesia. It has the fastest induction and recovery profile. It is also considered one of the safest because it does not slow breathing or blood flow to the brain.

The intravenous medications used for general anesthesia can also be used for conscious sedation and will be covered in greater detail in the "Conscious Sedation" section on the next page.

## REGIONAL ANESTHESIA

Regional anesthesia is the abolition of painful impulses from any region of the body by temporarily interrupting the sensory nerve conductivity, and motor function may or may not be involved. Under regional anesthesia, the patient does not lose consciousness. Regional anesthesia is often coupled with sedation.

Local infiltration is defined as the introduction of a local anesthetic drug into subcutaneous tissue or one that is applied topically. These agents are not considered conscious sedation.

Local anesthetics include procaine, chloroprocaine, tetracaine, cocaine, lidocaine, mepivacaine, bupivacaine, etidocaine, prilocaine, and ropivacaine. The differences between these agents are their duration of action and how they are metabolized. Also, sensory or motor nerves can be affected preferentially.

Peripheral blocks are defined as the introduction of a local anesthetic drug near a peripheral nerve. These blocks are used for anesthesia, postoperative analgesia, and diagnosis and/or treatment of chronic pain syndromes.

Epidural blocks are defined as the introduction of local anesthetic drug into the space around the spinal cord.

Spinal blocks are defined as the introduction of local anesthetic drug inside the dura mater. These are injected into the lumbar region.

Combined epidural/spinal blocks are the combination of the two. Spinal anesthesia is given first followed by placement of an epidural catheter for continuous or bolus administration of anesthetic solution.

Bier block is used for placement of local anesthetic into a limb. A double cuff is used on the extremity and inflated. Following this lidocaine is infused in an IV, which allows for anesthesia of the limb for as long as the cuff remains inflated.

## MONITORED ANESTHESIA CARE

The monitoring of a patient for a procedure ranges from no intervention to heavy sedation. There appears to be some controversy with MUA; some believe that it should only be done under general anesthesia, as per CPT code 22505. This is a problem that is still battled and should be changed. General anesthesia is not the safest route for MUA because the patient's protective reflexes are abolished. Damage has been done in the past due to secondary overstretching of the patient's joints and muscles beyond the end range. MUA should be performed under "conscious sedation," which allows the patient's own protective reflexes to respond, thus giving the MUA practitioner tactile feedback to limit the stretch and thus prevent overstretching. The main controversy today revolves around the level of consciousness necessary to provide the MUA procedure; it relates to the response the doctor desires from the patient and the safety of the patient. At what level does general anesthesia begin, and at what level is the patient considered "conscious"? The MUA procedure is better rated using guidelines established by the American Society of Anesthesiologists (ASA) for "monitored anesthesia care." Under monitored anesthesia care protocols, this procedure is provided only by board-certified anesthesiologists or under their direct supervision by certified registered nurse anesthetists (CRNA). This also follows guidelines established by the National Academy of MUA Physicians (NAMUAP). Because of that, this type of anesthesia may be classified as conscious sedation or may be more "general" in nature. By using this standard, the level of consciousness can be light or deep, depending on the requirement of the doctor performing the procedure, the comfort of the anesthesiologist, and patient safety. True conscious sedation may be too light for what is necessary to obtain the desired results. It is at this juncture that additional medications commonly used in the MUA procedure might place the patient in the "general anesthesia" category. A simple change from lighter anesthesia to a deeper anesthesia would also place the patient in a slightly more "unresponsive" state which would be required to achieve the desired results. A more correct approach to MUA today would be to use monitored anesthesia care and determine the level of anesthesia as needed during the procedure. This allows for what is commonly seen in MUA, where end range is maintained, the patient continues to breathe on their own, the patient responds to pain but the response is slowed down, and the patient does not remember the procedure. Control is maintained by the anesthesiologist throughout the procedure, and continued administration of medications allows the procedure to go smoothly while keeping the patient comfortable yet still responsive physiologically.

## CONSCIOUS SEDATION

Conscious sedation is produced by the administration of pharmocologic agents. A patient undergoing conscious sedation has a depressed level of consciousness, but retains the ability to independently and continuously maintain a patent airway. The patient can respond appropriately to physical stimulation and/or verbal commands. The medications and dosages utilized for conscious sedation are not intended to produce deep sedation or loss of consciousness. General anesthesia is not a form of conscious sedation. Practitioners of conscious sedation should be trained in advanced cardiac life support (ACLS) and comfortable with airway management and resuscitation.

The objectives of conscious sedation entail altering the level of consciousness and mood, providing relaxation and amnesia, elevating the pain threshold, and having minimal variation of the patients vital signs while maintaining consciousness and cooperation. The patient should be easy to arouse from sleep and have purposeful responses to verbal communication and tactile stimulation. The patient should be able to return to ambulation in a short period of time. The duration of amnesia should match the duration of the procedure.

The undesirable effects of conscious sedation are deep unarousable sleep, respiratory depression, airway obstruction, apnea, decrease in vital signs (i.e., bradycardia, hypotension, etc.), agitation, combativeness, and loss of pain reflexes.

## PHARMACOLOGY OF COMMONLY USED SEDATING AGENTS

Benzodiazepines provide sedation and amnesia, but are not analgesic or anti-emetic. These agents are potentiated by narcotics. The common medications in this class in order of duration are midazolam (versed), diazepam (valium), and lorazepam (ativan). The adverse effects of these drugs are respiratory depression, hypotension, bradycardia, and hypoventilation.

Narcotics provide analgesia. If given before a painful stimulus, the effect is more pronounced. The common medications in this class are alfentanil, sufentanil, fentanyl (sublimaze), remifentanil, meperidine (demerol,) and morphine. The adverse effects are respiratory depression, apnea (potentiated by benzodiazepines), bradycardia, hypotension, pruritus, nausea/vomiting, and urinary retention.

Barbiturates provide sedation and hypnosis. The common medications in this class are propofol (diprivan), methohexital (brevital), thiopental (pentothal), and ketamine (dissociative agent). The adverse affects are respiratory depression, apnea, tachy/bradycardia, hypotension, and pain on injection.

There are two reversal agents in use: one for narcotics and one for benzodiazepines. The duration of action of these reversal agents is usually shorter than those medications being reversed. Close monitoring of the patient is necessary because resedation can occur. Naloxone (narcan) is used in the reversal of narcotics, and flumazenil (romazicon) is used in the reversal of benzodiazepines. No reversal agents for barbiturates currently exist.

Pre-procedural evaluation of each patient is mandatory. This should be done by a primary care physician and/or anesthesiologist. Acute, unforeseen medical problems can arise before the procedure or the day of the procedure. These unforeseen problems may necessitate postponement of the procedure. However, standard pre-operative practices should allow for the identification of chronic conditions or significant items (i.e., coronary artery disease, hypertension, diabetes, etc.) in the patient's medical history. Should any issues arise they can be addressed prior to the day of surgery. The patient should have a complete medical history and physical. The medical history should include drug allergies, previous experience with sedation and/or anesthesia, pertinent laboratory and x-ray results, and medications.

Patients are given an American Society of Anesthesia (ASA) classification, which ranges from Class 1 to Class 6, with most patients falling between Class 1 and Class 3 (1 = normal healthy, 2 = mild systemic disease, 3 = severe systemic disease, 4 = severe systemic disease that is a constant threat to life, 5 = a moribund patient who is not expected to survive without the operation, and 6 = a declared brain-dead patient whose organs are being removed for donor purposes.)

The day of surgery, the patient is seen by the anesthesia provider and all data are reviewed (including the patients nothing by mouth [NPO] status). If everything is in order, the patient is taken to the operating or procedure room and placed on the procedure table. Monitors are used for measurement of blood pressure, EKG, heart rate, and oxygen saturation. IV access is established so sedating agents can be administered. After baseline vital signs have been established, the patient is sedated and the procedure begins. The sedation is usually accomplished by a combination of benzodiazepines, narcotics, and ultrashort-acting hypnotic agents. Pain tolerance and medication requirements vary. The range of responses to the various medications can be dramatic; therefore, titration of the various agents is the key to optimum sedation.

The post-operative course should be short if sedation is titrated and shorter-acting agents are used. With a combination of versed and propofol, most patients are awake and alert within 5 minutes after the procedure. Typically patients are able to be discharged within one half hour, depending on the facility.

So why is anesthesia used for MUA or MUJA? The reason relates to the muscles and ligaments, which stabilize joints. When muscles spasm, the doctor of chiropractic/osteopathy may not be able to put joints through a normal range of motion. Under anesthesia, the postural tone of muscles and muscle spasms is abolished, allowing the chiropractor/osteopath to gently manipulate joints by putting joints through a normal range of motion. The end result is to reduce the restrictive adhesions and reduce the misalignments of the involved vertebrae. This procedure works well for many patients who have pain and do not wish to undergo surgery. Some patients are in too much pain or have muscle spasms that are too severe and chronic to benefit from chiropractic/osteopathic care without anesthesia.

So why is conscious sedation used? An intravenous sedative is administered by a medical doctor (anesthesiologist) or CRNA. The patient is not subjected to the dangers of general anesthesia and is awake enough to preserve protective reflexes; however, the sedative allows for the adequate mobilization of the joints and vertebrae. The patient is sedated for 5–10 min, rather than for hours as during back surgery and usually recovers within 5–10 min after an MUA is finished.

In my practice, propofol is my preference for sedation because it provides all of the benefits needed for MUA with the least amount of side effects and a speedy maximum return to normal function.

# Choice of Anesthesia (From a Nonanesthesiologist's Perspective)

*Robert C. Gordon*

The choice of anesthesia is based on the comfort zone of both the anesthesiologist and the patient. The most widely used anesthetics for this procedure are diprivan (also called propofol) and versed.[1]

Brevitol and sodium pentothal (which were the drugs of choice in the early days of MUA) are barbiturates and can cause nausea and are very seldom used any longer. Diprivan has become more popular in recent times because it is the newer of the short-acting anesthetics, and has considerably fewer side effects and is metabolized by the body at a much higher rate.

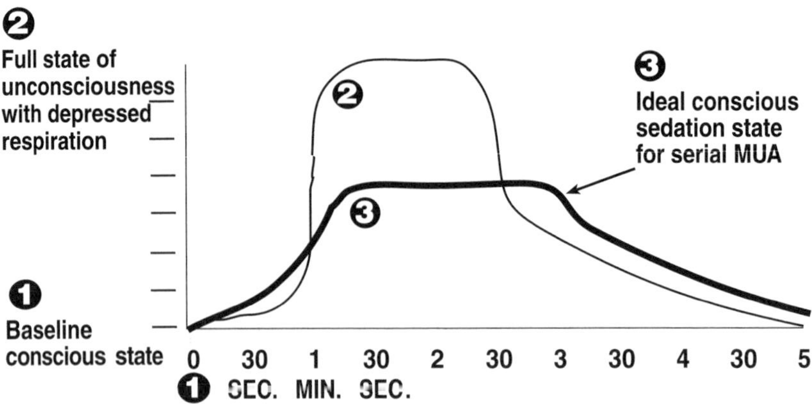


**FIGURE 10.2**

The anesthetic is usually administered depending on the patient's weight, and their titration usually varies with each patient's ability to metabolize the drug.

Of considerable interest with the use of diprivan has been the slight increase in titer in multiple or serial MUA as the patient is treated from the first day to the third. The patient continues to metabolize the diprivan so that the drug is completely gone by the next treatment, and by midday of the treatment, the patient feels very few, if any, side effects from the drug. This is extremely important because you can usually see a true picture of patient progress during the office visit later on that same day. When a barbiturate such as pentothol is used instead, the patient continues to have drug effects far into the day of the procedure and accurate determination of progress is harder to confirm.

All of these drugs are considered ultra-short-acting or rapidly acting anesthetics. If the drug were micrographed for compilation, there would be a short delay in response followed by a rapid effect on the central nervous system (CNS), which causes the patient to fall into a semi-conscious state (called conscious sedation) as respiration slightly declines. Almost immediately, there is a rise in the metabolic reaction so that the patient begins to move into the post-operative stage, or full consciousness.[3] Graphically, this effect might resemble the one shown in Figure 10.2.

The return to a conscious state is determined by the titration that is used and the metabolic effect the body has on the titer (amount of drug used). With the short-acting effect, the anesthesiologist works as a team member with the chiropractor/osteopath so that the desired effect on the patient is established and maintained until the procedure can be completed. The action of the drugs over a period of time is called pharmacokinetics and is divided into five phases:[4]

1. Absorption
2. Distribution
3. Tissue response
4. Biotransformation (metabolism)
5. Excretion

Once the proper titer or dosage is completed, the return to consciousness is rapid. However, waking does not mean that the anesthetic has completely worn off. Some anesthetics are better than others, especially when doing same-day post-MUA. Under no circumstances are patients allowed to operate any machinery or make important decisions following MUA at least for that day, and should be strictly monitored during recovery and accompanied by someone when leaving the facility. (See Figure 10.3 and Figure 10.4.)

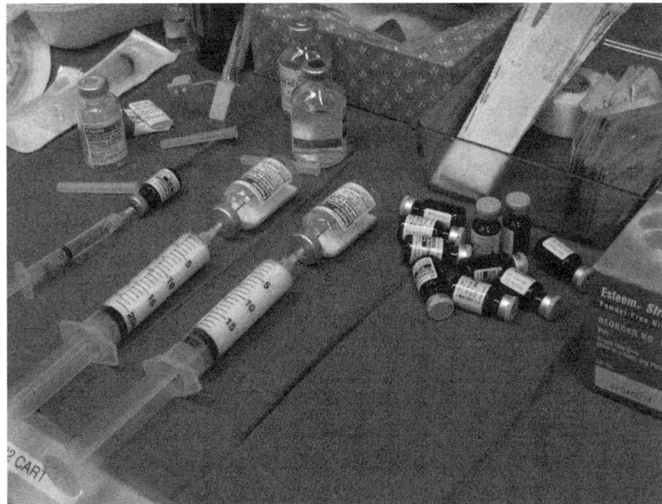

**FIGURE 10.3**

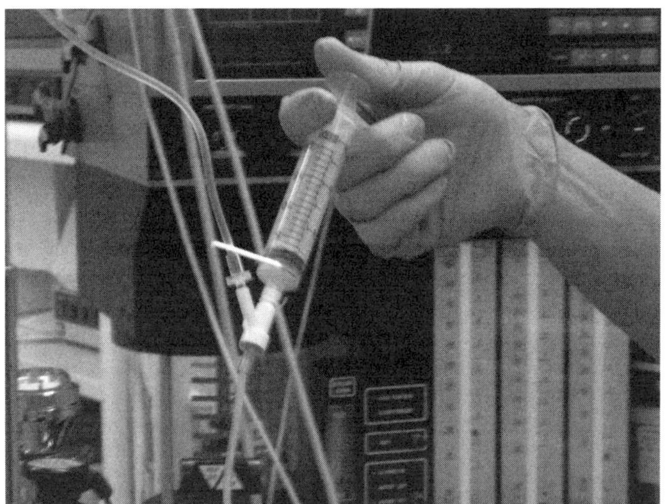

**FIGURE 10.4**

# Guidelines for the Use of Monitored Anesthesia Care (For the Nonanesthesiologist)

*Anthony Rogers*

Monitored anesthesia care (MAC) is a technique whereby the patient is given intravenous diprivan and versed by titration methods until the desired level of anesthesia is achieved. As presented earlier in this chapter, MAC can range anywhere from IV sedation or what is called conscious sedation to early general anesthesia. Here are the steps involved:

1. A history and physical are completed on every patient, with special attention given to age, history of heart disease, and drug and alcohol use.[4,5]
2. MAC/general anesthetic is administered only by a trained anesthesiologist or supervised CRNA with training in cardiac advanced life support. It is imperative that this individual be trained in airway management and IV fluid administration in the event of adverse reactions. A chiropractic physician is not licensed to even assist in the administration of drugs.
3. Qualified personnel must be present in the room with the patient at all times throughout the procedure and until the patient has returned to baseline alertness with reflexes present and is transferred to recovery.
4. Nurses trained to assist in anesthesiology should be educated and trained by the anesthesia department in pulse oximetry and patient monitoring.
5. A patient who has been given a general anesthesia should never be left unattended until fully recovered. The patient's oxygenation, ventilation, and circulation must be continually evaluated and documented to include, but not be limited to:
   a. Oxygenation – the patient's color
   b. Ventilation – respiratory rate, rhythm; the use of pulse oximeters is strongly recommended
   c. Circulation – the continuous use of EKG; BP monitoring should be continuous; an IV line should be in place at all times for emergency medications and replacement of body fluids
6. The following equipment and supplies in the surgery and recovery areas should include, but not be limited to:
   a. Oxygen
   b. Ambu-bag/mask system
   c. Intravenous equipment and fluids
   d. Crash cart with defibrillator
   e. Automatic blood pressure monitor
   f. Pulse oximeter
   g. EKG monitor

**Note:** All of these monitors plus the various anesthesia gases are required to be incorporated into the anesthesia cart that is present in a fully licensed ambulatory surgical center or hospital OR.

**Special note:** As a chiropractic/osteopathic physician, it is your responsibility as the patient's doctor to know that proper procedures are being followed, and if you feel they are not being followed properly, it is your responsibility to inform the people who control the situation to protect the safety of your patient.

# Emergency Life Support

*Anthony Rogers*

The chiropractic physician involved in the MUA program is going to be part of an environment where they could be involved in a life support situation. Many chiropractors today are involved with sports medicine and, as such, are responsible for on-field injuries and are potentially caught in a situation where life support could be required; but on the average, most chiropractic physicians, although trained in CPR, are not called on to administer life support techniques.

CPR, as we know, stands for cardiopulmonary resuscitation. Although the patient undergoing MUA is under constant monitoring by the anesthesia department, the chiropractic/osteopathic physician needs to be aware of the status of his or her patient at all times.

The most important consideration with a patient who is under sedation is to maintain an airway, and to make sure that the airway is not compromised. The reason for the blood tests, EKG, and chest films prior to putting a patient to sleep is to assist the anesthesiologist in knowing whether the patient is a candidate for anesthesia. Even then, the body can have an adverse response to the medication used and cause side effects that could cause the compromise of the patient's oxygen supply. Obviously when this happens, the primary response is to stop any other procedures and give immediate care to restore the airway and oxygen supply. The brain has about 4 min of sustained oxygen life before damage occurs, so respiration and resuscitation must be started immediately should the patient stop breathing.

The anesthesiologist will respond to all of these problems and is highly trained to handle these situations. If an emergency were to arise it is recommended that life support techniques be left up to the operating room staff.

The following signs of oxygen/airway compromise should be observed:

1. Color — A blue or gray facial color indicates lack of oxygen.
2. Pupil dilation — With the use of brevitol, most times the eyes are open, and pupils that are fixed and dilated indicate oxygen deprivation.
3. Nail beds turning blue — Indicates loss of oxygen supply.
4. Muscle rigidity — Onstead of muscular relaxation, indicates lack of oxygen getting to the muscles from blood source.

# Manipulation Under Joint Anesthesia/Analgesia (MUJA)

*Robert C. Gordon*

This textbook would not be complete if the secondary field of MUJA were not mentioned. This is a field that is somewhat of an offshoot of the MUA procedure. Those who practice MUJA exclusively, however, would probably argue that MUA is an offshoot of MUJA.

MUJA is a procedure that incorporates manual therapy with injection of the joint(s). It has been successfully used for many years as an adjunct to synovial joint dysfunction when there is biomechanical articular dyskinesia with accompanying pain. Rather than the manual therapist trying to force an articulation through a fixed range of motion, they refer the patient out first for an injection of an anti-inflammatory, usually a corticosteroid, with an analgesic and then an adjustive procedure is completed. This method has been found to be successful in helping to complete the specific adjustive maneuver.

Over the years this form of treatment has evolved into an office-based procedure in some cases and in other cases the patient has been treated at an ambulatory surgical center. The choice of treatment area for the procedure is also one of the controversies surrounding MUJA. Is it an office-based procedure, or should it be performed in a facility where life support is readily available?

If we use the methods that are being used more frequently today with this procedure, the MUJA procedure should be performed in an ambulatory surgical center or a procedure room in a hospital. If the procedure is performed as an office-based procedure, then it has to be performed in a multidisciplinary facility. This is not a procedure that can be performed in a chiropractic office. This procedure has to include the use of an injection into the joint, and, under the umbrella of the chiropractic office, this procedure falls outside the scope of practice even if a D.O. or an M.D. comes into that chiropractic office and performs the procedure. This regulation is well recognized by state chiropractic boards. If a chiropractic physician desires to incorporate MUJA into their practice, the procedure must be completed in an office that is not part of the regular chiropractic office or in a facility such as an ambulatory surgical center or hospital procedure room. The use of monitored anesthesia care and stretching as an adjunct to the injection and then incorporating the adjustive procedure adds MUA to the equation. If a local injection is done in a pain practice, the patient is then referred out for an adjustment.

It is this author's experience that the addition of monitored anesthesia care, such as using versed and propofol with the injection and the fibrosis release procedure followed by the adjustive procedure or MUA, is what is changing the old MUJA approach and actually making the outcomes better.

Several years have past since Dreyfuss et al.[6] first presented the clinical presentation of MUJA that has been referenced by many as a source for justifying the use of injection and adjustive or manual therapy. Although the concept has been adhered to by many, the protocols for the direction this procedure has taken have been enhanced considerably with the newer approaches that we are using with the MUA procedure being performed today. Dreyfuss et al.[6] were concerned with the use of a "general anesthesia," which at the time of their presentation was used with the MUA technique. We no longer place the patient in a position where the end range and painful ranges are beyond response. Controversies still exist as to what level of sedation/anesthesia should be used with the MUA technique, but the general consensus of patient safety and response remains the goal of the newer forms of MUA.

Our concept of MUJA today is the use of an injection as a part of the total MUA procedure. While it is agreed that MUJA remains one of the most logical and definitive methods of identifying pain of synovial origin, the combination of using progressive fibrosis release technique (stretching) procedures as an adjunct to the injection of the joint is more appropriate and has been shown to have a greater impact on patient response to the articular movement. Because of this we are incorporating this technique into the MUA field by adding the injection sequence to a serial MUA if the case calls for the injection. Our experience today with MUJA has not changed much from the types of cases that were presented by Dreyfuss and his colleagues. Sacroiliac problems, facet injections, and discogenic corticosteroid injections are still the stalwarts of the MUJA procedure. However, adding this to a serial MUA procedure has in recent years been shown to be a better approach, but it certainly has not eliminated the results of the injection with properly selected cases of MUJA. Certainly, there is a great deal of room for continued research into what constitutes the best cases for MUJA and which are better for simply using MUA, but the overall impression from cases being completed today with the suggested combination of procedures is that there is definitely room for using both modalities either separately or in conjunction with each other. Cases completed using MUA as the primary modality that were responding at a slower rate than anticipated have been noticeably improved with the addition of the injection. Cases such as saroiliac dysfunction and disc cases seem to be the most prominent that this author has seen used. Facet blocks and other synovial joint injections have also been used successfully with MUA. The outcome has been related to a form of diffusion of the medication when used in combination with the fibrosis release procedures that are used with MUA.

This author feels that there is definitely a place for the use of MUA and MUJA. At present, there are several clinical trials being completed that will hopefully give us definitive answers as to which procedure is better for a particular condition. As with all procedures that have shown improvement in patient outcomes, as these two procedures have, continued investigation is needed. Until all of that research is completed, however, there is documented evidence that the use of MUJA has validity and, in conjunction with MUA, has been very effective in relieving patient pain from prominent synovial joint articular dysfunction and dyskinesia.

## REFERENCES


1. Morey, L.W., Manipulation under general anesthesia, *Osteopathic Annals,* 127–35, March 1975.
2. Siehl, D., Manipulation of the spine under general anesthesia, *J. Am. Osteopath.,* vol. 62, 35–39, June 1963.
3. Hill, D.K., Tension due to interaction between the sliding filaments in resting striated muscle. The effect of stimulation, *J. Physiol.,* 199: 637–55, 1968.
4. Malseed, R.T., Pharmacology, drug therapy and nursing considerations, intravenous agents used in anesthesia, Library of Congress, 109–18, 1982.
5. U.S. Pharmacology Directory for Physicians, Anesthetics, Barbiturates, 243 –47, 1991.
6. Dreyfuss, M, Michaelsen, M., Horne, M., Manipulation under joint anesthesia/analgesia: A treatment approach for recalcitrant low back pain of synovial origin, *J Manipulative Physiol. Thera.,* vol. 8, Oct. 1995.
7. Frymayer, J., *The Adult Spine, Vol. 1.* Hagerstown, MD: Lippincott, Williams & Wilkins, 2003.

# 11 Preanesthesia Evaluation

*Ramona Carter*

## CONTENTS



## INTRODUCTION

Preanesthesia evaluation can be defined as the clinical assessment of the patient prior to the delivery of anesthesia for the purpose of identifying pertinent information to guide anesthesia plans as well as minimize anesthesia risks and adverse outcomes. This evaluation applies to anesthesia delivered for both surgical and nonsurgical procedures. The intent of this chapter is to familiarize the reader with common practice parameters of the preanesthesia evaluation. Recommendations are based on literature review, consensus opinions, and expert proposals and should not be interpreted as "standards of care" or "clinical practice guidelines" as there are insufficient data or evidence-based studies to support this interpretation.

## LEVELS OF ANESTHESIA

Anesthesia is categorized into four levels dependent on depth of sedation achieved. They are as follows: (1) minimal sedation (anxiolysis), (2) moderate sedation/analgesia (conscious sedation), (3) deep sedation/analgesia, and (4) general anesthesia. Spinal manipulation under analgesia (MUA)

**TABLE 11.1**
**Contrasting Differences between Minimal and Moderate Sedation Used in MUA**

|  | Minimal Sedation | Moderate Sedation |
| --- | --- | --- |
| Responsiveness of patient | Normal verbal responses | Purposeful responses to verbal or tactile stimuli* |
| Airway status | Unaffected | No intervention required |
| Spontaneous ventilation | Unaffected | May be affected but remains adequate |
| Cardiovascular function | Unaffected | Maintained |
| Cognitive function | May be impaired | Is usually impaired to some degree |

*Note that withdrawal reflex to painful stimulus is not considered a purposeful movement.

is performed typically at the level of moderate sedation. See Table 11.1 for a comparison of the differences between minimal and moderate sedation.

Anesthesia depth levels are a continuum and patients sometimes may respond inadvertently to the given analgesic resulting in a deeper level of sedation than solicited.[1] The provider should therefore be prepared to rescue a minimal or moderate sedation patient from deep sedation where spontaneous ventilation may be inadequate and airway intervention possibly required.

Minimal and moderate sedation is often performed in the office setting for minor outpatient procedures. Typically patients are generally healthy and at low risk of adverse outcomes. Patient expectations for a favorable anesthesia experience are very high, and poor outcomes are generally unexpected in this situation.[2,3] There have been concerns raised regarding the safety of office-based anesthesia, especially now that it is becoming a more common practice due to multiple financial influences and both provider and patient convenience.[4]

Risks for office-based anesthesia commonly measure outcomes affecting morbidity and mortality. Major complications include but are not limited to death, emergent intubation, ventilator requirement, surgical airway requirement, moderate to severe hypotension, cardiac events (including myocardial infarction or cardiac arrest), thromboembolic events, and pneumonia. Major adverse reactions are infrequent and usually predictable during the pre-anesthesia evaluation. Minor complications occur more frequently and, therefore, tend to cause the most patient distress. These minor adverse outcomes include protracted nausea and vomiting, dyspnea, anxiety and pain related to the planned procedure, and discomfort with intravenous (IV) insertion.[5,6]

Adverse outcome measurements have shown that there is still room for improvement in decreasing morbidity and mortality associated with office-based anesthesia. Frequently encountered problems include a lack of appropriate accreditation for the facility, substandard office equipment and maintenance, providers who are unfamiliar with dealing with rare emergency situations, a limited office pharmacy, a lack of emergency support and transport plans, inadequate patient monitoring, and insufficient patient evaluation prior to anesthesia.[4] The provider should consider these factors when determining the most appropriate location to deliver anesthesia and perform the selected procedure for any individual patient. The provider also needs to be familiar with current practice advisories where they exist, and be aware of any hospital, local health department, or state regulations concerning the delivery of anesthesia in their area of practice.[2]

The remainder of this chapter will focus on the constituents of an effective preanesthesia evaluation. As previously stated, the main purpose of the preanesthesia evaluation is to assess the patient's current medical status and minimize potential anesthesia risks accordingly. This begins with obtaining pertinent historical information, evaluating current health status and stability of medical conditions, and possibly uncovering unknown health problems. Standard practice suggestions recommend reviewing old medical records, collecting an accurate history and physical, reviewing prior anesthesia history, and determining the necessity for selected preprocedure labs and consults.[7,8]

---

**TABLE 11.2**
**Highlights from ASA Report on Practice Advisory for Preanesthesia Evaluation[8]**

1. Determine ASA classification, ASA 3 and 4 warrant complete evaluation and consultation with anesthesiologist.
2. Assess medical condition determined by history, physical, and labs.
3. History should be current, <30 days, and reassess on day of procedure.
4. Perform selected labs based on medical condition.
5. List specific factors to consider when assessing risk of complications and need for consultations.

---

## TIMING OF EVALUATION

The evaluation should be performed far enough in advance of the procedure to allow for interventions if necessary. Accreditation agency standards require the evaluation to be performed within 30 days of the procedure and that the patient be reassessed with documentation noting any changes of medical status on the day of the procedure.[7] This evaluation does not have to be performed by the provider delivering the anesthesia.

Anesthesia plans are most frequently changed for the following conditions: gastroesophageal reflux, insulin requiring diabetes mellitus, asthma, heart disease, or suspected difficult intubation.[9] Optimally treating chronic medical problems prior to anesthesia minimizes risk and leads to better outcomes.

## REASONS FOR SCREENING

The preanesthesia evaluation provides the opportunity to choose anesthesia plans with the patient. Discussions on patient education, developing anesthesia expectations, and obtaining informed consent are commonly done at this time. This enables the provider to achieve more efficiency in patient care, and creates higher levels of patient satisfaction with the service provided.

In summary, effective practices quantify risks of anesthesia to the patient and minimize this risk through preprocedure treatment when possible. The main determinants of anesthesia risk arise from the patient's medical status, procedure planned, and anesthesia utilized. For procedures of low invasiveness in a patient with low severity of disease, the evaluation can be performed before or on the day of the procedure. Otherwise, if a patient has more significant severity of disease or an invasive procedure is planned, the evaluation should be performed in advance, allowing enough time to evaluate potential risk factors. See Table 11.2 for selected highlights of suggested preanesthesia evaluation practices reported in detail in the Practice Advisory for Preanesthesia Evaluation, American Society of Anesthesia Report.[8]

## MEDICAL EVALUATION

The medical history is perhaps the most critical portion of the preanesthesia evaluation. It will direct the priorities in the following sections on the physical exam and preprocedure lab studies. The medical status and degree of stability of the patient is usually determined by the questions asked here. The medical history typically reviews elements regarding current medical illnesses, prior hospitalizations and surgeries, medications used and any known drug allergies, pregnancy risk, and history of tobacco, alcohol, or substance use. Specifically, the medical history should search for history pertaining to cardiovascular, pulmonary, hepatic, or renal disease, bleeding disorders, and musculoskeletal or neurological problems.

The most important anesthesia risk related to the patient's history is related to cardiopulmonary status.[7] Cardiovascular conditions such as angina, coronary artery disease, myocardial infarction, symptomatic arrythmias, uncontrolled hypertension, or congestive heart failure may warrant further preanesthesia testing before the procedure. Representative questions to assess the patient for cardiovascular disease include: Have you ever had a heart attack? Do you have a heart murmur? Do you become short of breath after walking? Do you have chest pains or a skipped heartbeat? Do your ankles swell? Have you been told to take antibiotics prior to routine dental work? Have you fainted recently? Has your blood pressure been elevated in the past year or are you being treated for high blood pressure? Similarly, respiratory conditions including asthma or chronic obstructive pulmonary disease, history of airway surgery, upper or lower airway tumor, oxygen usage at home, or history of respiratory distress will warrant a review to consider whether further testing prior to anesthesia is needed. Questions to ascertain presence of potential respiratory problems are suggested as follows: Have you been hoarse for more than one month? Do you snore? Have you ever had pneumonia? Do you have difficulty breathing? Wheezing? Chronic cough? Have you been told you have emphysema? Asthma? Have you ever smoked? If a patient has a history of significant lung disease, he or she should be specifically asked about prior need for intubation, and any recent exacerbations of the disease. This is also an excellent opportunity to discuss smoking cessation prior to anesthesia with the patient. Patients should be counseled to stop smoking 4–8 weeks prior to anesthesia. The usage of dental appliances could interfere with airway management, and patients should be specifically asked about dentures, partial plates, bridges, or crowns.

## PRIOR ANESTHESIA HISTORY

The preanesthesia history differs from the typical medical history in a few key areas that are designed to specifically assess anesthesia risk. History regarding prior anesthesia experiences and complications should be documented. Family history should query the patient for anesthesia experiences in close relatives including thrombotic, hemorrhagic, or hyperthermia complications. These findings could suggest clotting disorders or malignant hyperthermia syndrome (MHS). Family history of delayed recovery from paralysis under anesthesia can be secondary to hereditary pseudocholinesterase deficiency.[7]

Assessment of psychological and support systems may be investigated if there are anticipated assistance needs for recovery after the planned procedure. Assessment of functional status and exercise tolerance may reveal that a patient has a low level of activity. Symptoms of serious illness such as claudication/angina/dyspnea are commonly absent in these patients, limiting the examiner's ability to detect certain associated illnesses that could pose serious anesthesia risk. A medical history must be documented prior to anesthesia unless performed in an emergency situation.

A summary of recommended preanesthesia history components is listed in Table 11.3.[7–11]

Many medications have possible interactions with anesthetic agents or side effects that could have a negative effect during anesthesia. The anesthesia provider needs to review the patient's medications prior to the procedure, allowing enough time to discontinue medications with potential risk. Pharmacologic agents that are commonly used for MUA with moderate sedation include opiods, benzodiazepenes, barbiturates, and miscellaneous drugs such as chloral hydrate, propofol,

---

**TABLE 11.3**
**Medical History to Be Documented Prior to Anesthesia**

1. Previous medical illnesses
2. Previous surgical procedures
3. Medication history and drug allergies
4. Previous anesthesia experiences and complications
5. History of alcohol, tobacco, or substance abuse
6. Family history of anesthesia problems

---

**TABLE 11.4**
**Herbal Supplements that May Affect Anesthesia (list is limited review only)**

| Herb Supplement | Used For | Potential Anesthesia Risk |
| --- | --- | --- |
| Ephedra/Ma Huang | Appetite suppressant | Elevations in blood pressure or heart rate |
| Feverfew | Migraines, arthritis | May increase bleeding |
| Garlic | Lowering cholesterol | May increase bleeding |
| Ginger | Nausea, vomiting | May increase bleeding |
| Gingko biloba | Improving memory and circulation | May increase bleeding |
| Ginseng | Improve energy and concentration | May increase bleeding |
| St John's Wort | Depression or anxiety | May prolong anesthesia effects |
| Valerian | Sleep aid | May prolong anesthesia effects |
| Vitamin E | Slow aging, antioxidant | May increase bleeding |

and ketamine. The anesthetic drugs are all potentiated by sedatives/CNS central nervous system depressants, and caution should be used to prevent oversedation and the concurrent risk of respiratory depression and apnea. Barbiturates, benzodiazepenes, opiods, tricyclic antidepressants, antihistamines, and phenothiazines are common CNS depressants, and dose reduction of anesthetic should be considered in patients taking these medications. Debilitated and elderly patients are also more sensitive to the effect of anesthetics. Propofol is contraindicated in patients with egg or soybean oil allergy.

On the other hand, some medications are useful to continue and are beneficial to reduce anesthesia-related complications. Treatment with inhaled bronchodilators, certain antiarrythmics, antiepileptics, specific antihypertensives, and medications used for the treatment of gastroesophageal reflux, H2 blockers, and proton pump inhibitors reduce risks associated with the disease that they were prescribed for, and patients are usually advised to continue taking them on the day of anesthesia.[7]

The medication history should be sure to include herb, vitamin, and nutritional supplement usage. Many of these natural medications have serious drug interactions that could increase anesthesia risk. The patient will need to be educated regarding this and purposefully questioned regarding usage as patients frequently omit this information for various reasons, including concern of giving a negative impression to the medical provider, and belief that these supplements are natural and therefore "safe." Table 11.4 lists common supplements, indications for use, and potential side effect or interaction.[12–14]

## PHYSICAL EXAM

Following the history-taking part of the evaluation, the examiner usually performs the physical exam. A minimal physical exam as determined by the American Society of Anesthesiology (ASA) task force will include documentation of vital signs/blood pressure, airway assessment, pulmonary exam with auscultation of the lungs, and cardiovascular exam.[11] The physical exam is expanded to include further assessment as directed by the medical history. Additional physical exam findings to look for are skin exam to evaluate for jaundice, cyanosis, easy bruising; extremities for presence of edema; nervous system exam to discern neurological impairments; and musculoskeletal exam, particularly to assess head and neck mobility for limitations that could affect airway management.[7,11,15,16]

The airway assessment is a unique part of the preanesthesia exam. The goal is to identify patients at risk for having a difficult airway. This assessment is derived from the medical history such as previous problems with difficult airway during procedures, stridor, snoring, sleep apnea, and history of deforming rheumatoid arthritis. The physical exam should note marked obesity, facial malformations, small mouth opening, or short neck.[10,17,18] If there are findings that cause the examiner to be concerned about potential airway problems, plans regarding location of where the procedure will be performed and available emergency access should be reviewed.

## ASA CLASSIFICATION

The history and physical exam are used to determine the ASA physical status classification. Each patient should be given the proper ASA classification as part of the routine pre-procedure screening.[10] It gives the practitioners a common language in referring to the severity of systemic disease in various patients. Patients who are classified as a ASA-3 level or higher will generally need a consult with their primary physician prior to moderate levels of sedation. It should be understood that the classification is not a risk assessment system.

### ASA Physical Status Classification[10]

ASA-1 — A normal, healthy patient

ASA-2 — A patient with mild systemic disease that results in no functional limitations. Examples: controlled hypertension, diabetes mellitus, chronic bronchitis, obesity.

ASA-3 — A patient with severe systemic disease that results in functional limitation. Examples: poorly controlled diabetes with vascular complications, angina pectoris, prior myocardial infarction, pulmonary disease that limits activity.

ASA-4 — A patient with severe systemic disease that is a constant threat to life. Examples: unstable angina pectoris, advance pulmonary, renal or hepatic dysfunction.

ASA-5 — A moribund patient who is not expected to survive without the operation. Examples: ruptured abdominal aortic aneurysm, pulmonary embolus, head injury with increased intracranial pressure.

ASA-6 — A declared brain-dead patient whose organs are being removed for donation.

E (emergency operation) — Any patient for whom an emergency operation is required.

## DIAGNOSTIC TESTING

The final information-gathering step in the preanesthesia evaluation is reviewing available lab data and determining need for further lab studies. Many articles have been published in recent years debating the issue of routine preanesthesia/preprocedure lab studies, and there is an overall consensus that it is not a valuable tool.[15,19–22] Traditionally, routine preoperative lab tests were ordered for the following reasons: (1) to detect unsuspected abnormalities that might influence anesthesia risk, (2) to establish baseline labs that may need further monitoring after the procedure, and (3) for medico legal reasons. These rationales have been deemed invalid in the literature and the practice highly discouraged.[22]

Laboratory studies should be viewed as a supplement to the history and physical, which is the most effective way to screen for disease. Lab studies are overall not useful in screening asymptomatic patients for disease unless disease is suspected due to findings on the history and physical.[8,15,19] Where they are of the most value is in evaluating current medical illnesses, detecting unknown progression of disease state, optimizing the patient's condition, and confirming suspected diagnoses.

The reasons not to order routine preanesthesia lab studies are more compelling. It is estimated that the examiner ignores approximately 30%–60% of abnormal lab test results done routinely for screening in asymptomatic patients.[21] Additionally, there is a lack of documentation to support the provider's reasoning on the decision not to pursue an abnormal test finding with follow-up studies. Failure to pursue abnormal findings and concurrent lack of documentation to support this is a common practice, which can unfortunately increase medicolegal risk. When considering pursuing an abnormal test, the health-care provider needs to determine the harm/benefit ratio of follow-up testing. False positive test results create significant anxiety and can lead to harmful or invasive procedures that are not otherwise indicated. The unnecessary cost to society has negative implications as well. In this era of diminishing medical resources and increasing patient need, the cost of performing unindicated tests results in further depleting resources and creating additional medical cost, thereby reducing available resources to provide care for others. In conclusion, the rationale not to order routine preoperative testing is based on the fact that abnormal tests usually do not influence anesthesia management plans, providers commonly ignore abnormal tests in asymptomatic patients, and nonselective testing incurs significant cost with minimal benefit to the patient.[15,20,21,22]

Laboratory tests should be obtained when they meet the following requirements: the result will represent a significant health risk that can be modified by preanesthesia treatment, the condition being tested for cannot be determined adequately by appropriate history and physical exam, and the disease has a level of prevalence with a sufficiently sensitive and specific test to have a likelihood ratio warranting follow-up studies if an abnormality is found.[8] Labs to consider selectively for preanesthesia evaluation include but are not limited to hemoglobin/hematocrit, platelets, serum chemistries, renal function tests, liver function tests, coagulation studies, urinalysis, pregnancy test, chest x-ray, and electrocardiogram. Specialized studies to assess cardiac disease such as stress testing or respiratory function through spirometry of pulmonary function tests frequently require consultation with a specialist to determine anesthesia risks.

Next we list specified lab tests and common indications for testing.[8,9,15,16,22,23]

## HEMOGLOBIN/HEMATOCRIT

This test is recommended when the planned procedure is likely to involve significant blood loss (e.g., vascular procedures). Consider if the patient has a medical history of anemia or conditions frequently associated with anemia: myeloproliferative disease, cancer, renal disease, abnormal bleeding, or anticoagulant usage. It is also recommended if the physical exam suggests anemia with findings of pallor or resting tachycardia.

## PLATELETS

This test is recommended when the planned procedure is likely to involve significant blood loss (e.g., vascular procedures). Consider if the patient has a medical history of thrombocytopenia, recent exposure to drugs known to decrease platelets, or conditions associated with thrombocytopenia (myeloproliferative disease, cancer, abnormal bleeding, easy bruising) or is taking anticoagulants.

## COAGULATION STUDIES, PT/PTT/INR

These tests are not ordered routinely because, even when they are abnormal, they are not good predictors of post-operative hemorrhage. They are ordered typically if the planned procedure is likely to involve significant blood loss (e.g., vascular procedures). Consider these tests if the patient has a medical history of abnormal bleeding, chronic liver disease, malnutrition, or chronic antibiotic usage causing clotting factor deficiency, or is taking anticoagulants.

## BLOOD UREA NITROGEN (BUN)/CREATININE (CR)

Consider these tests in patients with a medical history of renal disease or a high likelihood of renal disease: age >64 years, diabetes mellitus, liver disease, cardiovascular disease, hypertension. Medications that are excreted by kidneys can result in abnormalities as well. Common culprits include diuretics, nonsteroidal antiinflammatories, ace inhibitors, and digoxin.

## LIVER FUNCTION TESTS (LFTs)

Consider performing these tests in patients with a medical history of liver disease, hepatitis/jaundice, alcohol abuse, bleeding/bruising abnormalities, or history of vomiting blood (hematemesis/coffee ground emesis). Routine screening not recommended as elevations of LFTs without symptoms do not usually influence management. Of note, low levels of serum albumin are known to be associated with adverse perioperative outcomes in major surgery; unfortunately, there is no effective treatment for this.

## CHEST X-RAY (CXR)

CXRs are routinely done if the procedure planned is invasive of the thorax. Consider testing if the patient has symptoms of a pulmonary infection, is at high risk of tuberculosis, or has a history of cardiovascular disease, pulmonary disease (also consider pulmonary function tests), or cancer. If the trachea is abnormal on physical exam, a CXR should be done to further evaluate the anatomy for risk assessment of airway compromise.

## ELECTROCARDIOGRAM (EKG) IN NONCARDIAC SURGERY ASSESSMENT

EKGs should be obtained in patients with symptoms of chest pain, palpitations, shortness of breath, or congestive heart failure (uncompensated). Also consider if the patient is over 50 years of age or has a medical history of hypertension, diabetes, cardiovascular disease, or tobacco use. A history of myocardial infarction, angina, congestive heart failure, diabetes mellitus, or findings of Q-waves on an EKG are common indications for cardiac stress testing.[24,25]

It is interesting to note that either an abnormal BUN/Cr or H/H is more likely to identify patients at risk for adverse post-procedural outcomes when compared to other tests. However, the CXR and EKG are the most likely tests to have abnormal findings. It is prudent to not unnecessarily order these tests as it can result in further testing for evaluation of these abnormalities.[22]

The decision to order laboratory tests is also heavily influenced by the assessment of inherent procedural risk. This risk is typically indexed to one of the following categories:[20]

1. *Low-Risk Procedure* poses minimal physiologic stress and risk to the patient independent of medical condition.
2. *Moderate-Risk Procedure* poses moderate physiologic stress with risk of minimal blood loss, fluid shift, or post-op change in normal physiology.
3. *High-Risk Procedure* poses significant perioperative and post-operative physiologic stress.

It is usually not necessary to obtain most of these tests if the procedure planned is low risk and the patient will be under minimal/conscious sedation. This would be the typical scenario encountered in patients undergoing MUA.

## SUMMARY

The ultimate goal in performing a preanesthesia evaluation is to provide the examiner with the necessary tools to render an accurate interpretation of risk including both the patient's medical status and inherent procedural risks, to protect patients from undergoing anesthesia/procedures where risk outweighs benefit, and to minimize known risks whenever possible. Recall that the main determinants of anesthesia risk are the patient's medical status, procedure planned, and anesthesia utilized.

Medical status risk is optimally minimized by obtaining pertinent medical history, an adequate physical exam, and laboratory studies as indicated. The most critical medical risks of anesthesia are, in general, related to cardiopulmonary status. A review of known medical illnesses, previous surgical procedures, medication history, drug allergies, and alcohol, tobacco, or substance abuse are common to most health-care providers. The preanesthesia history differs slightly from the typical medical history as it includes prior anesthesia experiences and complications. Essential physical exam components to be documented include vital signs/blood pressure, pulmonary exam, cardiovascular exam, and limitations that could affect airway management.[8] The medical history and physical exam are reviewed in conjunction to assign the patient an overall medical status as outlined in the ASA classification system.[10] The value of this tool is in guiding the provider in determining when preprocedural consultation with the patient's primary care provider or specialist should be considered and acknowledging that ASA classification should not be used to assign risk.

In summary, MUA should typically be considered a low-risk procedure when performed under minimal/conscious sedation. Risk is further minimized if the patient is in ASA classification ASA-1 or ASA-2, denoting healthy or mild chronic stable disease state. Providers of MUA should be readily able to recognize most predisposing health factors that could increase this risk by performing a thoughtful and attentive preanesthesia evaluation.

## REFERENCES


1. Green, S.M., Krauss, B. Procedural sedation terminology: Moving beyond "conscious sedation," *Ann. Emerg. Med.*, vol. 39 (4), 2002.
2. Twersky, R.S., Springman, S, Philip, B.K., Considerations for anesthesiologists in setting up and maintaining a safe office anesthesia environment, *Office-Based Anesthesia*, 2000.
3. Iverson, R.E., Sedation and analgesia in ambulatory settings, *Plast. Reconstr. Surg.*, vol. 104 (5), 1559–64, 1999.
4. Arens, J.F., Anesthesia for office-based surgery: are we paying too high a price for access and convenience? *Mayo Clin. Proc.*, vol. 75 (3), 225–28, 2000.
5. Bitar, G. et al., Safety and efficacy of office-based surgery with monitored anesthesia care/sedation in 4778 consecutive plastic surgery procedures, *Plastic Reconstruct. Surg.*, vol. 111 (1), 150–56, 2003.
6. Kopp, V.J., Preoperative preparation, value, perspective and practice in patient care, *Anesthesiol. Clin. North Am.*, vol. 18 (3), 2000.
7. Litaker, D., Preoperative screening, *Medical Clinics of North America*, vol. 83 (6), 1999.
8. Pasternak, L.R. et al., Practice advisory for preanesthesia evaluation, *Anesthesiology*, vol. 96 (2), 2002.
9. Roizen, M.F., Foss, J.F., Fischer, S.P., Preoperative Evaluation, in Miller, R.D., Ed. *Anesthesia*, vol. 1, 4th ed., New York: Churchill Livingstone, 827–82, chap. 23, 1994.
10. Smart, T., Sedation and Analgesia Training Module, available online at http://www.sedationtraining.com.
11. Gross, J.B. et al., Practice guidelines for sedation and analgesia by non-anesthesiologists, *Anesthesiology*, vol. 96 (4), 1004–17, 2002.
12. American Society of Anesthesiologists: What you should know about your patients' use of herbal medicines and other dietary supplements, available online at http://www.ASAhq.org.
13. Ang-Lee, M.K., Moss, J., Yuan, C.S., Herbal medicines and perioperative care, *J. Am. Med. Assoc.*, vol. 286, 208–16, 2001.
14. O'Hara, M.A., Kiefer, D., Farrell, K. et al., A review of 12 commonly used medicinal herbs, *Arch. Fam. Med.*, vol. 7, 523–36, 1998.
15. King, M.S., Preoperative evaluation, *Am. Fam. Phys.*, 2000.
16. Roizen, M.F., Anesthetic implications of concurrent diseases, in Miller, R.D., Ed., *Anesthesia* 903–1015, chap. 25, 1994.
17. Mallampati, S.R., Gatt, S.P., Gugino, L.D. et al, A clinical sign to predict difficult tracheal intubation: a prospective study, *Can. Anesth. Soc. J.*, vol. 32, 429, 1985.
18. Samsoon, G.L.T. and Young, J.R.B., Difficult tracheal intubation: a retrospective study, *Anesthesia*, vol. 42, 487, 1987.
19. Roizen, M.F., Kaplan, E.B., Schreider, B.D., Lichtor, L.J., and Orkin, F.K., The relative roles of the history and physical examination, and the laboratory testing in preoperative evaluation for outpatient surgery: the "Starling" curve of preoperative laboratory testing, *Anesthesiol. Clin. North Am.*, vol. 5, 15–34, 1987.
20. Pasternak, L.R., Preoperative screening for ambulatory patients, *Anesthesiol. Clin. North Am.*, vol. 21 (2), 2003.

21. Roizen, M.F., More preoperative assessment by physicians and less by laboratory tests, *N. Engl. J. Med.*, vol. 342 (3), 204–5, 2000.

22. Smetana, G.W., Macpherson, D.S., The case against routine preoperative laboratory testing, *Med. Clin. North Am.*, vol. 87 (1), 2003.

23. Kaplan, E.B., Sheiner L.B., Boeckmann, A.J., Roizen, M.F. et al., The usefulness of preoperative laboratory screening, *J. Am. Med. Assoc.,* vol. 253, 3576–81, 1985.

24. Karnath, B.M., Preoperative cardiac risk assessment, *Am. Fam. Phys.*, 2002.

25. Schroeder, B.M., Updated guidelines for perioperative cardiovascular evaluation for noncardiac surgery, *Am. Fam. Phys.*, 2002.

# 12 MUA Procedure Protocol

*Robert C. Gordon*

## CONTENTS



"No amount of experience in the office will qualify a physician for manipulation of the patient under a general anesthetic. No hospital should permit the physician to perform such manipulation until he has been observed and has received supervision and the approval of an experienced operator who himself has been previously approved by certification and hospital proficiency standards." [1]

The procedure for manipulation under anesthesia has been divided into three important phases: the pre-op testing proper patient selection and medical clearance examination, the actual technique itself, and the follow-up care.

The patient will go for pre-op testing and medical clearance, and the anesthesiologist will see the patient 2 or 3 days prior to the procedure to certify that the patient is okay to be anesthetized. The anesthesia clearance is sometimes completed on the same day as the procedure.

On the day the MUA is performed for the first time, the patient will be required to arrive an hour or so early to fill out the proper paperwork.

"The number of MUAs and frequency will be left up to the primary practitioner's discretion, based on the severity of the condition and the patient response. It is possible that the patient will require multiple MUA procedures in order to accomplish maximal results." [2,3,4]

Following the MUA, and after the patient has been discharged, it is recommended that the patient receive physical therapy. This should include interferential therapy or electrical stimulation, as well as cryotherapy. Gentle range of motion (ROM) stretching is also recommended. Physical therapy would be the same if more than one MUA were required. The patient would then be seen for 7–10 days following the final MUA to prevent the remodeling of the collagen adhesions (see Chapter 2). This is then followed by the prescribed rehabilitation program (see Chapter 13).

## TRACTION STRETCHING WITH MUA

Traction stretching is an integral part of the cervical, thoracic, lumbar, and pelvic adjustive techniques when the patient is under anesthesia. When the patient is in the relaxed state of twilight sedation, the muscles that support the spinal areas of involvement can be tractioned into full elongation. A muscle that has been traumatized becomes inflamed. In the case of the muscle, fibro-adhesions will be laid down in a matrix between the muscle fibrils. This abnormal fibrous tissue causes the muscle to stay shortened in length. Since the muscle is also probably not used properly, the length of the muscle is also affected by disuse.

Guyton speaks of the muscle fibrils as being made up of filaments called actin and myosin, which are capable of sliding inward and outward in an interlocking mechanism as the muscle lengthens and shortens.[5,6] When there is disuse of a muscle from either immobilization, muscle splinting, or contracture, the muscle does not have its full capacity to contract and relax.[7]

Since muscle is connected to bone even though layered, a joint that is inflamed and immobile will have a shortened muscle because the muscle is not able to elongate during normal movement. Fibro-adhesions form in these areas of disuse as a protective mechanism for the purpose of preventing tears should the patient move quickly and abnormally lengthen a muscle that has been in a contracted state for prolonged periods of time.[5,7,8,9]

When stretching techniques are used prior to adjusting the anesthetized patient, the adhesions are altered in the muscle fibrils and we are attempting to elongate the muscle. In this way, the joint can be taken to its full range so that the adhesions in the joint and joint capsules are also capable of being altered. If the stretching technique was not done, the muscle fibril would be forced to work in a shortened state, causing the joint to be restricted and remain only slightly movable during adjustment. Multiple MUAs are necessary before joint adhesions are altered.

There are multiple mechanical functions required for spinal movement just as there are multiple impulses that create these movements. If the MUA is to benefit the patient, many of the adhesions that have formed in the muscles, joints, and joint capsules must be altered so that normal movement is allowed to return.

## STRESS–STRAIN CURVE

1. **Elastic range:** Initially the strain is directly proportional to the ability of the material to resist the force. The tissue returns to its original size and shape when the load is released.
2. **Elastic limit:** The point beyond which the tissue will not return to its original shape and size.
3. **Plastic range:** The range beyond the elastic limit extending to the point of rupture. Tissue strained within this range will be permanently deformed.
4. **Yield strength:** The load beyond the elastic limit that produces permanent deformation within the tissue. Once the yield point is reached, there is sequential failure of the tissue with permanent deformation (remodeling), and the tissue passes into the plastic range of the stress–strain curve. The deformation may be from a single load or the summation of several subcritical loads.[10]
5. **Ultimate strength:** The greatest load the tissue can sustain. Once the maximum load is reached, there is increased strain (deformation) without an increase in stress.
6. **Necking:** The region where there is considerable weakening of the tissue; less force is needed for deformation, and failure rapidly approaches.
7. **Breaking strength:** The load at the time the tissue fails.
8. **Failure:** Rupture of the integrity of the tissue.

Influences on the stress–strain curve include:

1. **Resilience:** The ability to absorb energy within the elastic range as work is accomplished. Energy is released when the load is removed and the tissue returns to its original shape.
2. **Toughness:** The ability to absorb energy within the plastic range without breaking (failing). If too much energy is absorbed with the stress, there will be a rupture. This is why linear (or continuous) force is used with MUA instead of a forceful ballistic stretch.

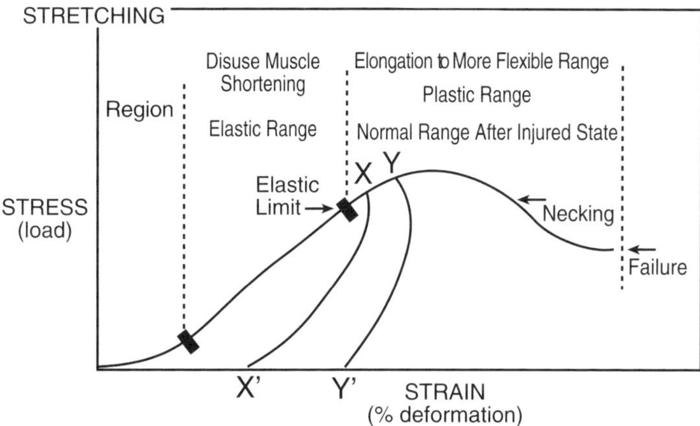


**Stress–Strain Curve**

3. **Creep:** When a load is applied for an extended period of time, the tissue elongates, resulting in permanent deformation. It is related to the viscosity of the tissue and is therefore time dependent. Deformation depends on the amount of force and the rate at which the force is applied. Creep occurs with low-magnitude load, usually in the elastic range, over a long period of time. The greater the load, the more rapid the rate of creep, but not in proportion to strain; therefore, a lesser load applied for a longer period of time will result in greater deformation. Increased temperature increases creep and therefore distensibility of the tissue.[7,10–12] During MUA the magnitude of the load is dependent on the practitioner's perception of the muscle tension. Continuous linear force stretching is used to overcome the Golgi tendon response to secondary muscle contraction, but it is also used to create a physiological change in the myofibril prior to muscle fiber damage. This stretch could be classified as being in the "disuse" plastic deformans range, and it is necessary to achieve this range with MUA so that permanent normal elongation of the muscle occurs.

4. **Structural stiffness:** Tissue with great stiffness will have a higher slope in the elastic region of the curve, indicating there is less elastic deformation with greater stress. Contractures and scar tissue have greater stiffness, probably due to a great degree of bonding between collagen fibers and their surrounding matrix.

5. **Heat production:** Energy is released as heat when stress is applied. It is depicted by the area under the curve (hysteresis loop) in the plastic range. As the tissue is heated, it more easily distends.

6. **Fatigue:** Cyclic loading of the tissue may cause failure below the yield point. The greater the applied load, the fewer number of cycles are needed for failure. A minimum load is required for this failure; below the minimum load an apparent infinite number of cycles will not cause failure. This is called the endurance limit. Examples of fatigue are stress fractures and overuse syndromes. Biologic tissue has the ability to repair itself after cyclic loading if the load is not too great and time is allowed before the cyclic loading is again applied. This is another reason why multiple or serial MUA procedures are recommended. By working in incremental stages the injured muscles and accompanying joint dysfunction can recover from the damage that stress and overexertion has caused. We hypothesize that we perform MUA in serial fashion to promote healing of injured tissue without causing additional stress to the muscle fibers, but we base this hypothesis on the above information, which is well recognized in the literature[10] (see Chapter 5).

## MUA TECHNIQUES

The adjustive technique used with manipulation under anesthesia is a specific diversified technique. The spinal motion unit is palpated and the specific spinal segment is localized. Full traction is accomplished to extend the elastic barrier, and a low velocity thrust is applied.

Conservative forces are generally applied in two areas:

A high-velocity, low-amplitude force (thrust) breaks up adhesions.
A low-velocity, high-amplitude force, passively taking a joint to its full range of motion, is
   particularly suited for stretching pariarticular tissue.

With MUA, when the vectors of force are applied discriminately and carefully, less force is required for the thrust to overcome restriction and produce normal motion. (See Chapter 5.)

## RESPONSIBILITIES OF THE FIRST ASSISTANT

The first assistant is a certified MUA physician with the same advanced manual therapy training as the primary practitioner. This procedure cannot be completed without a certified first assistant, and most facilities today will not allow MUA to be performed unless a certified first assistant is present for liability reasons. This has also been addressed by the National Academy of MUA Physicians and is part of the standards and protocols for MUA (see Chapter 7). The first assistant is responsible for

1. Assisting in the positioning of the patient to help with the manipulation/adjustment.
2. Assisting with stabilizing the patient so that certain stretching movements can be accomplished.
3. Assisting with the adjustment if assistance is necessary.
4. Helping monitor the patient's progress as the technique is being done.
5. Assisting with the movement of the patient to the gurney following the MUA procedure.
6. Helping ensure patient and practitioner safety.

Most malpractice carriers today recognize only a certified MUA practitioner as a first assistant since the first assistant must also be certified to perform MUA. It also becomes a liability issue for the facilities where MUA is performed if someone other than a certified MUA practitioner is performing any part of the MUA procedure. If an injury were to occur to a patient during the procedure and the facility were to become involved in litigation, having both the primary and the secondary providers certified in MUA would put the facility in a much better position to defend itself.

The National Academy of MUA Physicians addresses this issue in its standards and protocols under MUA safety and explains that, because the patient is in a semi-conscious state during the procedure it takes additional "assistance" to move the patient through the required positions for the procedure. According to the Academy: "The first assistant is responsible for helping the primary practitioner move the patient through the prescribed ranges of motion. The first assistant is present to insure that all movements are accomplished without injury to the patient or to the primary practitioner performing the procedure. As a result of the added weight of the patient in a semi-conscious state, there is a high risk of injury. A certified first assistant practitioner is the only safe way to perform this procedure. It is unsafe to perform an MUA without a certified first assistant."[4]

## THE MUA PROCEDURE

The patient is either taken to the procedure room by gurney or escorted by the nursing staff. The patient is asked to lie supine on the operating table, and the anesthesia monitors for the procedure are connected to the patient. When the anesthesiologist and the primary practitioner are ready, the procedure begins in the cervical spine. The procedure begins in the cervical spine because we have found over the years that the majority of anesthesiologists prefer for the cervical work to be completed so that an adequate airway is maintained throughout the whole procedure. Since the cervical area is most prominent for this purpose, most anesthesiologists prefer that the work in this area finishes first.

## THE CERVICAL SPINE

The patient is approached from the cephalad end of the table, and neutral axial cephalad traction is applied to the patient's cervical spine. Contact is at the base of the skull in the occipital area. The first assistant applies countertraction on the patient's shoulder while contacting the shoulders with an underhand grip bilaterally (Figure 12.1).

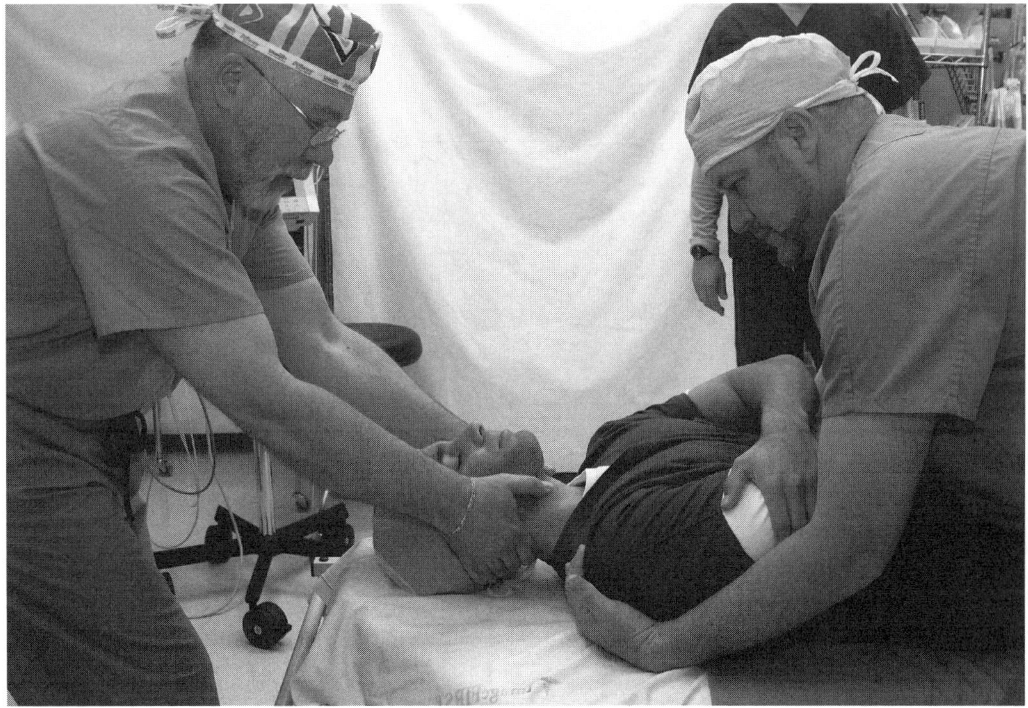

**FIGURE 12.1**

Goal: To achieve maximum end range and allow decompression of the discs and articulations.

Axial traction in the same manner is applied while taking the cervical spine into a lateral traction maneuver first to one side and then, maintaining traction, to the other (Figure 12.2 and Figure 12.3). The first assistant contacts the shoulders and continues countertraction as each side is tractioned by the primary practitioner.

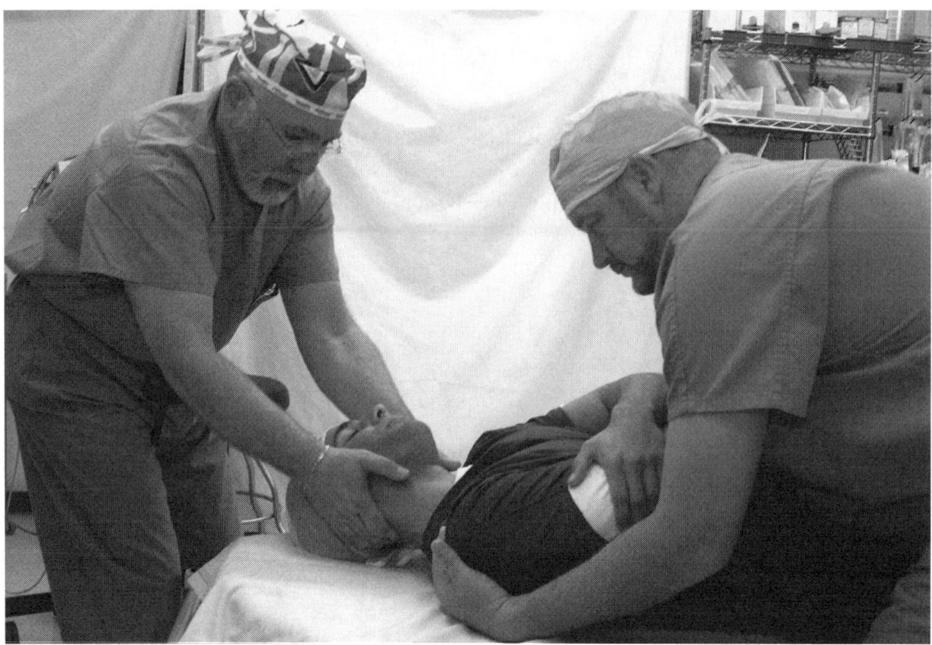

**FIGURE 12.2**

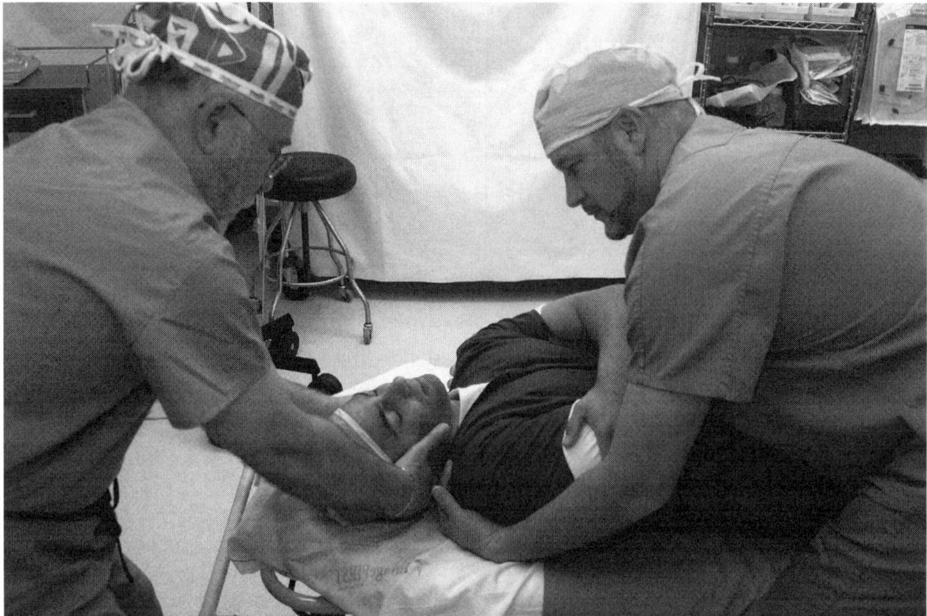

**FIGURE 12.3**

Goal: To achieve maximum end range and allow decompression of the discs and articulations.

Forward flexion is accomplished next by contacting the posterior skull and bringing the cervical spine forward into full available flexion (Figure 12.4). The first assistant is applying countertraction toward the table on the patient's shoulders as the forward traction is accomplished.

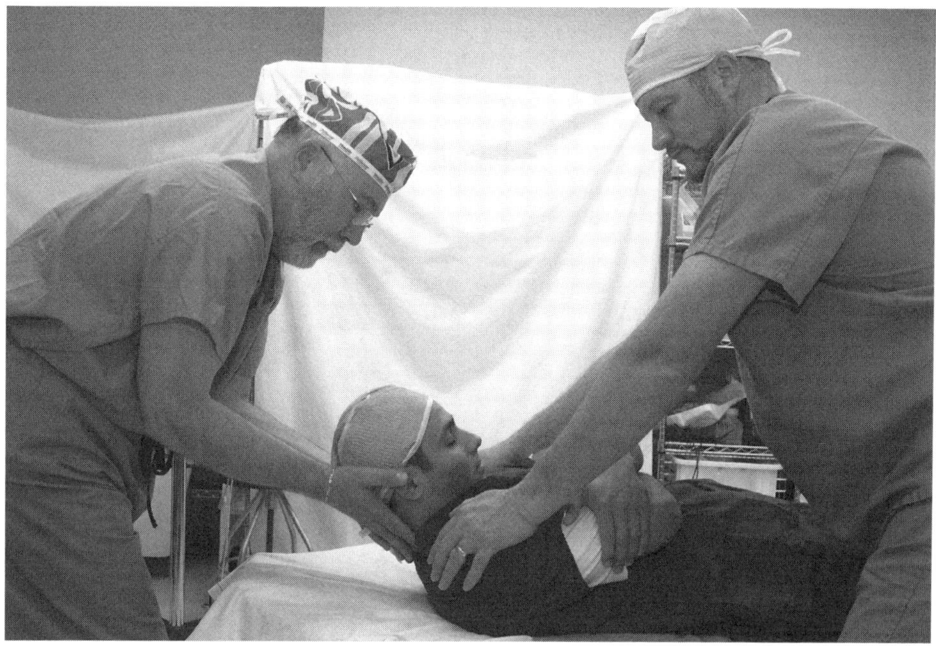

**FIGURE 12.4**

Goal: To achieve maximum end range.

The primary practitioner then crosses their arms under the patient's head and with the palms flat against the table tractions the patient's head into forward flexion (Figure 12.5). The palms are forced under the patient's shoulder to achieve maximum forward traction of the lower cervical spine and upper trapezius muscles. The first assistant countertractions the patient's shoulders.

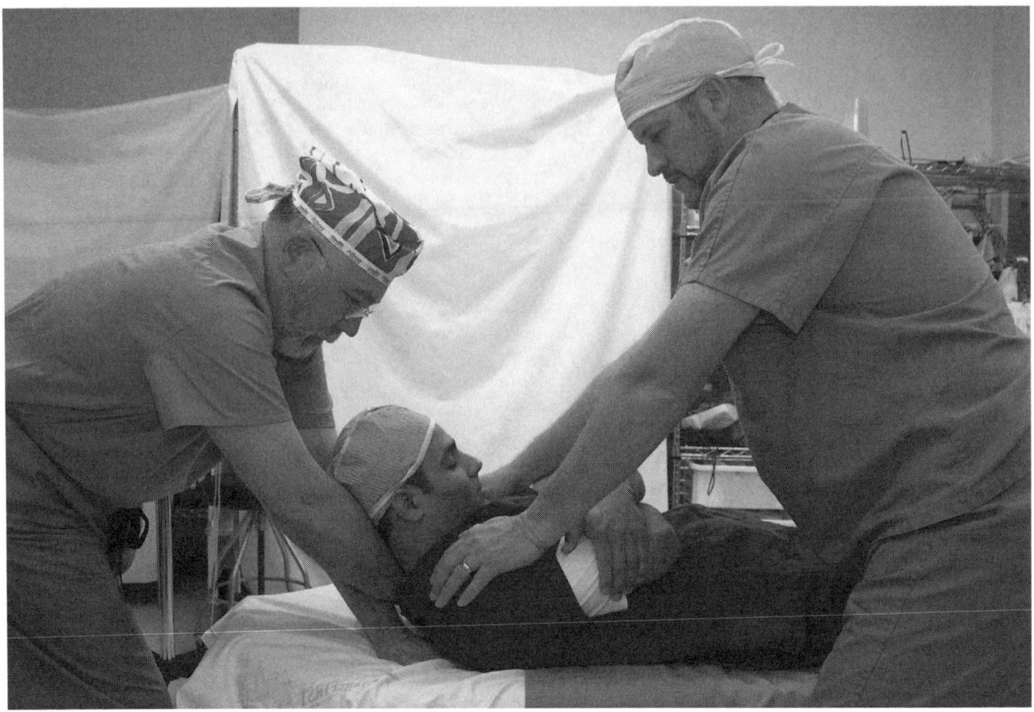

**FIGURE 12.5**

Goal: To achieve maximum end range and distract segmentally into the upper thoracic vertebrae.

A stair-stepping maneuver is accomplished by distracting the cervical spine cephalad, tractioning anteriorly, then applying forward/caudad pushing movements (Figure 12.6). This series of maneuvers is started in the lower cervical spine and, segment by segment, moved up toward the base of the skull. The first assistant is stabilizing the patient's shoulders by distracting as the stair-stepping maneuvers are completed.

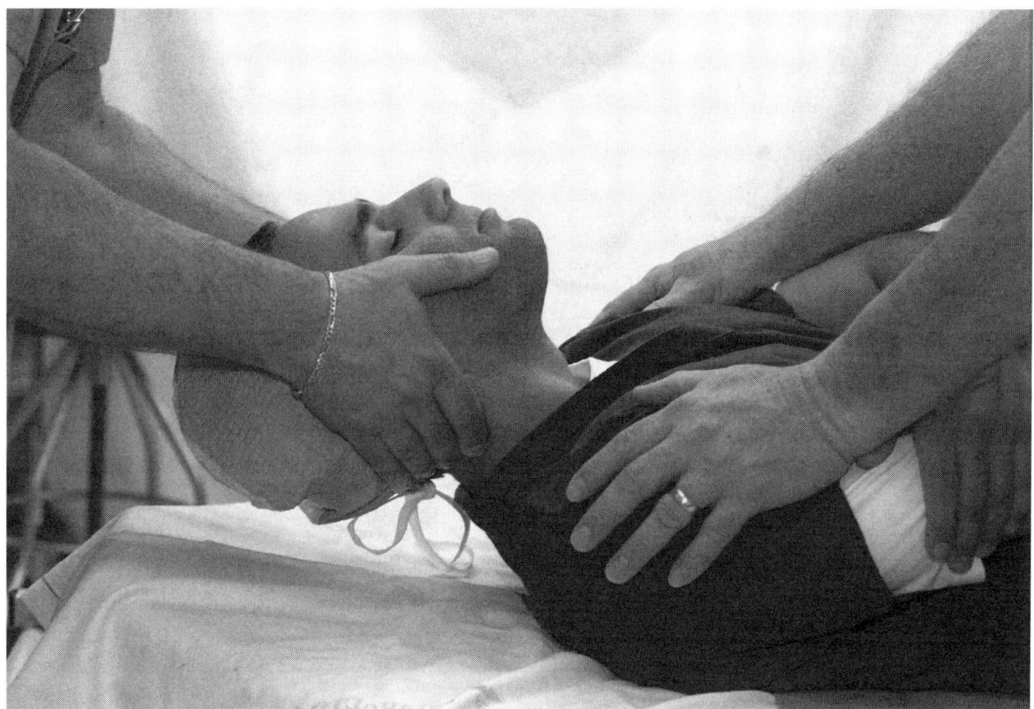

**FIGURE 12.6**

Goal: To achieve maximum end range and isolate facet decompression.

The patient's head is then rotated to one side or the other by the primary practitioner (Figure 12.7). Once complete rotation is accomplished, the primary practitioner reaches up under the patient's head from the contralateral side from rotation and flexes the patient's head in an oblique manner. The first assistant is countertractioning the shoulders posteriorly.

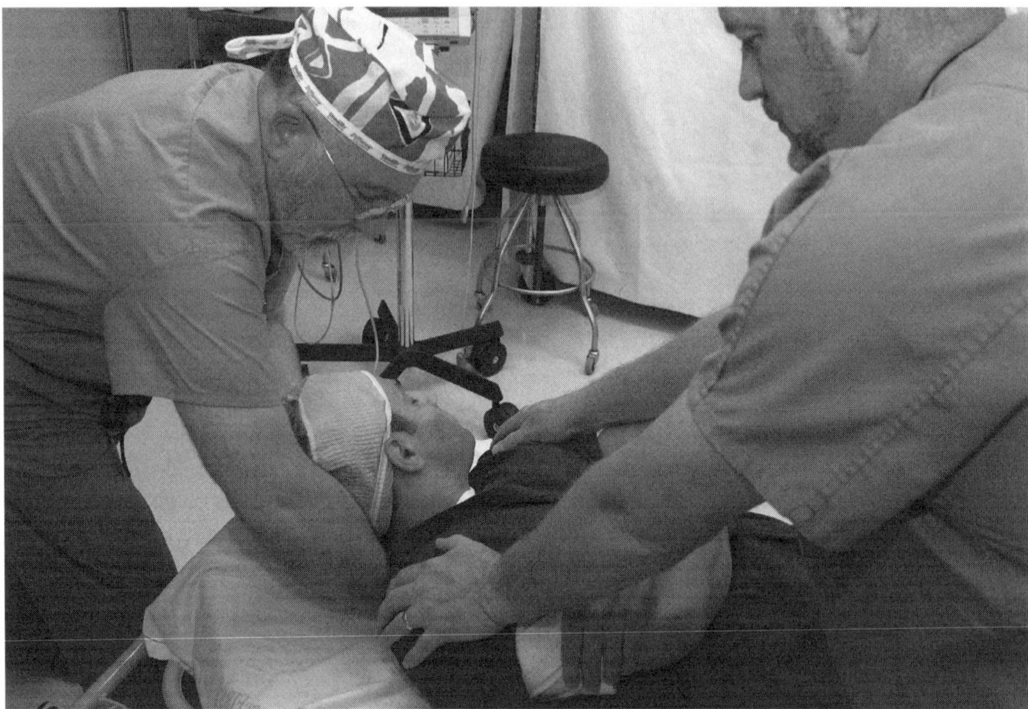

**FIGURE 12.7**

Goal: To achieve maximum end range.

The primary practitioner continues the lateral/oblique lift by placing the hand on the angle of the jaw to maximize oblique forward flexion (Figure 12.8). The first assistant continues the countertraction.

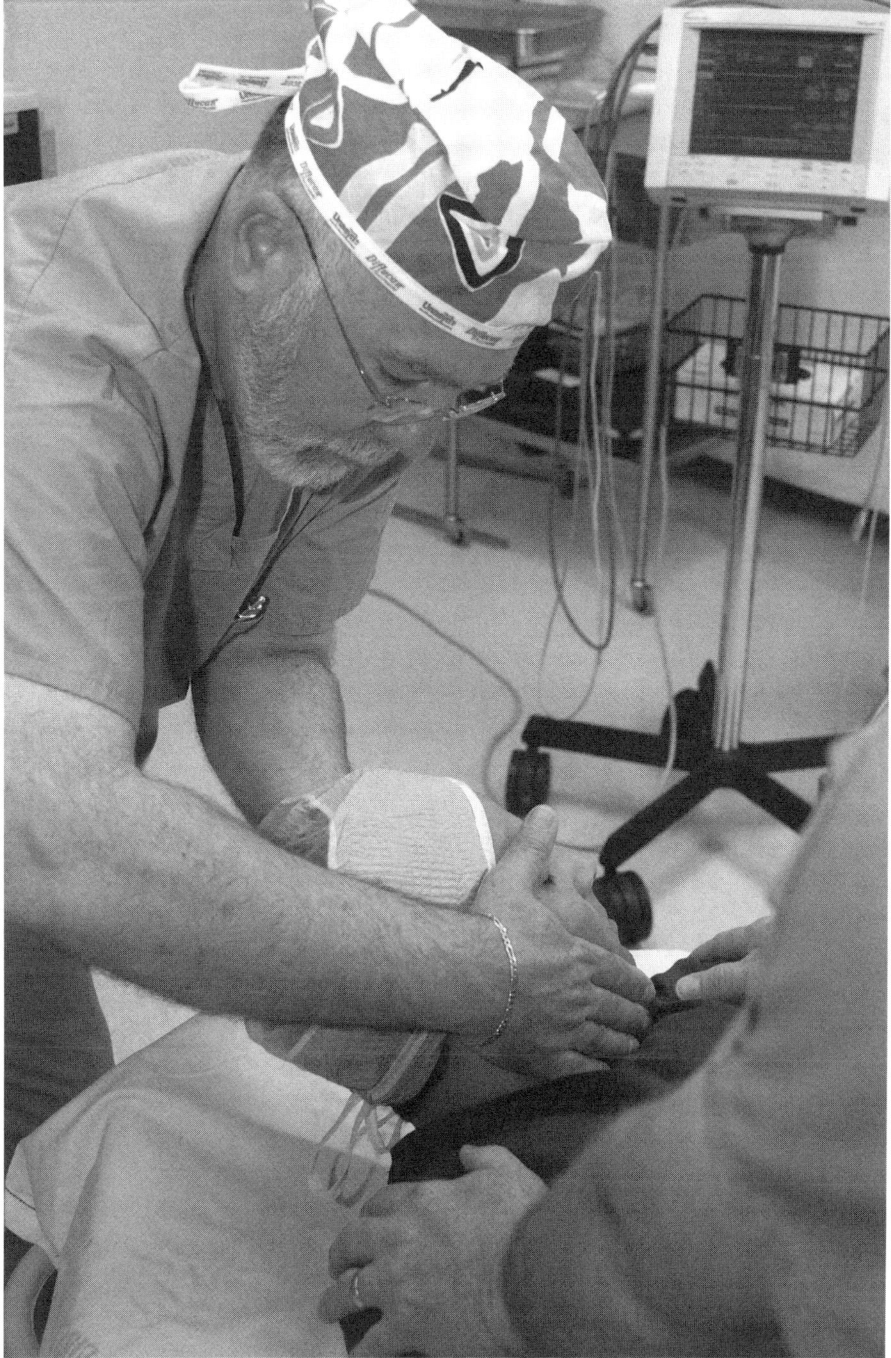

**FIGURE 12.8**

Goal: To achieve maximum end range in upper cervical muscles.

The procedure is then repeated on the lower side in the same manner (Figure 12.9 and Figure 12.10). The first assistant countertractions the patient's shoulders as in the previous maneuver.

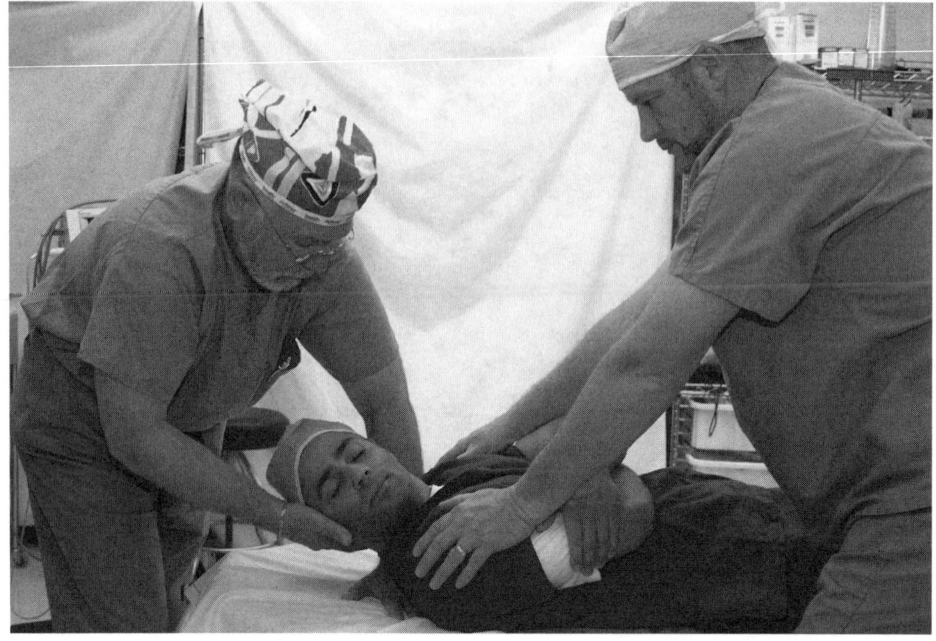

**FIGURE 12.9**

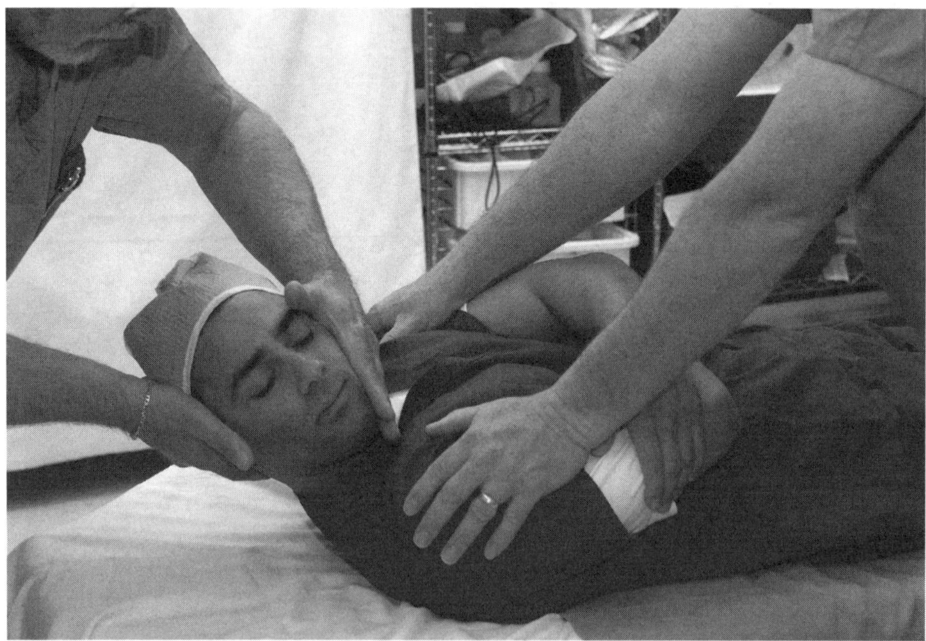

**FIGURE 12.10**

Goal: To achieve maximum end range.

All of these stretches are then followed by closed reduction segmental adjustive procedure(s) that the primary practitioner feels are necessary to achieve the desired results using a low-velocity impulse-thrust maneuvers (Figure 12.11). The first assistant countertractions the patient's shoulders with an underhand grip in order to allow for slight distraction of the segments as the adjustment is accomplished.

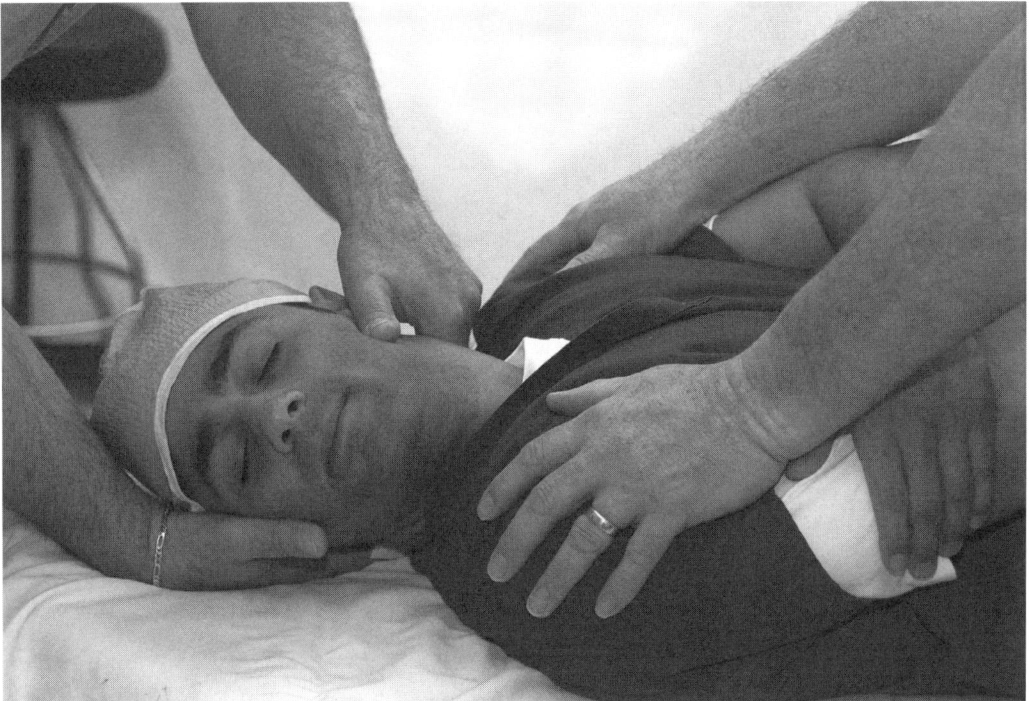

**FIGURE 12.11**

Goal: To correct fixated articulations and improve/enhance neurological/circulatory function.

## The Thoracic Spine

With the patient in the supine position on the operating table, the primary practitioner raises one of the patient's arms from the cephalad end of the table (Figure 12.12). Crossing over with the away hand for traction, the practitioner reaches into the lateral border of the latissimus dorsi and serratus group to distract these muscles toward the head, or cephalad. In this position, the patient's arm is distracted against the practitioner's arm for maximal traction. The traction starts as low as the practitioner can reach and moves cephald. The first assistant is stabilizing the patient at the level of the hips bilaterally.

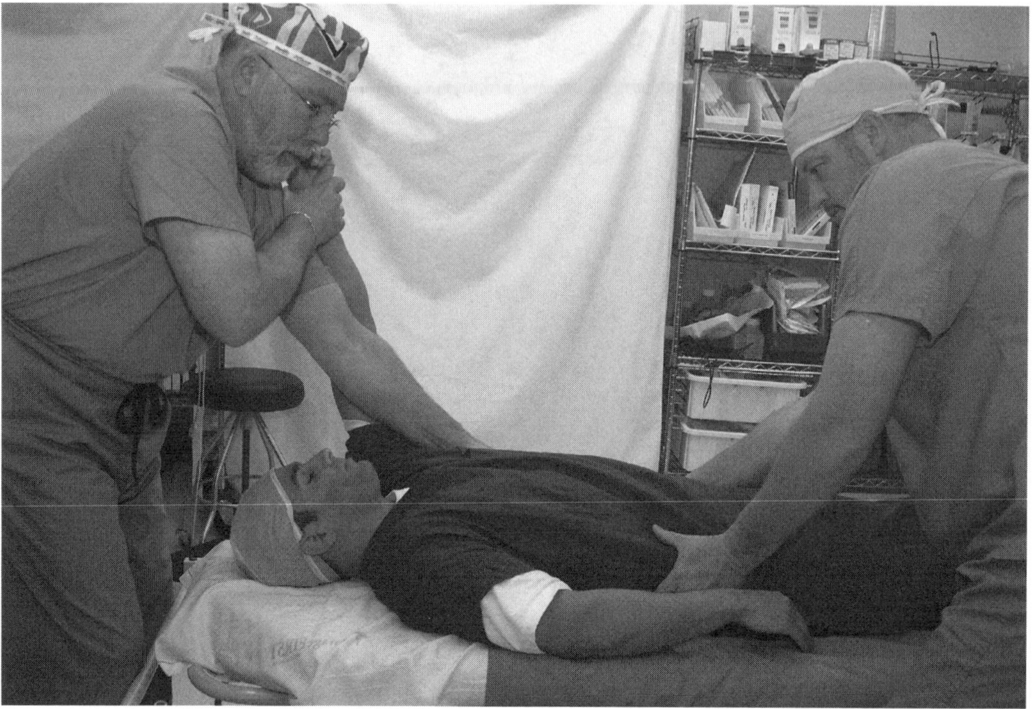

**FIGURE 12.12**

Goal: To achieve maximum end range with muscles affecting the thoracic area.

This traction procedure is then repeated on the opposite side by either the first assistant or the primary practitioner (Figure 12.13). This is left to the discretion of the primary practitioner.

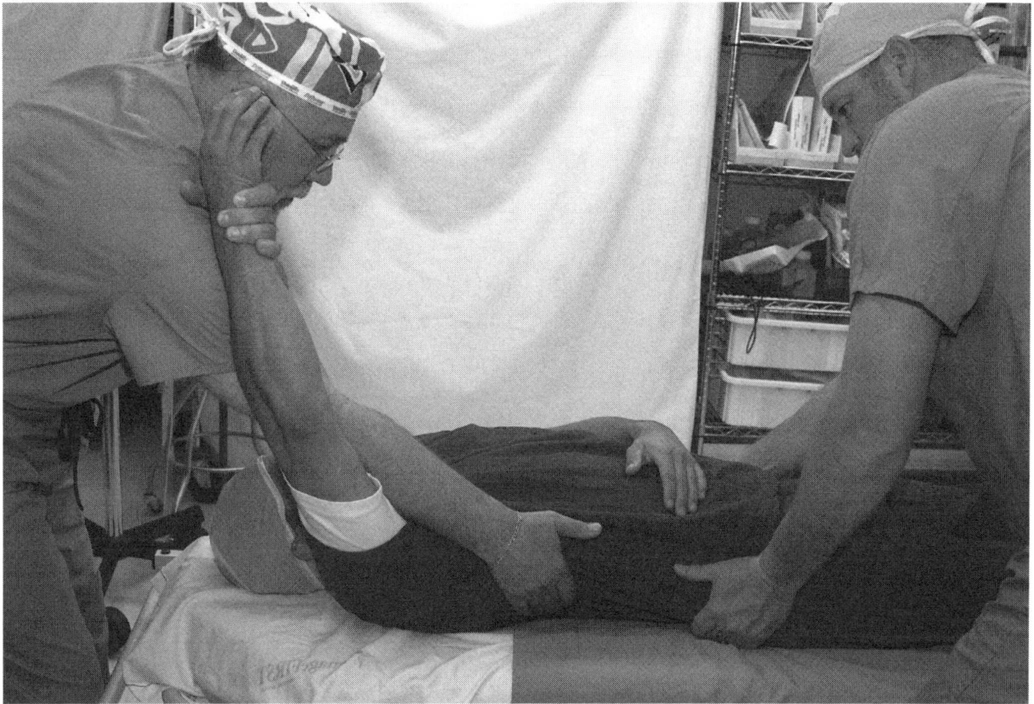

**FIGURE 12.13**

Goal: To achieve maximum end range with muscles affecting the thoracic spine.

The patient's arms are then crossed over the chest. With the help of the first assistant, a rolling maneuver is accomplished so that proper segmental contact is taken for closed reduction anteriority thoracic adjustment(s) by the primary practitioner using a low-velocity impulse-thrust (Figure 12.14 and Figure 12.15). This procedure is completed in all areas that are necessary to achieve the desired results.

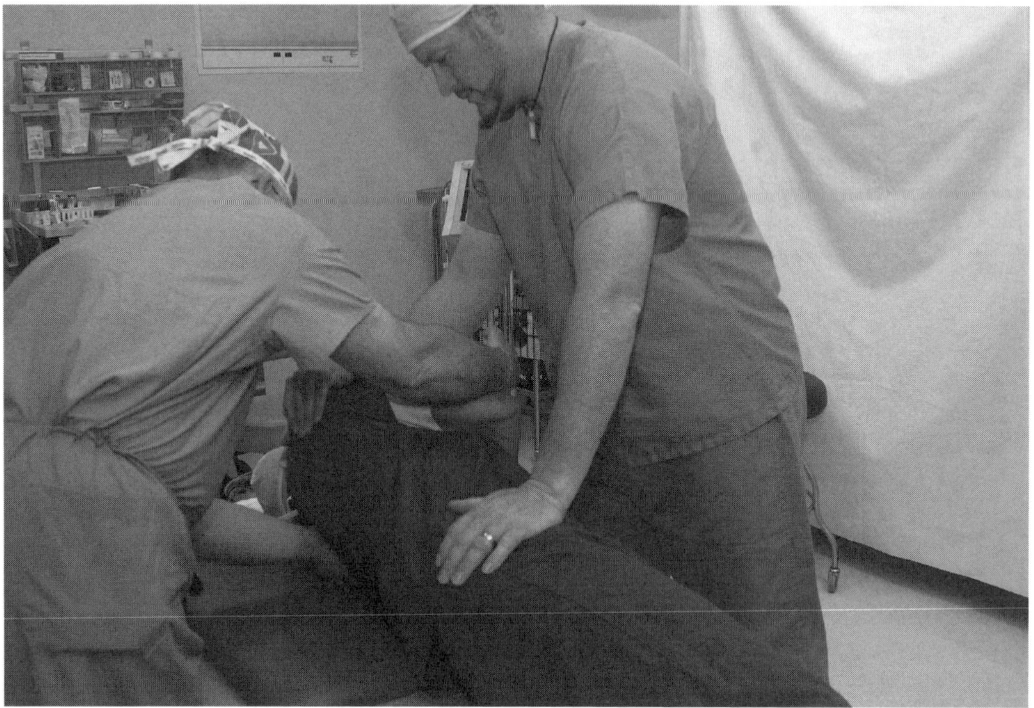

**FIGURE 12.14**

Goal: To reduce fixation and segmental dysfunction in the thoracic spinal vertebrae.

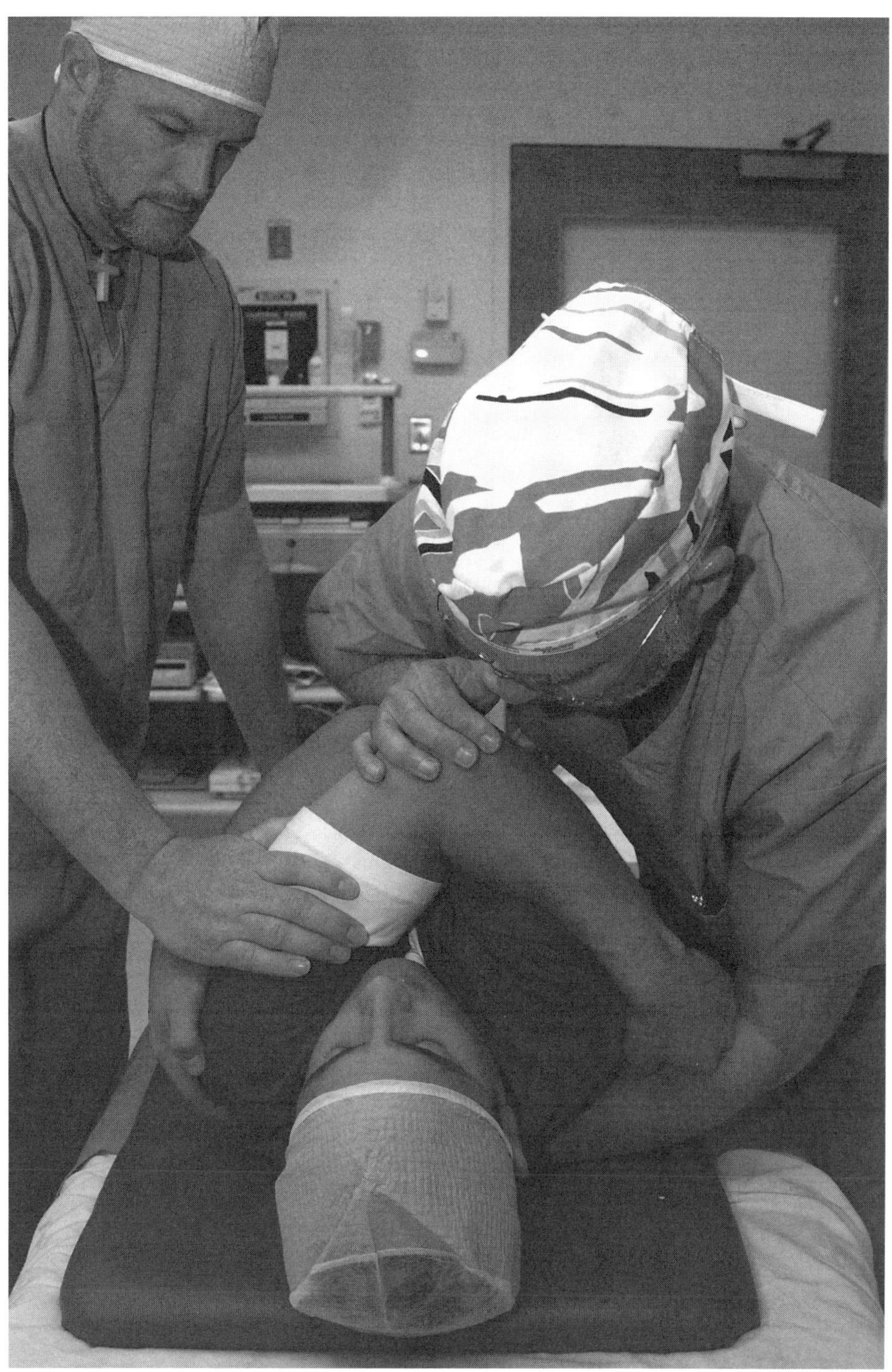

**FIGURE 12.15**

## THE LUMBAR SPINE

The lumbar spinal MUA procedures begin with straight leg raising (SLR) on the side of the primary practitioner (Figure 12.16). With the patient in the supine position on the operating table, the primary practitioner addresses the patient's lower extremity, which is elevated alternatively in a straight-leg raising maneuver to accomplish the patient's allowable ROM. The ROM is measured in degrees from the horizontal and taken to the point of resistance. Here linear force is applied for a period of time until the end range is achieved. (This may vary depending on the practitioner's assessment of the muscle tone, tightness, anatomical length, and injury involvement.) Hip flexion is increased gradually as the patient responds to the forces used. Simultaneously the first assistant applies a myofascial release procedure from the gastrocnemius to the hamstring muscles as the stretching continues.

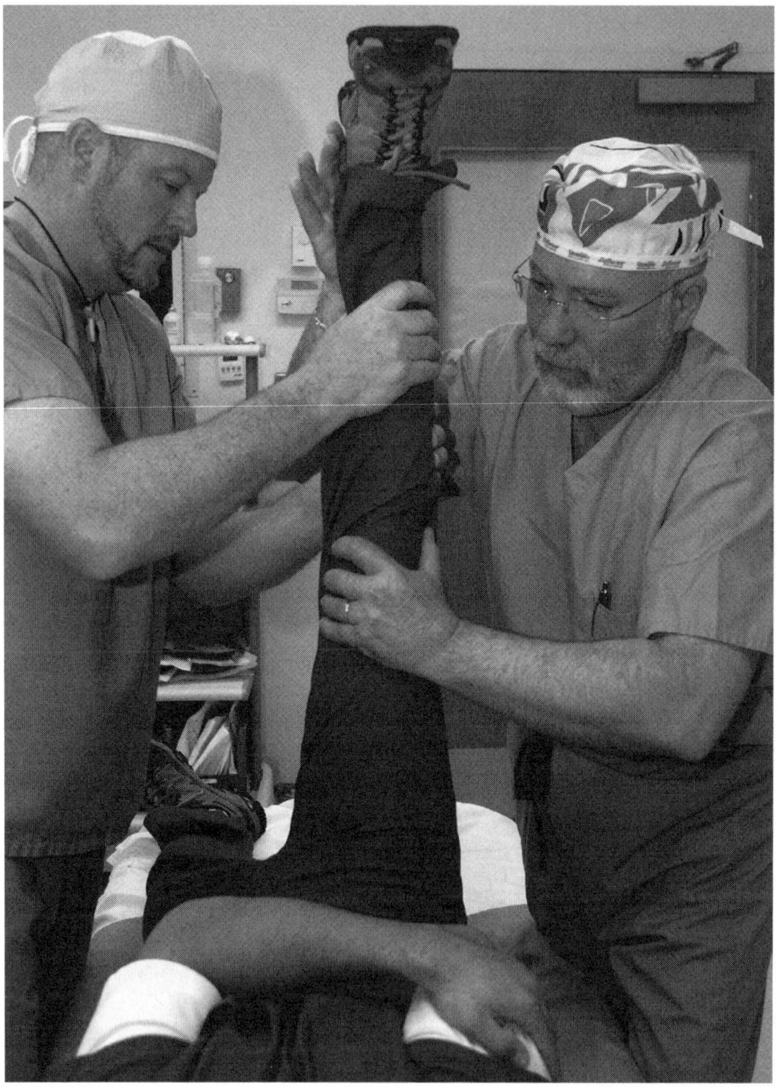

**FIGURE 12.16**

Goals: To achieve maximum end range of the hip flexors and to allow for stretching of the neurological component elements of the lumbar plexus.

The knee is then flexed for forward traction. In this manner each lower extremity is tractioned in a lateral oblique cephalad plane, a neutral sagittal plane, and a medial oblique cephalad plane traction maneuver (Figures 12.17, 12.18, and 12.19).

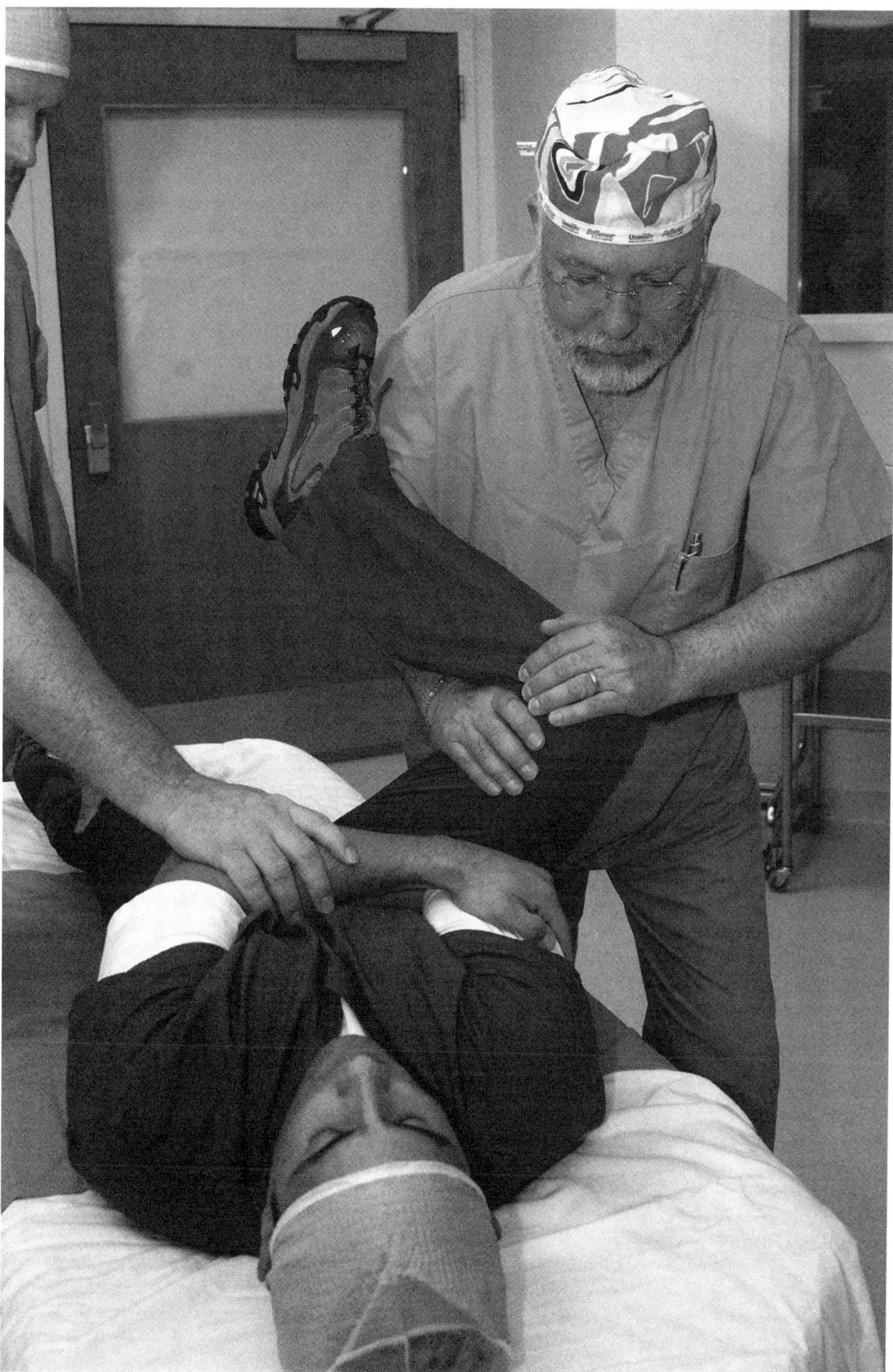

**FIGURE 12.17**

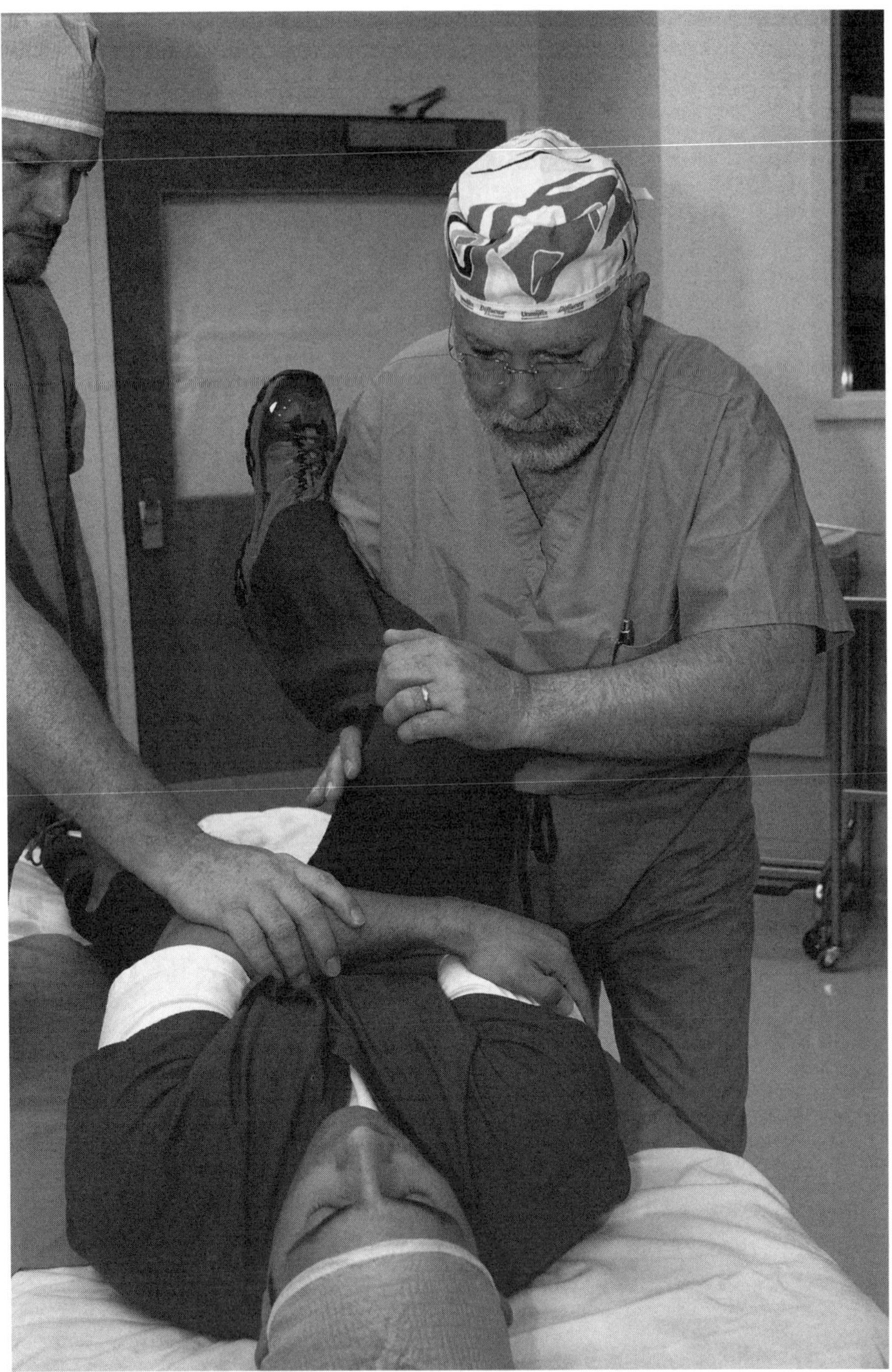

**FIGURE 12.18**

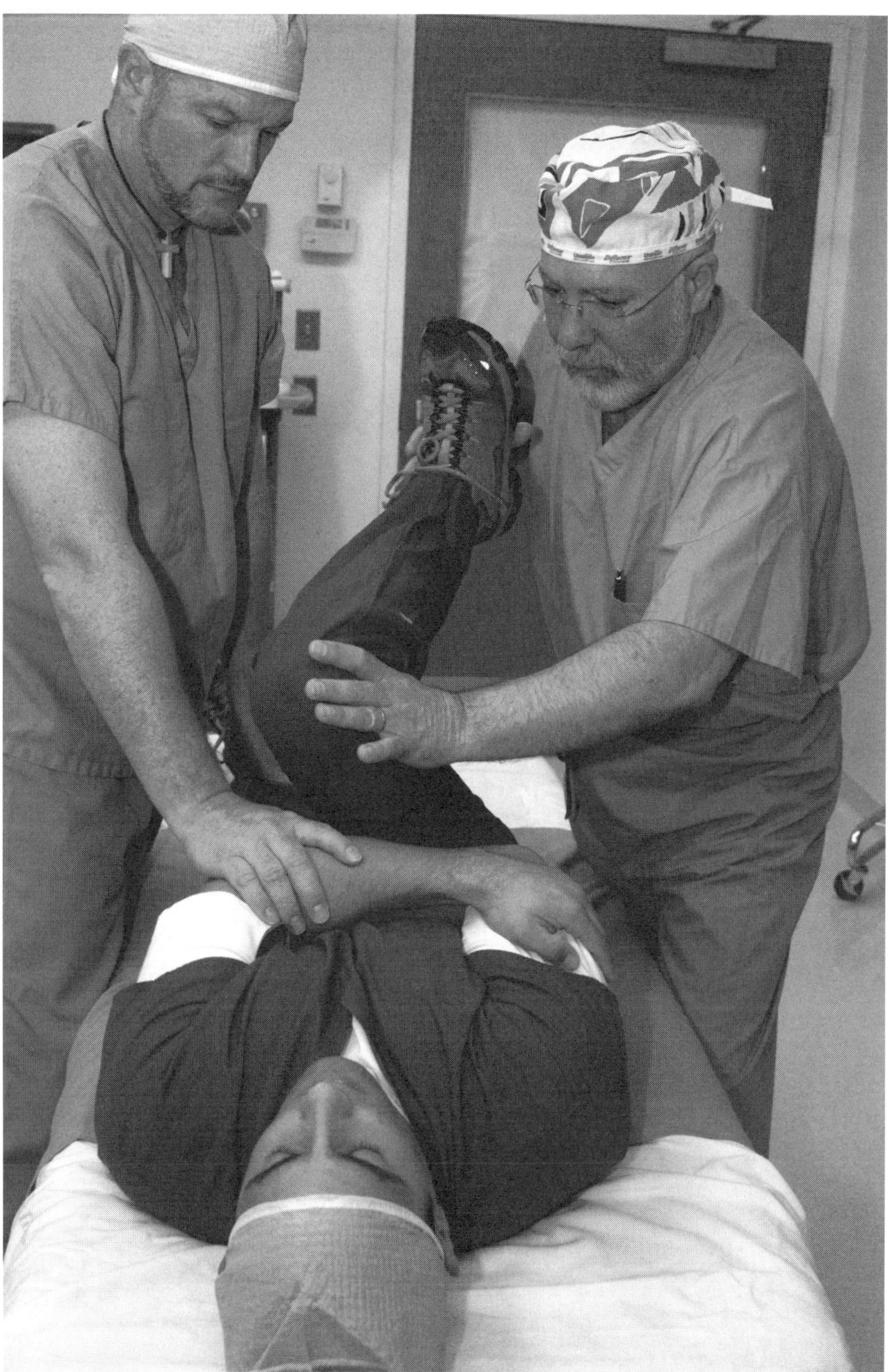

**FIGURE 12.19**

Goal: To achieve maximum end range of the hip flexors and lower lumbar holding elements.

The knee remaining in the bent position with the patient's foot down on the table is brought by the first assistant across the patient in an adduction move (Figure 12.20). Gentle downward rolling traction is accomplished.

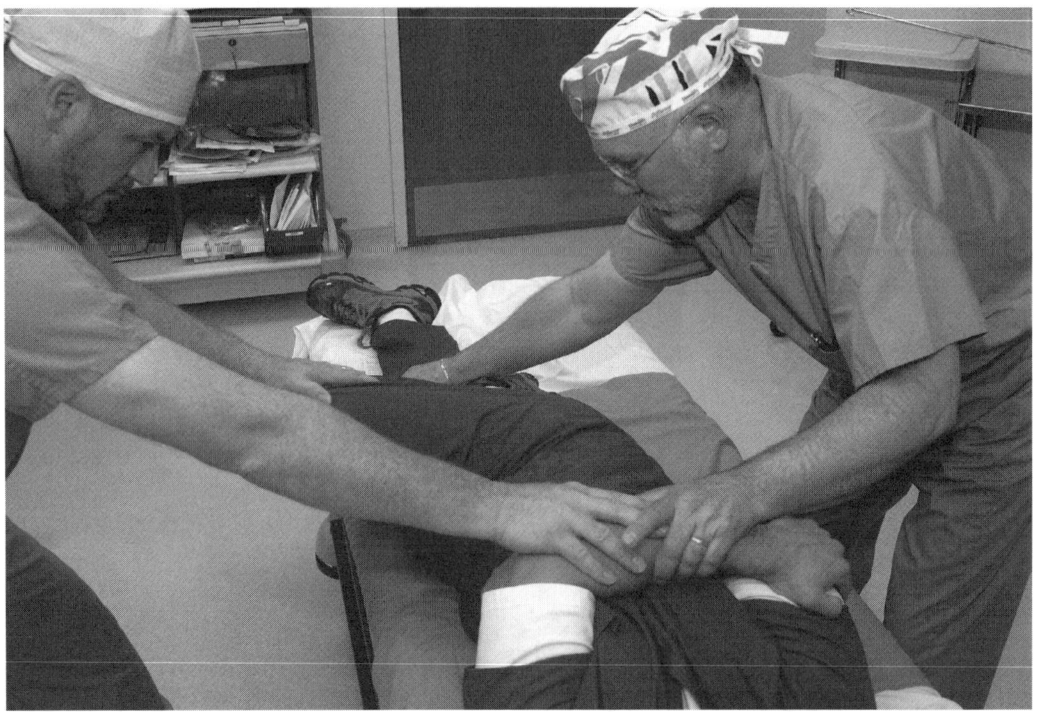

**FIGURE 12.20**

Goal: To reach maximum end range stretching the abductors of the hip.

If necessary the primary practitioner then takes the patient's bent knee back to a medial oblique position and completes a "piriformis bow string stretch" (Figure 12.21). This maneuver is explained thoroughly in the classroom setting during demonstration. It involves tractioning down toward the obturator foramen to release the piriformis muscle, which might be in spasm before performing a myofascial release procedure.

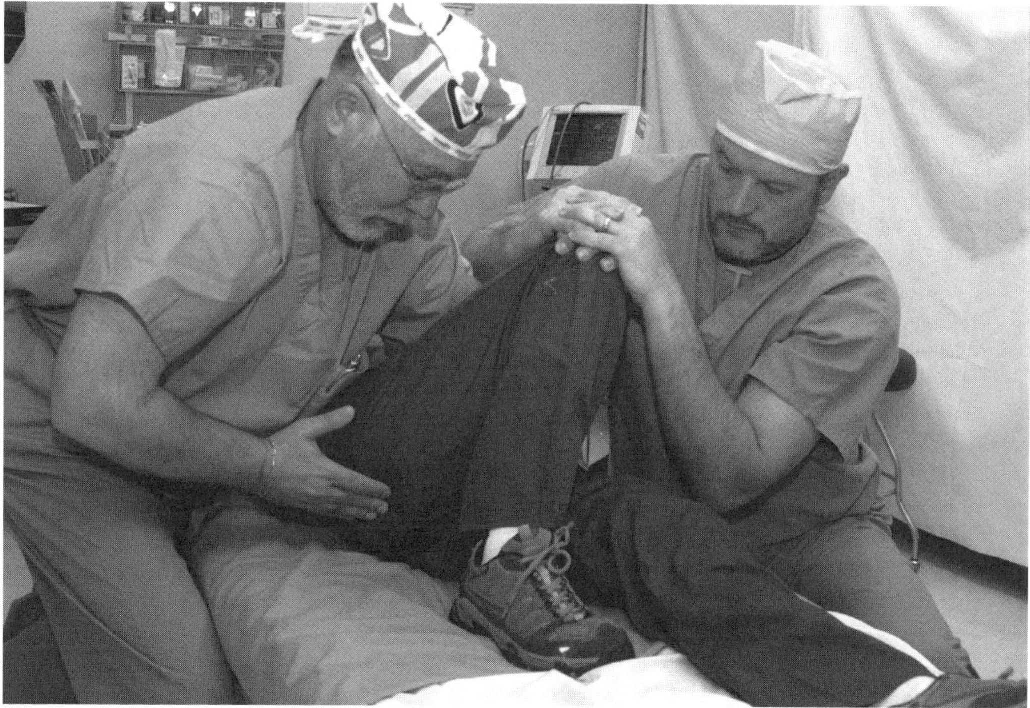

**FIGURE 12.21**

Goal: To release spasm in the piriformis muscle.

The patient's knee is then bent and laterally extended away from the body in the Patrick-Fabere, or figure of 4, maneuver (Figure 12.22). A gentle stretch is accomplished in this position. Do not apply too much pressure downward.

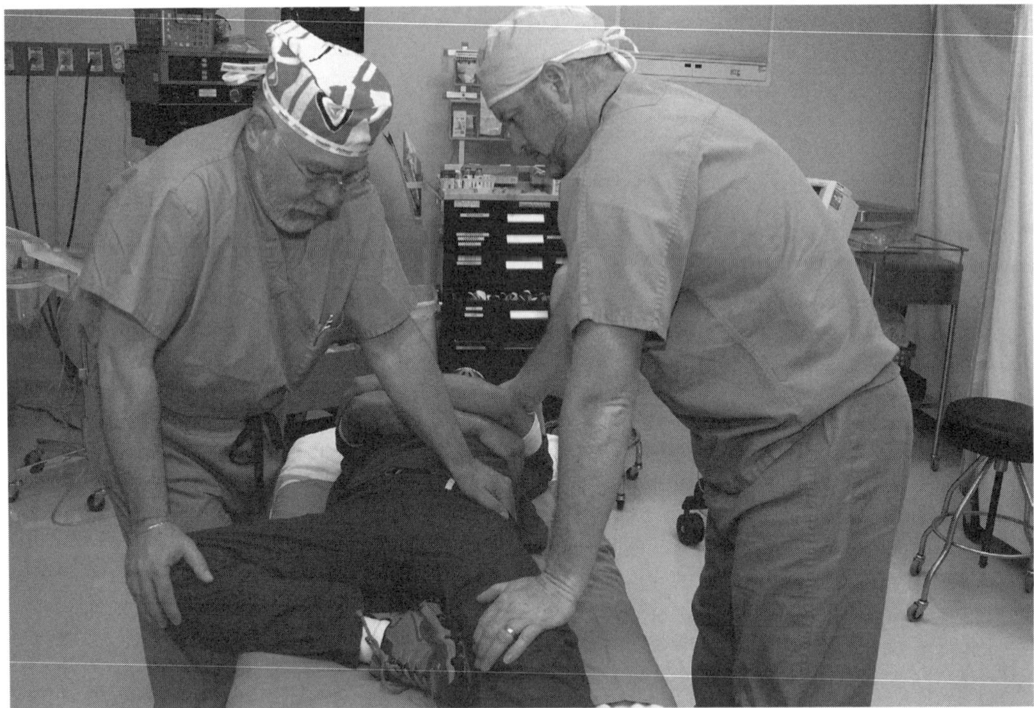

**FIGURE 12.22**

Goal: To reach maximum end range.

The patient's lower extremity is then tractioned. Both internal and external rotation with extension caudad traction is accomplished to about 30–35 degrees. Internal rotation followed by external rotation (it doesn't matter which is first) is accomplished, and the lower extremity is laterally tractioned to 30–35 degrees on the horizontal plane (Figure 12.23 and Figure 12.24).

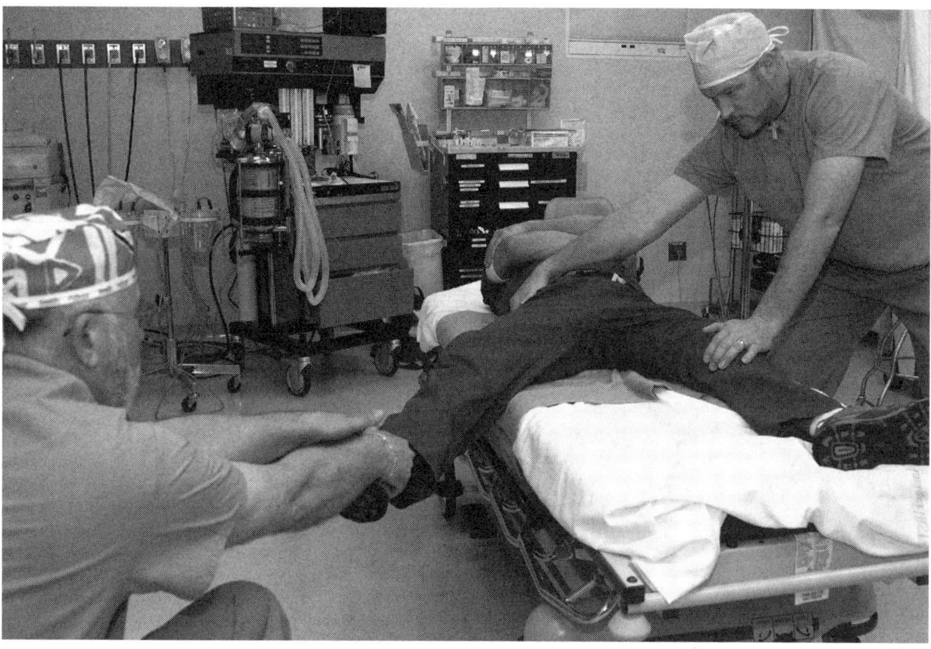

FIGURE 12.23

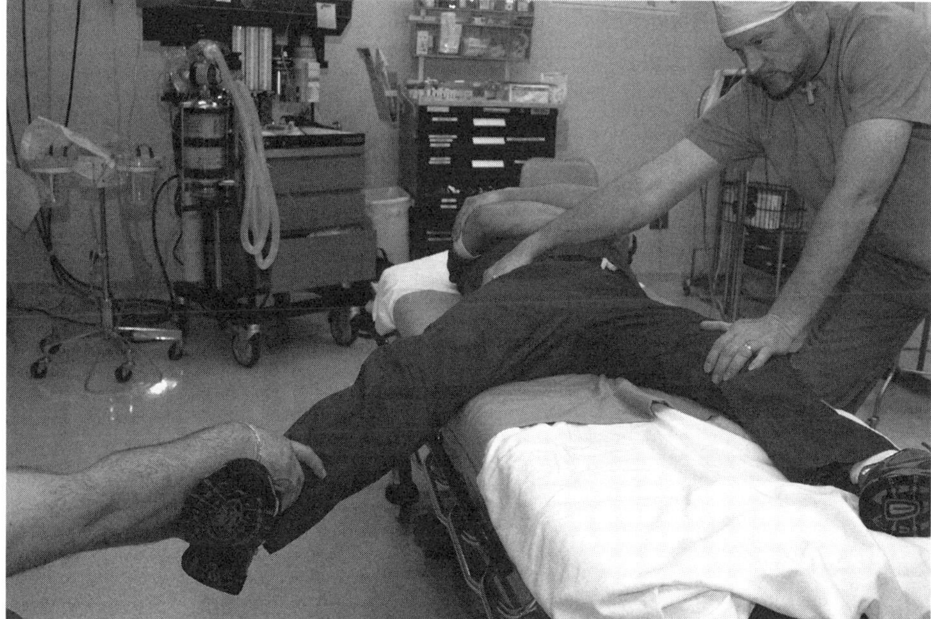

FIGURE 12.24

Goal: To reach maximum end range of the hip adductors and hip and lower extremity rotators.

The lower extremity is then tractioned out to 45 degrees in the neutral posture on a horizontal plane and a slight pulse thrust is completed (Figure 12.25).

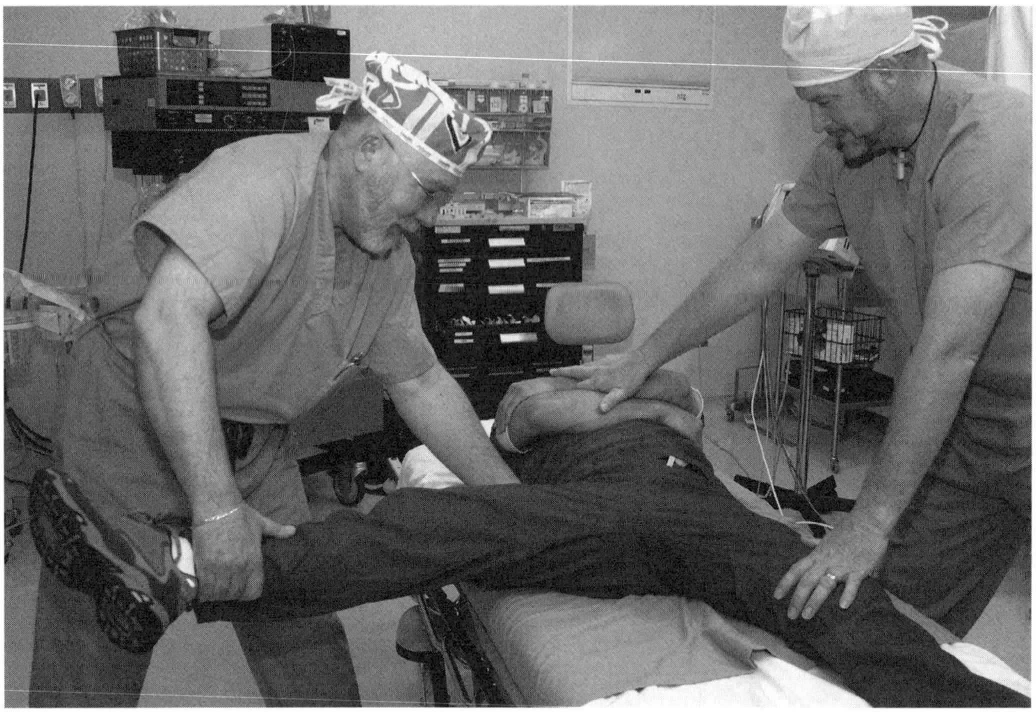

**FIGURE 12.25**

Goal: To reach maximum end range of the hip adductors and traction thrust the femoral-acetabular articulation.

The entire lower extremity stretching process is then accomplished by the first assistant on the opposite side (Figures 12.26 to 12.35).

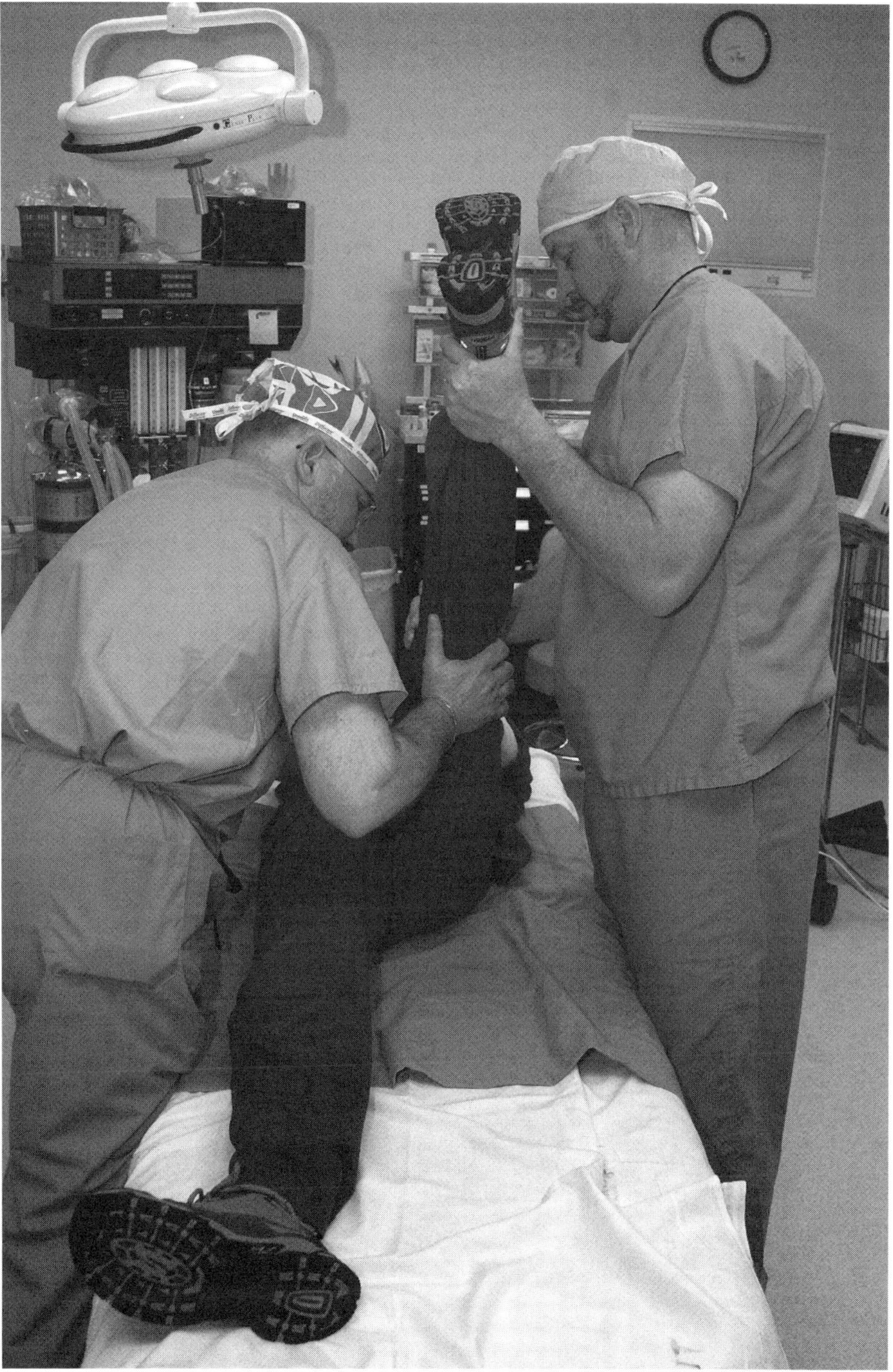

FIGURE 12.26

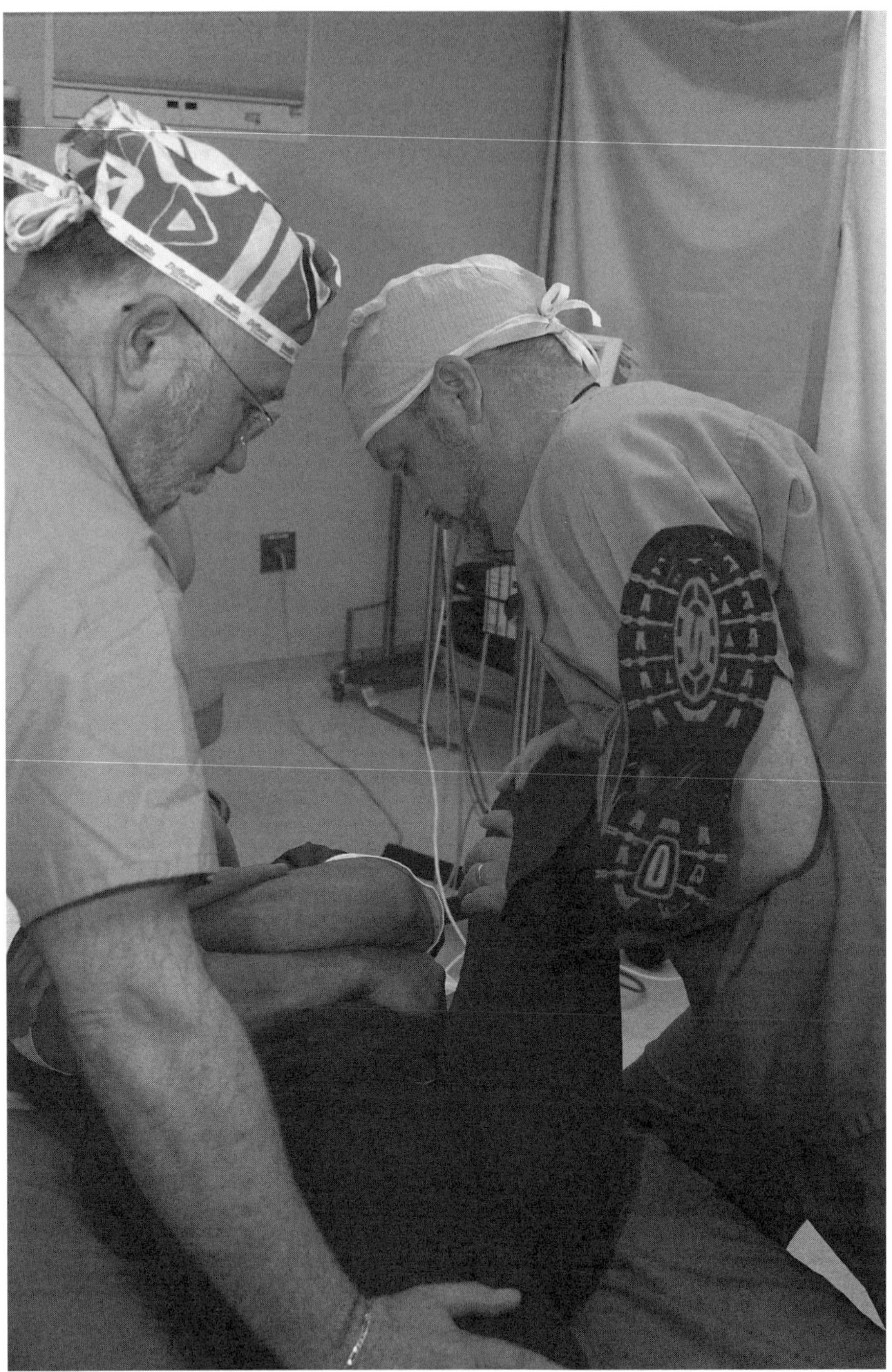

**FIGURE 12.27**

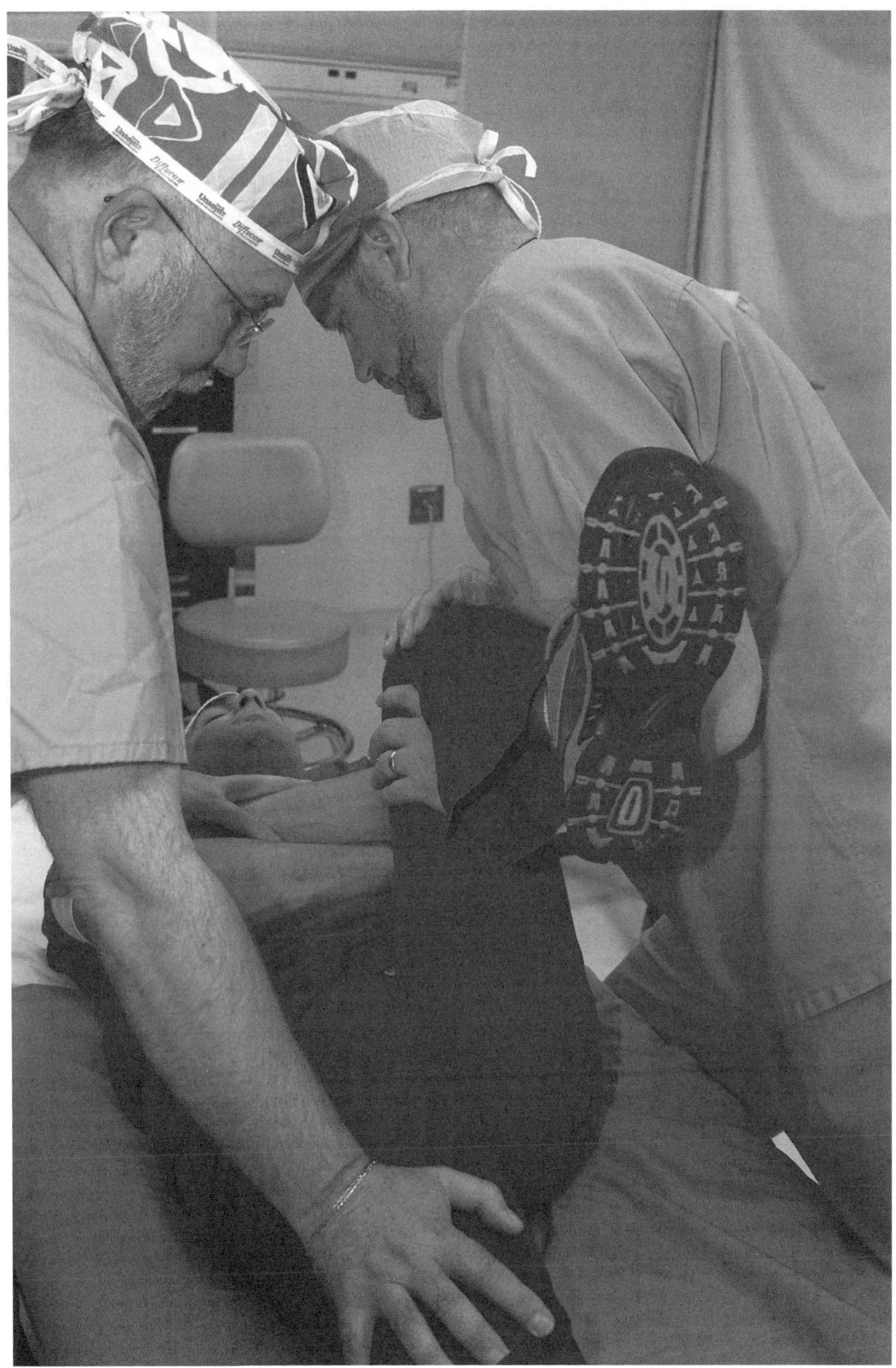

**FIGURE 12.28**

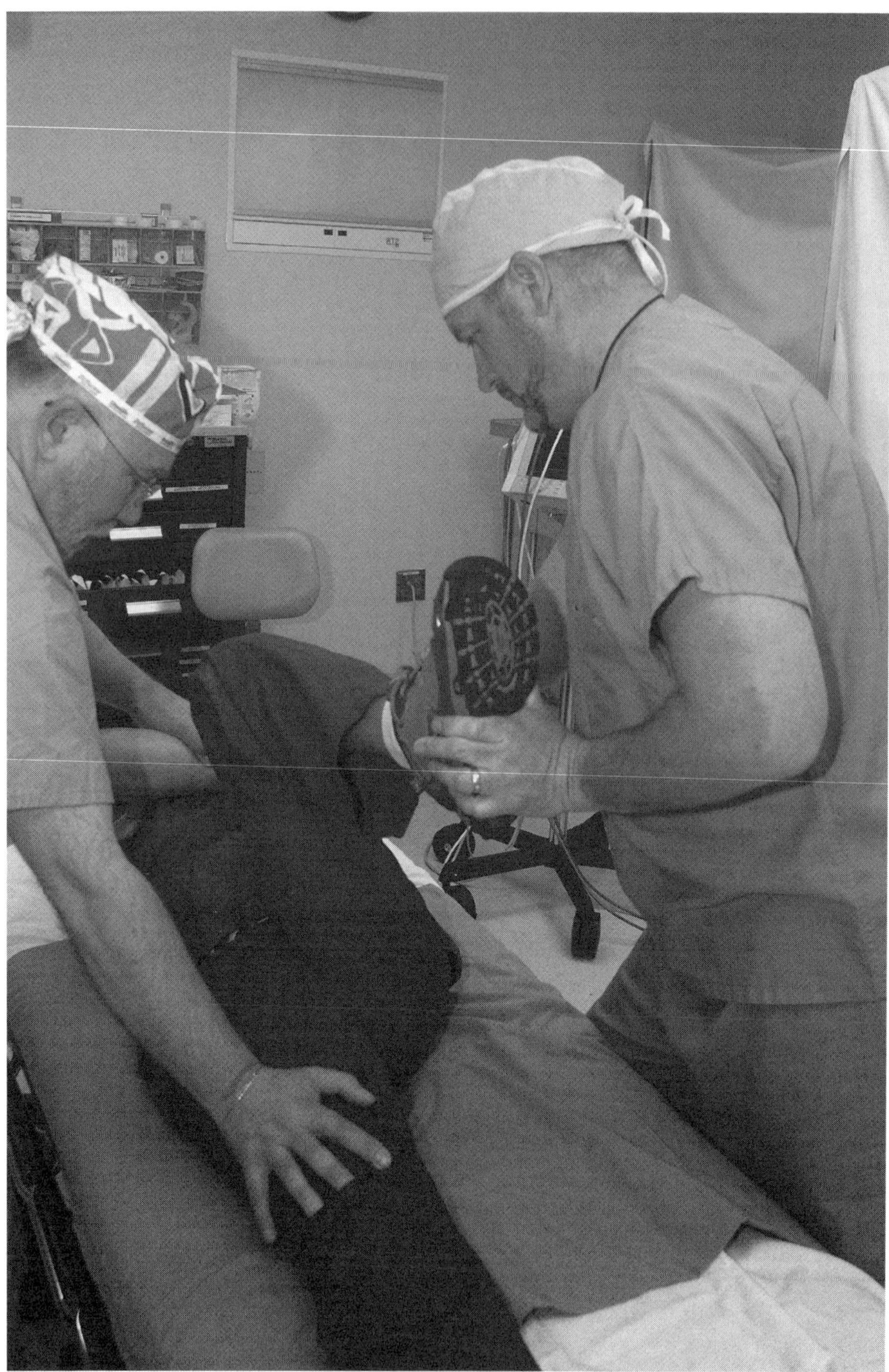

**FIGURE 12.29**

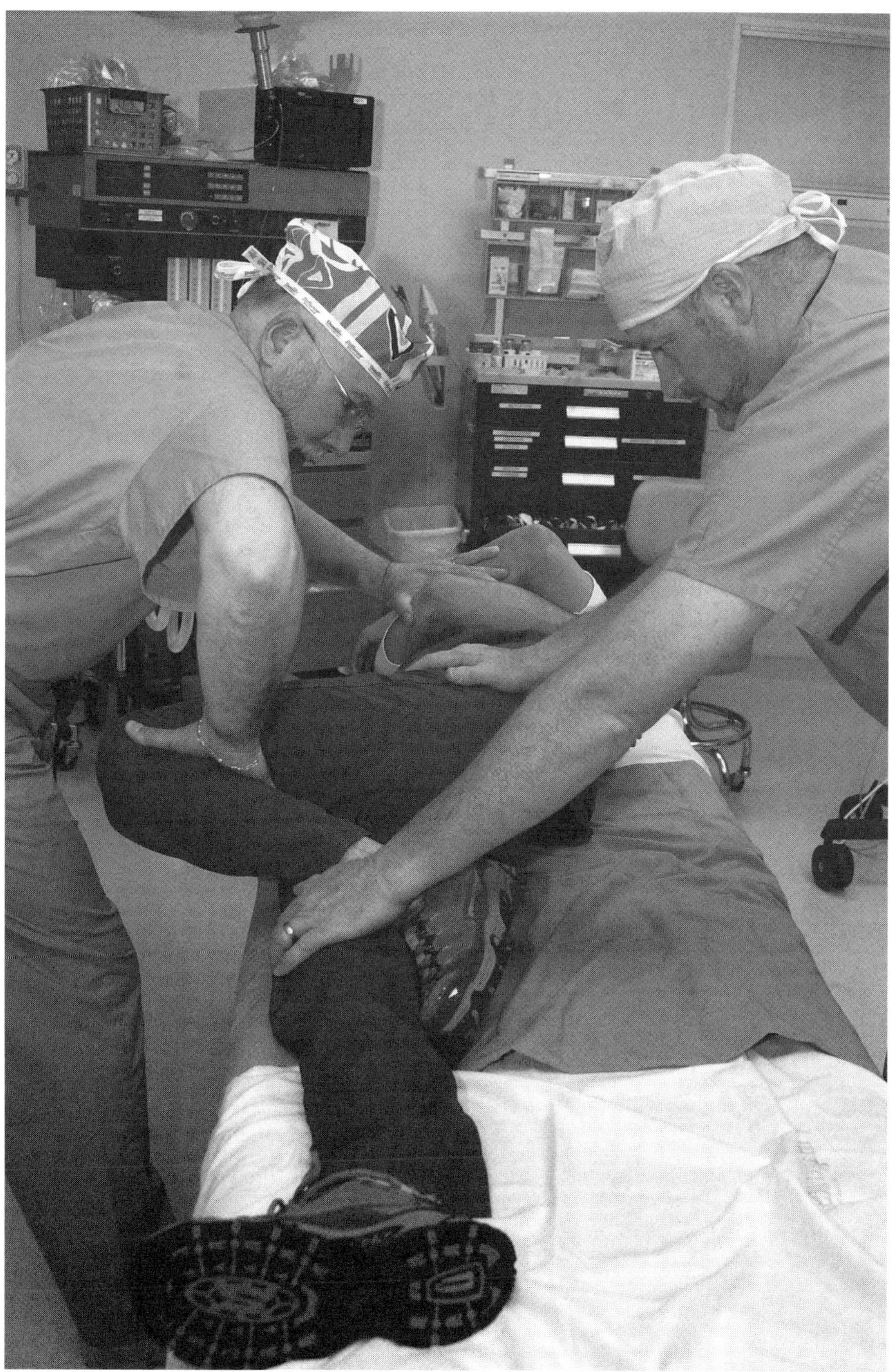

**FIGURE 12.30**

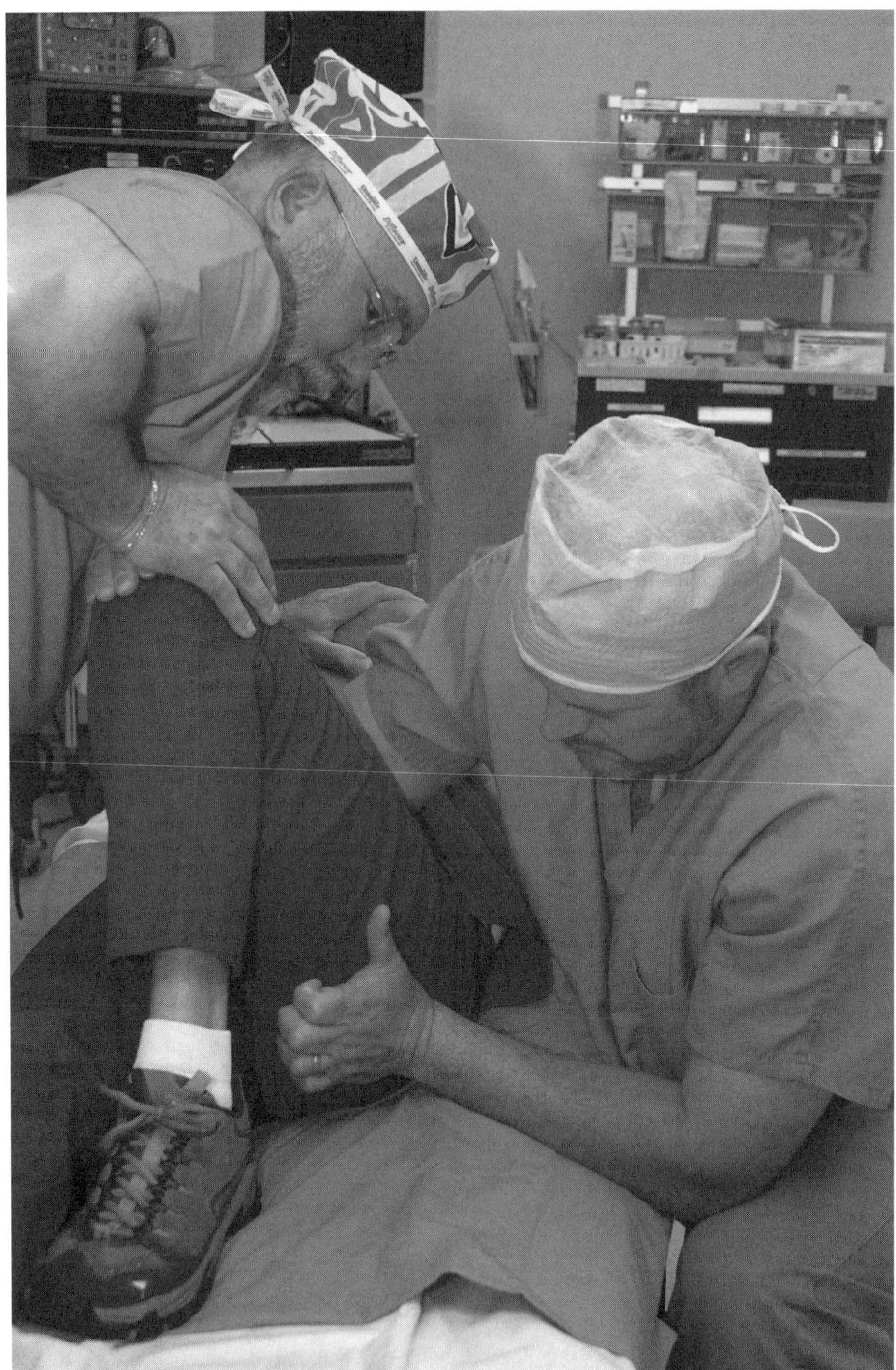

**FIGURE 12.31**

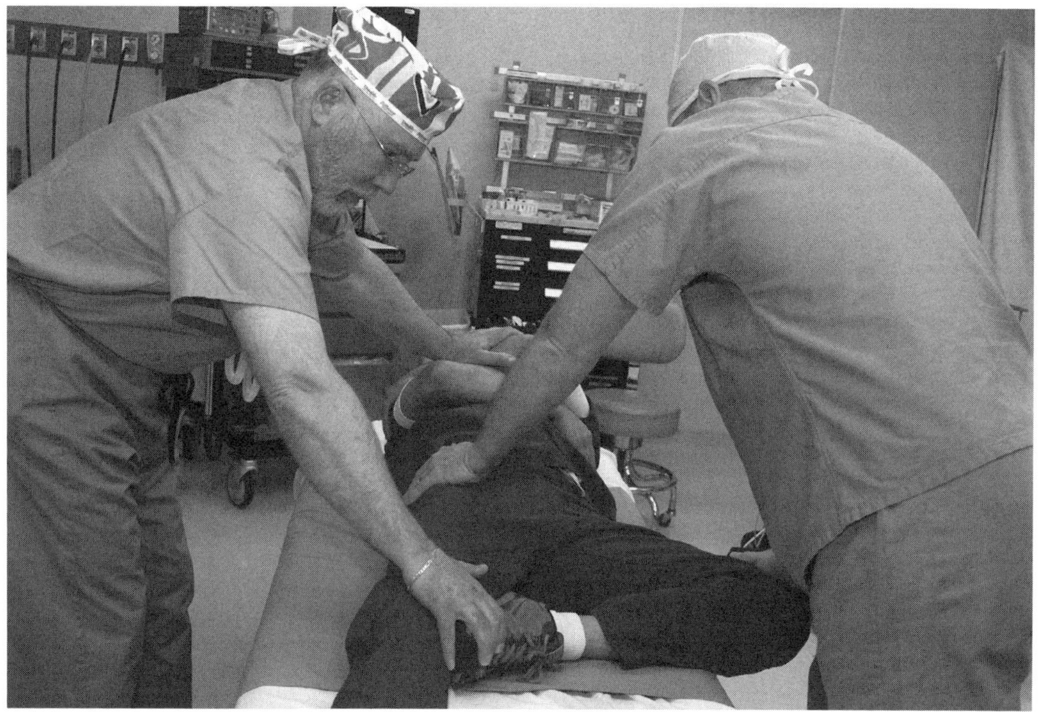

**FIGURE 12.32**

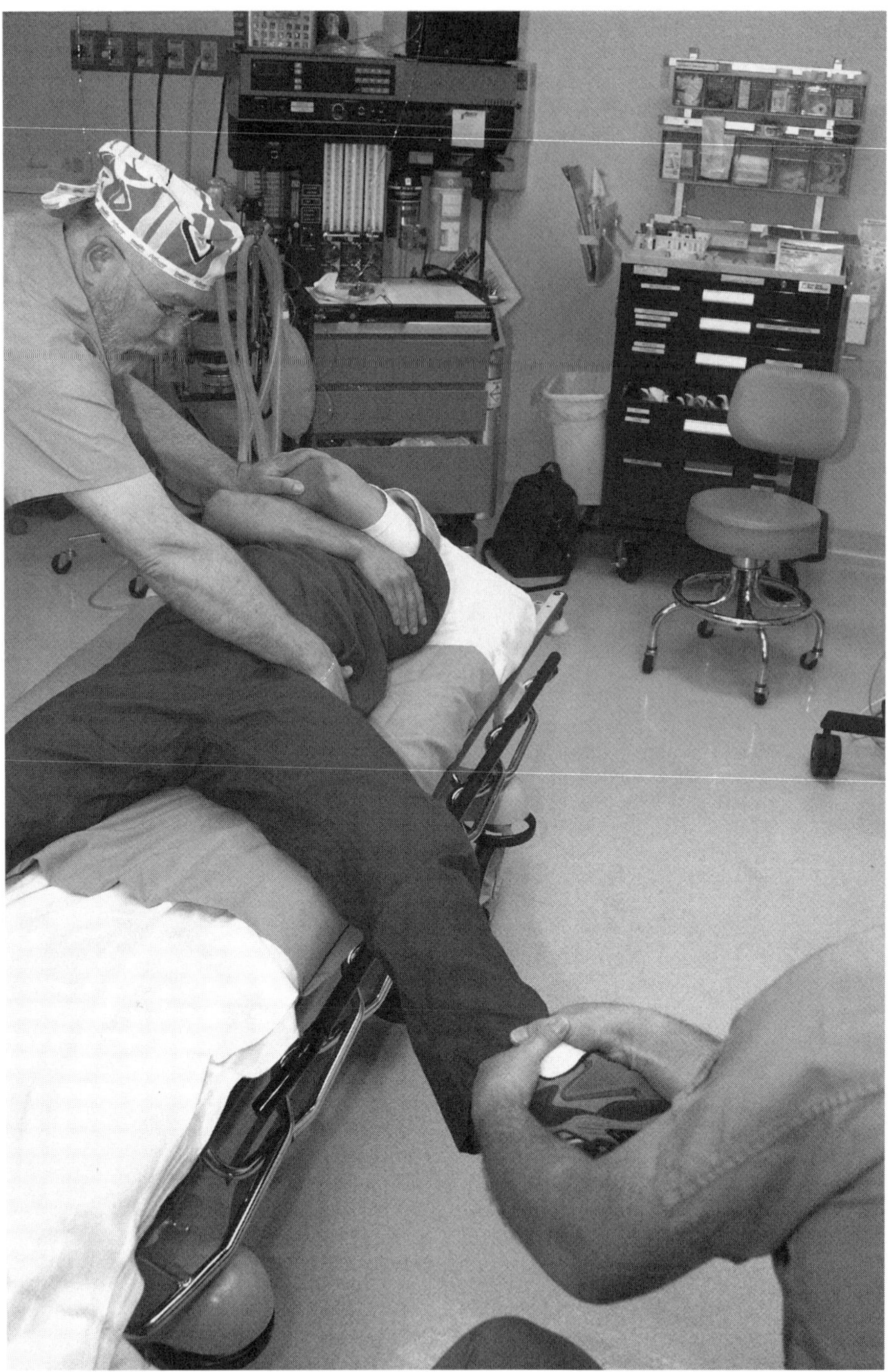

**FIGURE 12.33**

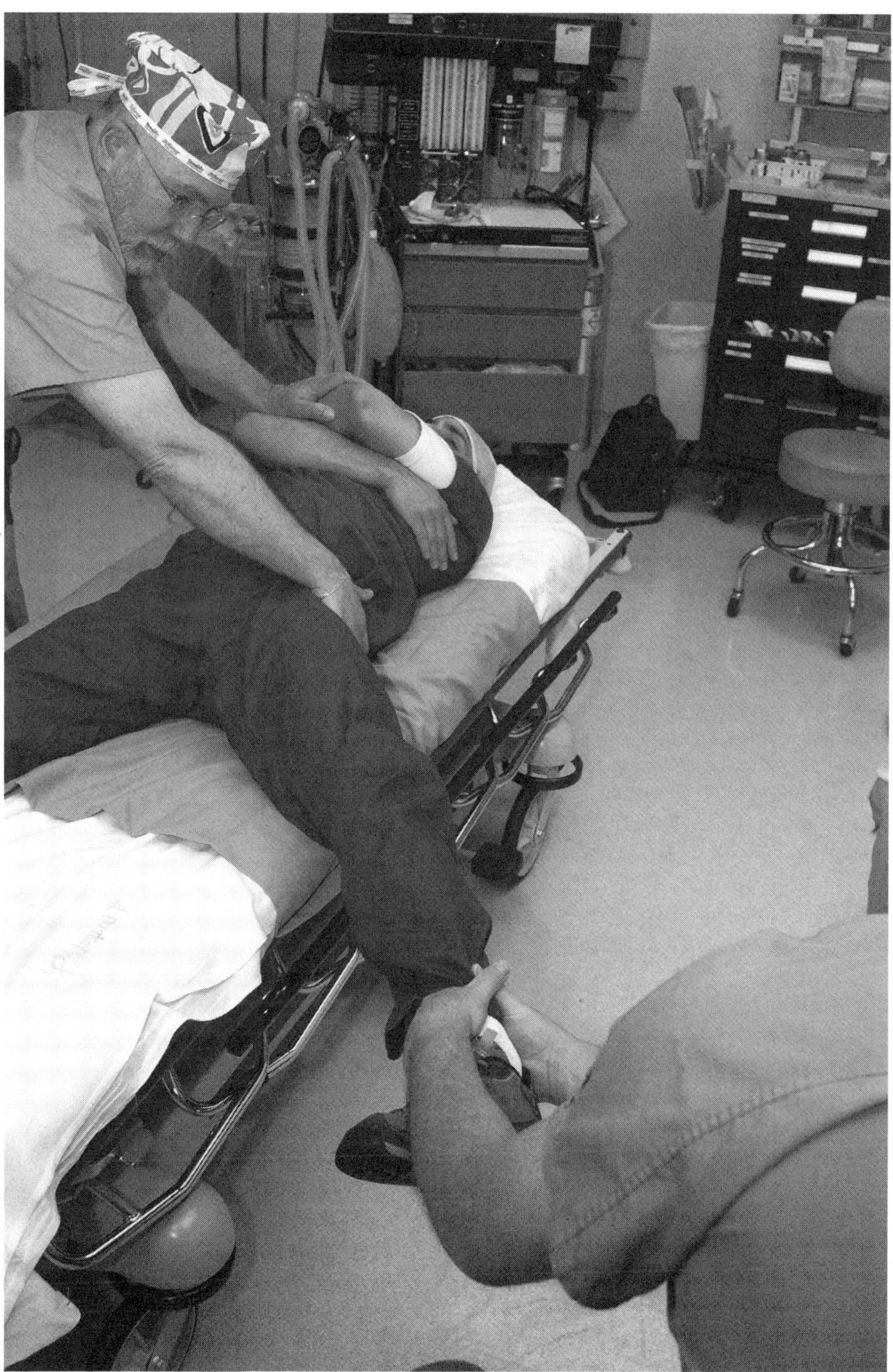

**FIGURE 12.34**

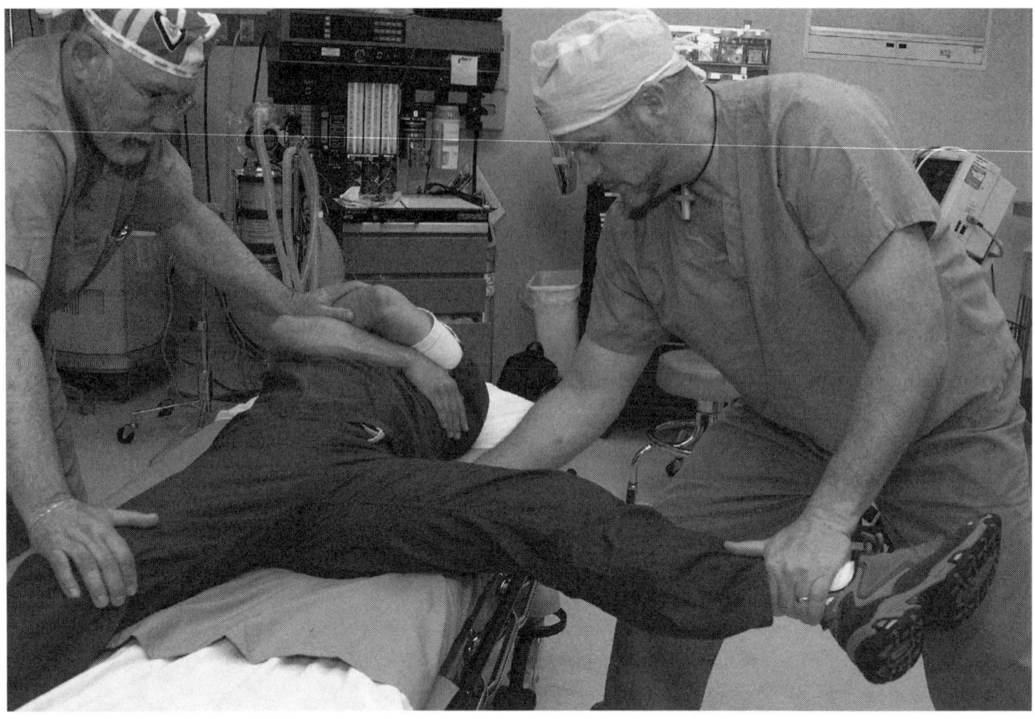

**FIGURE 12.35**

Goal: To reach maximum end range as above on the opposite side of the body.

The knees are then bent bilaterally by the primary practitioner and first assistant and by approximating the patient's knees to the abdomen in a knee-to-chest fashion, the lumbo-pelvic musculature is stretched in a sagittal plane (Figure 12.36). Controlled traction is gradually applied to the lumbar holding elements while the hip is lifted with contact on the sacral base by the primary practitioner and the first assistant. The knees of the patient must be held outside the torso in this maneuver to alleviate abdominal pressure, and the knees are only brought to the patient's nipple line in forward flexion.

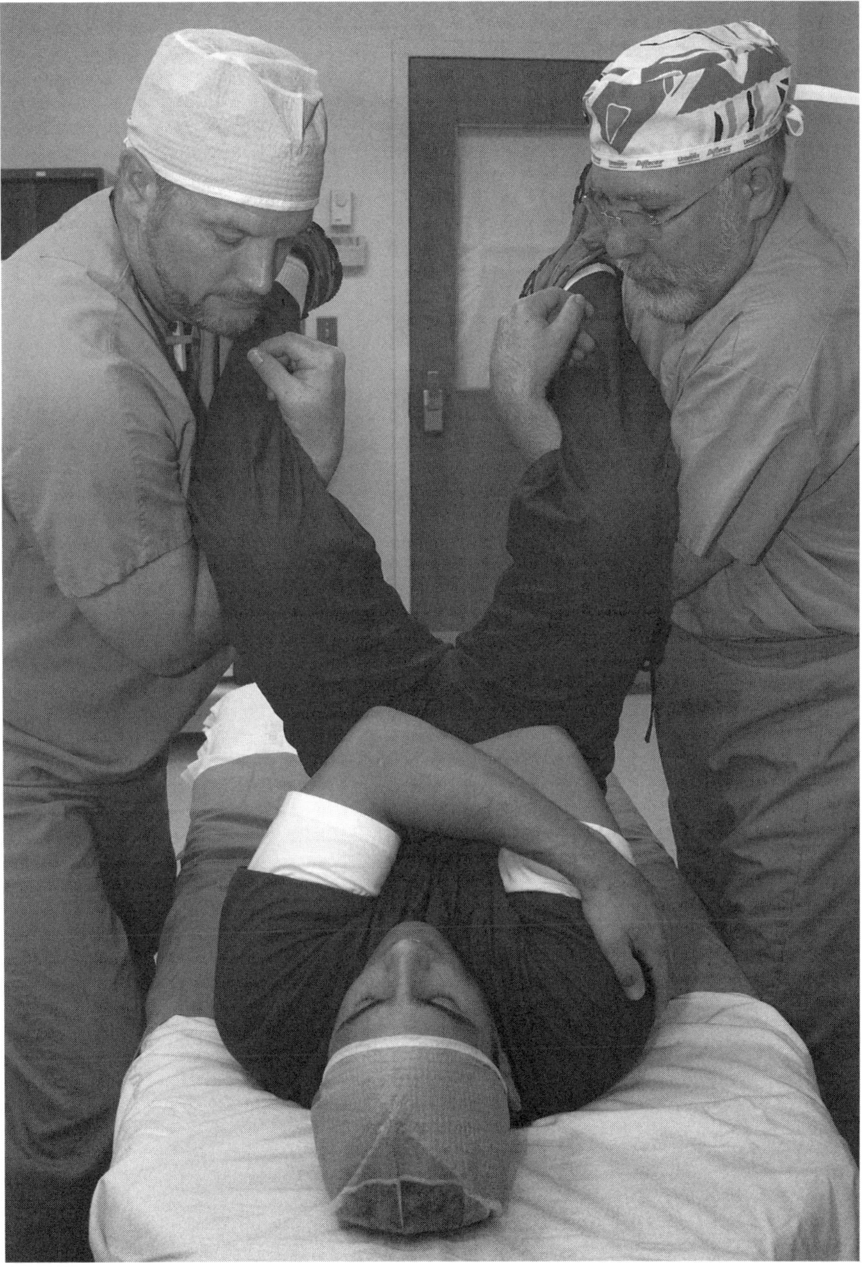

**FIGURE 12.36**

Goal: To reach maximum end range of the lower lumbar holding elements.

With the patient's lower extremities kept in a hip/knee flexion position, the primary practitioner rolls the patient obliquely lateral and downward to elongate the lumbar fasciae and musculature (Figure 12.37). The first assistant helps to stabilize the patient on the table.

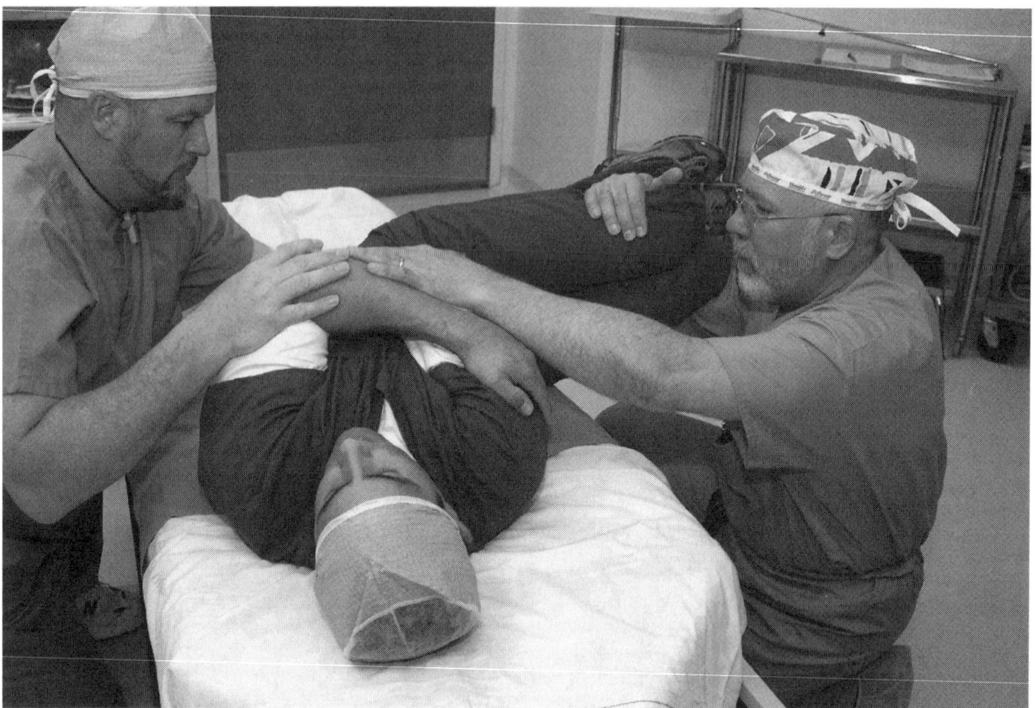

**FIGURE 12.37**

Goal: To reach maximum end range of the lower lumbar holding elements.

The primary practitioner then brings the knees in the hip-knee flexion position into his or her stomach and tractions cephalad and oblique, and then downward to achieve maximum traction (Figure 12.38). The first assistant stabilizes the patient on the table.

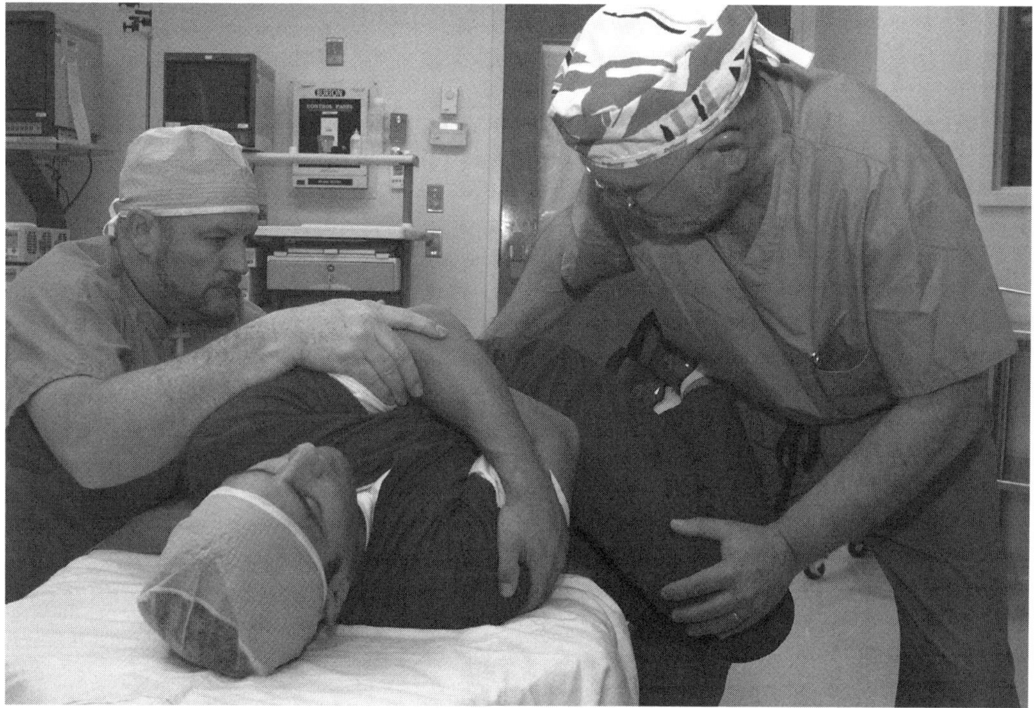

**FIGURE 12.38**

Goal: To achieve maximum end range of the mid to upper lumbar holding elements.

This process is then repeated on the opposite side by the first assistant while the primary practitioner acts as a stabilizer (Figure 12.39 and Figure 12.40).

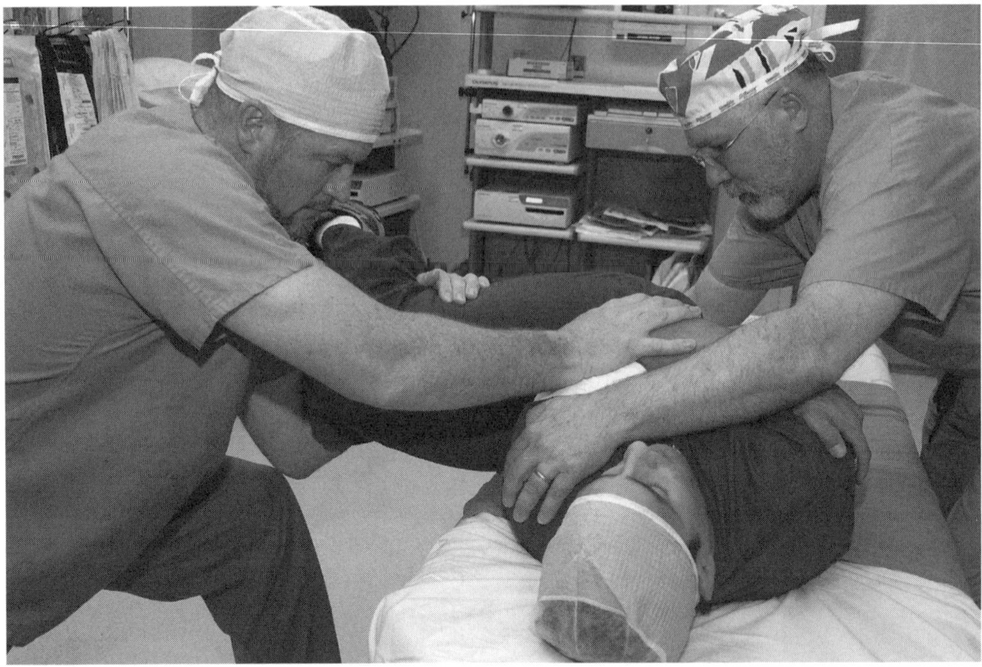

**FIGURE 12.39**

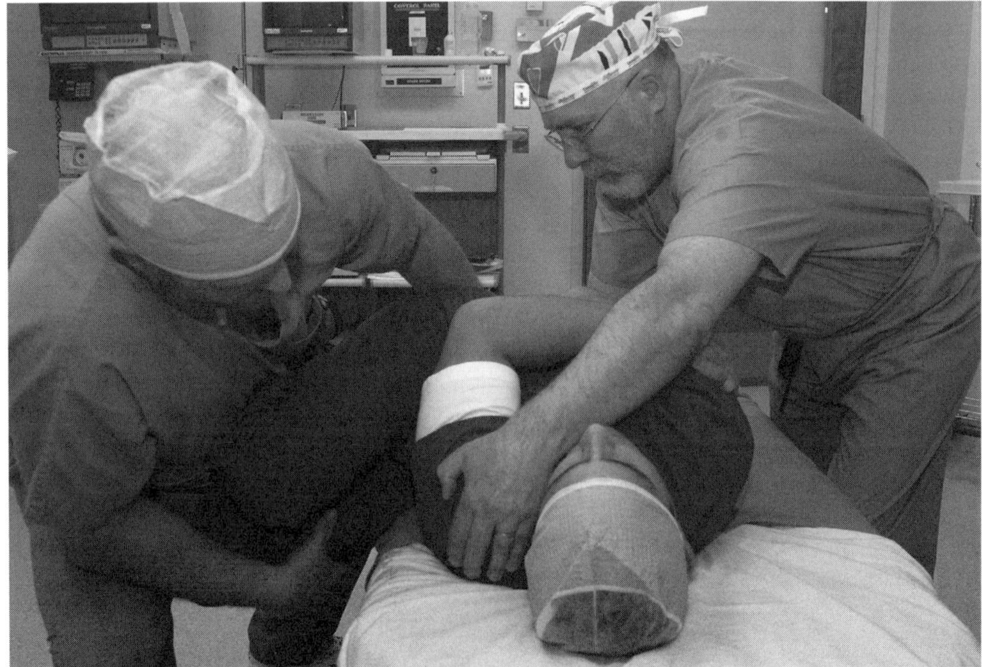

**FIGURE 12.40**

Goal: To achieve maximum end range of the lumbar holding elements bilaterally.

With the use of the undersheets, the patient is then carefully placed in the left/right decubitus position and positioned so that the lumbar spine is centrally located over the kidney plate to the point where the lumbar spine is attaining the horizontal, and derotated to avoid facet imbrication (Figure 12.41).

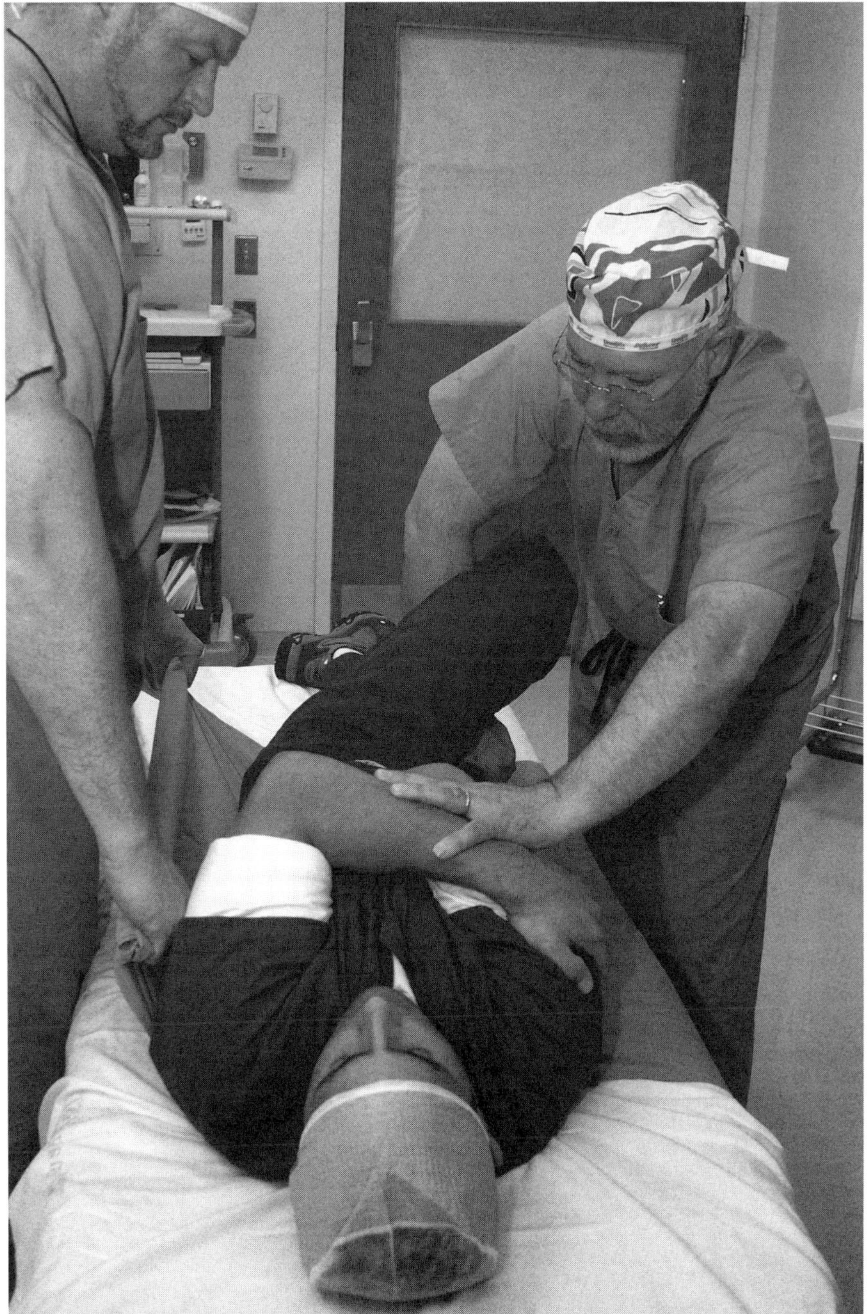

**FIGURE 12.41**

Goal: To reduce facet imbrication and disc stress for the lumbar adjustive procedure.

With the patient in the side-lying decubitus position and facing the primary practitioner, the first assistant contacts the sacral base and the patient's knee in an underhand position (Figure 12.42). The lower extremity is then extended and anterior traction is accomplished by the first assistant applying countertraction on the sacral base as he or she brings the lower extremity posterior in a horizontal arch. The top knee is kept in a bent position and the lower knee is slightly bent.

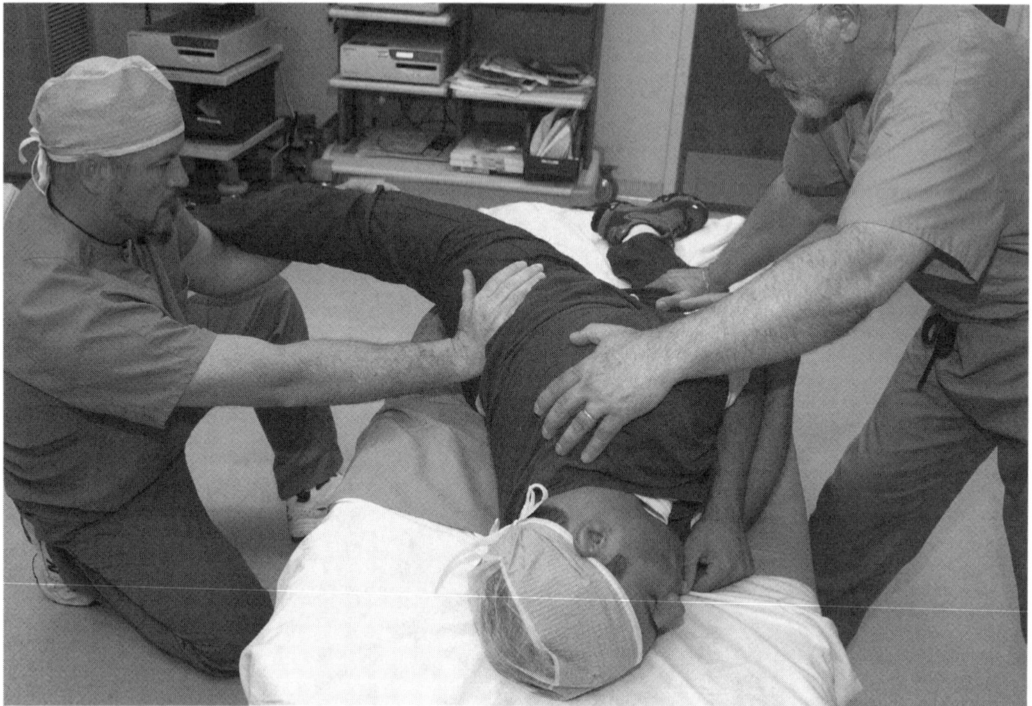

**FIGURE 12.42**

Goal: To reach maximum end range for the iliopsoas stretch.

The first assistant then straightens out the patient's knee from the position the patient was in previously, and brings the lower extremity more down toward the floor, tractioning away from the table in a hip extension maneuver (Figure 12.43).

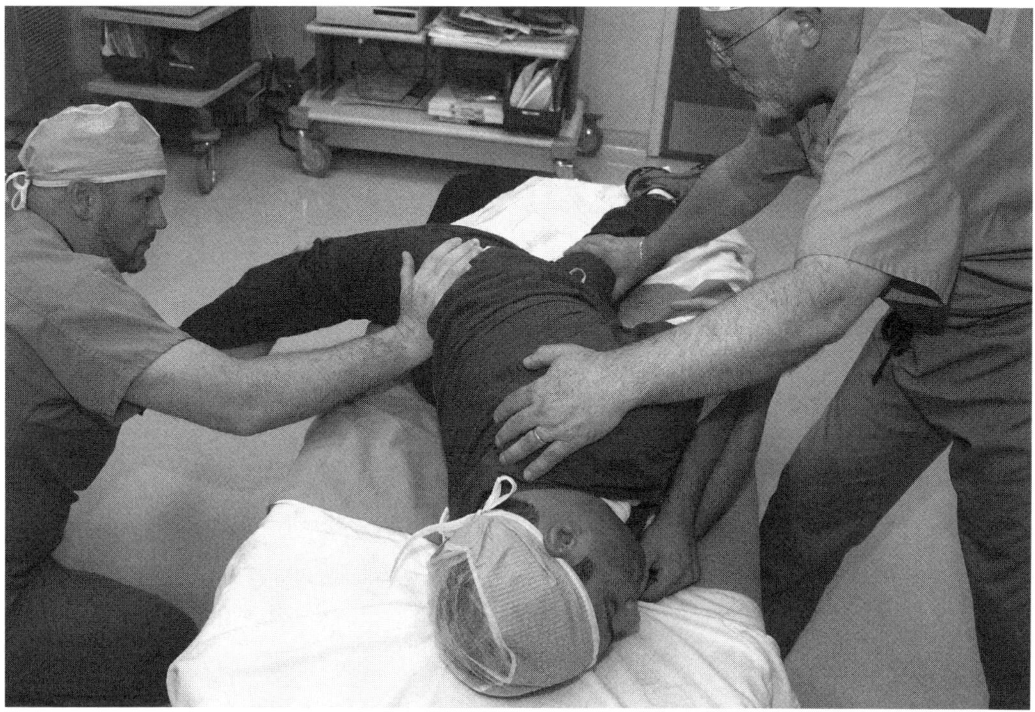

**FIGURE 12.43**

Goal: To reach maximum end range in stretching both the tensor fasciae lata (TFL) and the iliotibial band (ITB).

The primary practitioner then repositions the patient for closed reduction adjustment(s) of the lumbar vertebrae, which will complete the desired spinal segmental corrections using a low-velocity impulse thrust (Figure 12.44).

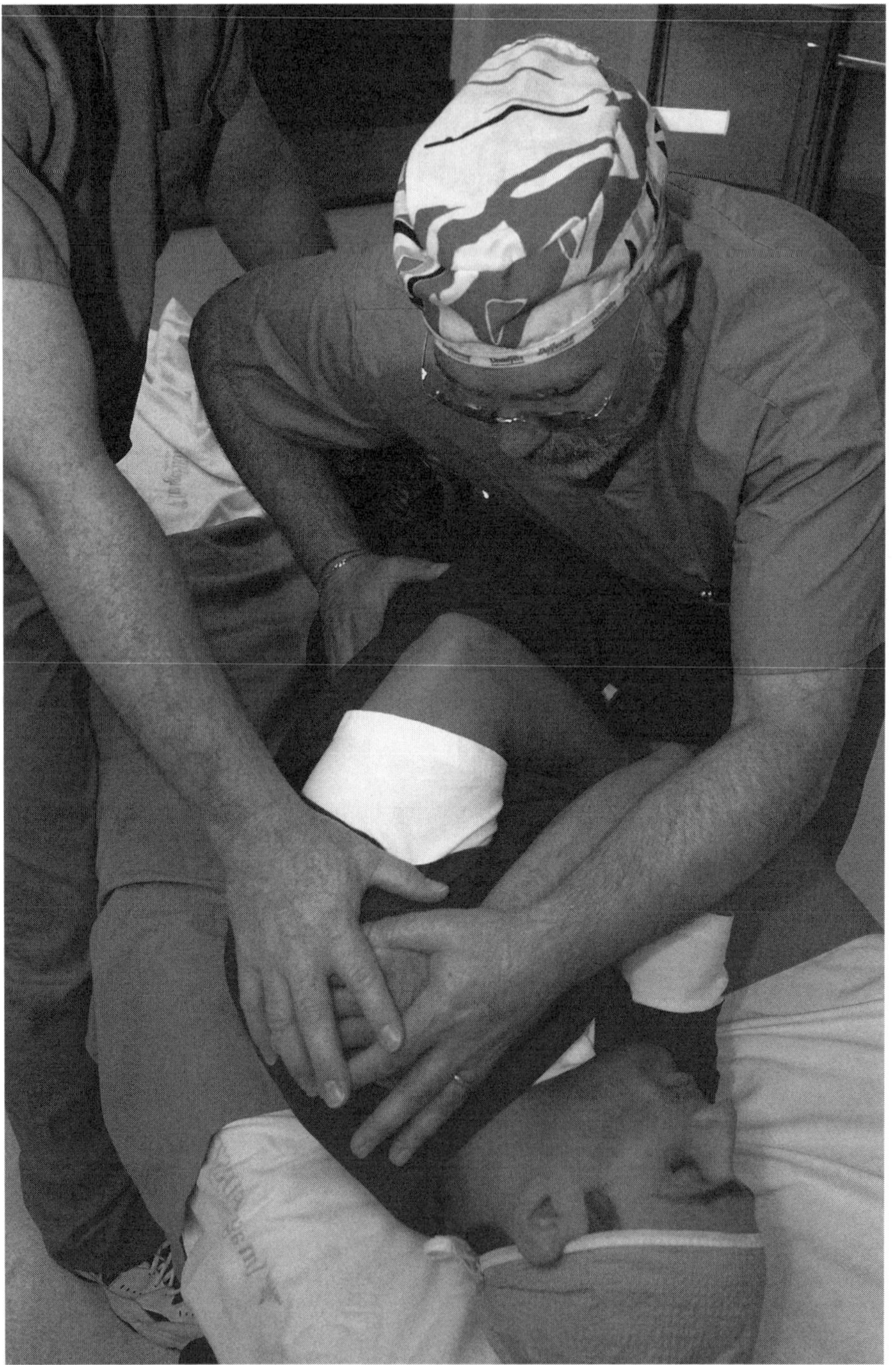

**FIGURE 12.44**

Goal: To correct the spinal segmental dysfunction necessary to achieve the desired results.

The patient is then repositioned on the table with the help of the undersheets. The first assistant then carefully rolls the patient to the opposite side into a sidelying decubitus position. The same procedures are then followed by the primary practitioner for the purpose of stretching the iliopsoas and the TFL (Figures 12.45, 12.46, and 12.47).

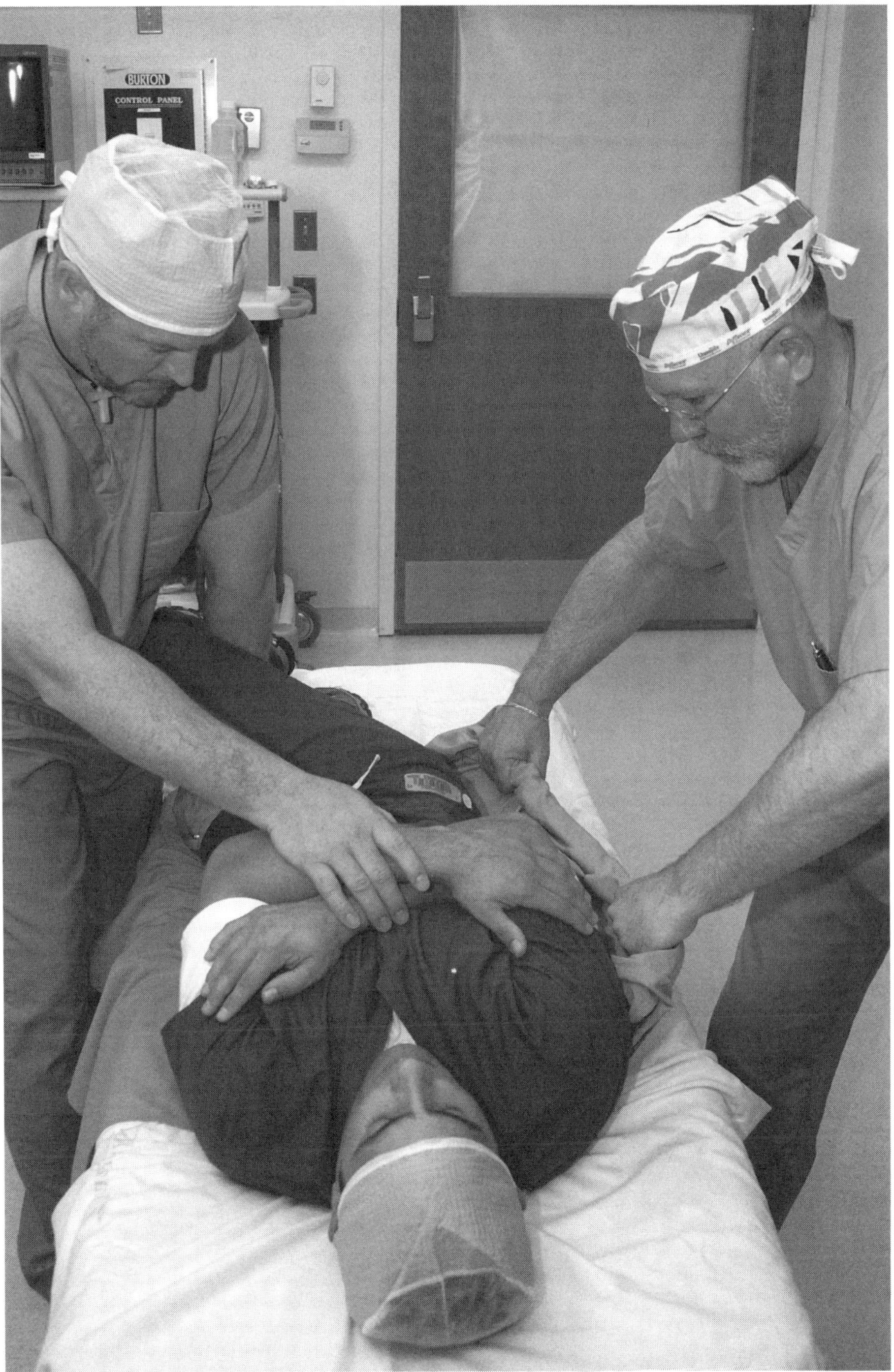

**FIGURE 12.45**

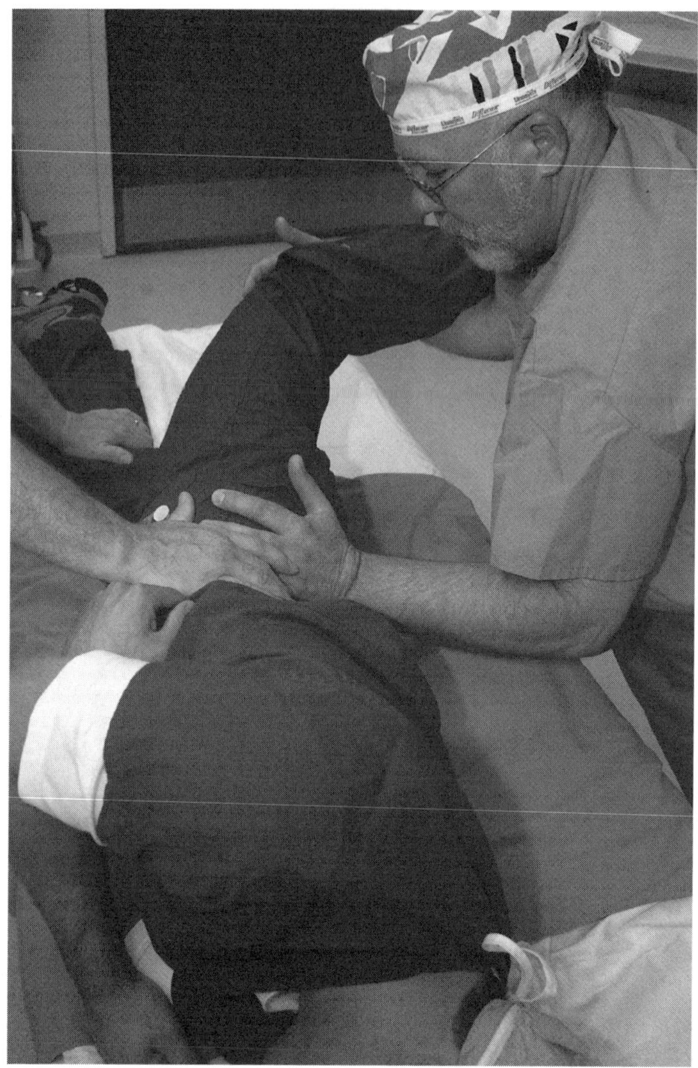

**FIGURE 12.46**

Goal: To achieve maximum end range necessary for stretching the iliopsoas and the TFL.

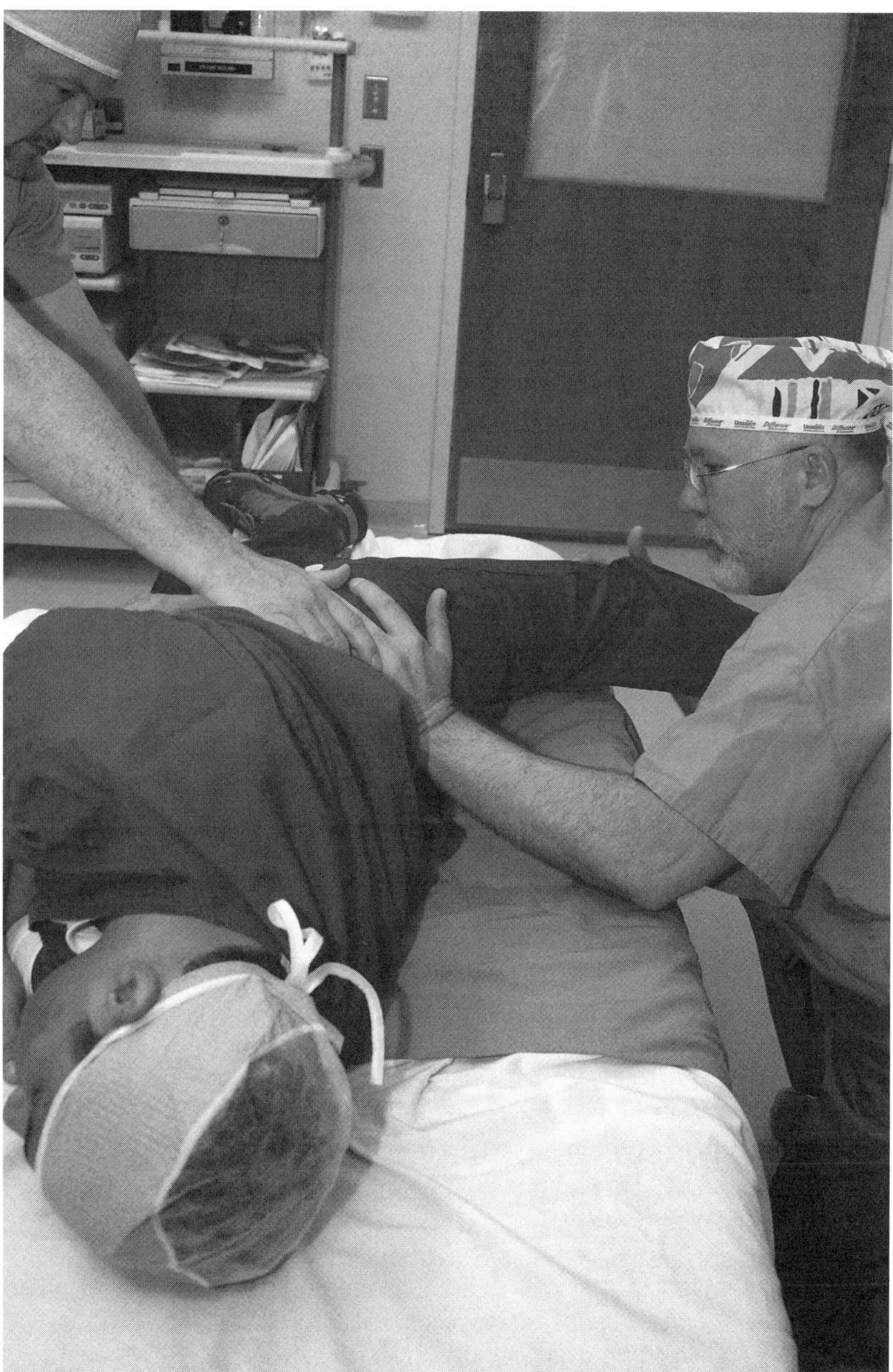

**FIGURE 12.47**

The first assistant then accomplishes a closed reduction adjustment of the posterior/superior iliac spine (PSIS) if necessary using a low-velocity impulse-thrust (Figure 12.48). The primary practitioner may prefer to have the patient stabilized in order to move to the opposite side so that the desired adjustive correction can be accomplished.

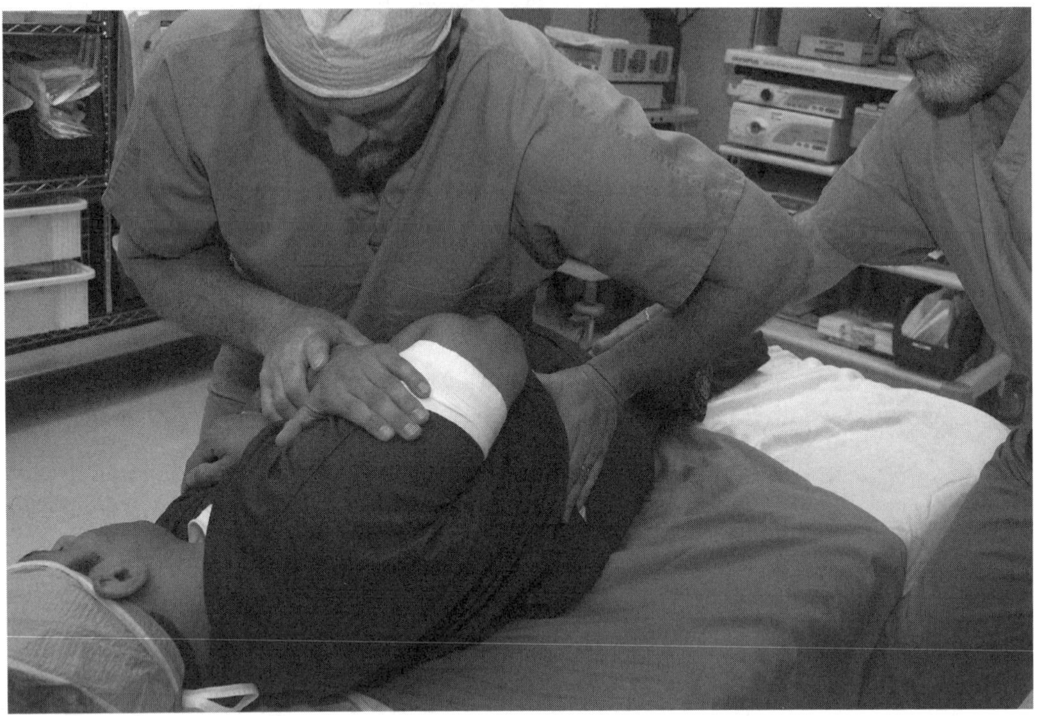

**FIGURE 12.48**

Goal: To complete the desired adjustive procedure for the spinal/pelvic segmental dysfunction.

The patient is then repositioned in the neutral supine position and the arms are brought to the side. The patient is transferred to the gurney (if the procedure was not performed on the gurney) and the guard rails are pulled up to prevent the patient's arms from falling. The patient is then transferred to the recovery area.

## PATIENT'S INFORMATION/INSTRUCTIONS
## FOLLOWING ANESTHESIA

1. Fluids and a snack will be provided in recovery.
2. Patient can have a light meal after 1 hour and resume a normal diet after 4 hours.
3. Patient should not drive the day of the procedure.
4. Patient is not to do any manual work the day of the procedure.
5. Patient should not make any major decisions the day of the procedure.
6. All patients should return to the practitioner's office following the MUA.
7. Any patient experiencing any adverse effects should contact their treating practitioner immediately.

## REFERENCES


1. Capps, S., Texas College of Chiropractic, syllabus: Manipulation under anesthesia; postgraduate course of study, 1992.
2. Gordon, R., Cornerstone Professional Education Inc., MUA course syllabus sponsored by the National University of Health Sciences, 5th ed., August 1998.
3. Gordon, R., with contribution from Furno, P., Cornerstone Professional Education Inc., MUA syllabus currently sponsored by the National University of Health Sciences, 5th ed., August 1998.
4. National Academy of MUA Physicians (NAMUAP): Standards and protocols for MUA, written 1995; rev. October 1996.
5. Guyton, A.C., *Textbook of Medical Physiology*, 4th ed., WB Saunders., Philadelphia, 1971: 113–16.
6. Guyton, A.C., *Textbook of Medical Physiology*, 7th ed., WB Saunders, Philadelphia, 1986: 113–16.
7. Kisner, C., Colby, L.A., Stretching, from *Therapeutic Exercise Foundations and Techniques*, 2nd ed., F.A. Davis, Philadelphia, 1990: 109–20.
8. Kotlke, F.J., Therapeutic exercise to maintain mobility, in *Handbook of Physical Medicine and Rehabilitation*, Kruser, Kotlke, Elwood (Eds.), Philadelphia, WB Saunders, 1971: 389–401.
9. Roy, S., Irvin, R., *Sports Medicine, Prevention, Evaluation, Management, and Rehabilitation*, Prentice-Hall, Englewood Cliffs, NJ, 1983: 125–28.
10. Alter, M., *The Science of Stretching*, 2nd ed., Champaign, IL, Human Kinetics Pub., 1988: 13–21, 23–31, 33–41.
11. Hill, A.V., The transition from rest to full activity in muscle: the velocity of shortening, *Proc. Roy. Soc. B.*, 1951: 138: 329–32.
12. Hill, A.V., *First and Last Experiments in Muscle Mechanics,* Cambridge University Press, Cambridge, U.K., 1970.

# 13 Post-MUA Physical Therapy and Rehabilitation Guidelines

*Fred E. Russo*

The scope of this chapter is designed to offer the physician some insights into the varied physical therapy modalities and their applications for the post-MUA patient. Since the author advocates the use of interferential current (IFC) with cryotherapy initially (in acute and subacute stages) and then with thermotherapy in the chronic stage (days 10 and on) of the rehabilitation process, the applications and theory of thermotherapy and cryotherapy as they relate to the post-MUA physical therapy regime will be the main focus of this discussion. This chapter will not provide in-depth detail over which electrical modality to choose, the advantages and disadvantages of each modality, or how it is to be applied.

As noted in the MUA protocols (NAMUAP), physical therapy is to be carried out daily, beginning after the first MUA and continuing 7–10 days thereafter, with the rehabilitation portion continuing on through day 35.

The rehabilitative process begins in the acute and subsequent subacute stage of healing days 1–5. The goals of these stages are to[1]

1   Control inflammation
2.  Create analgesic environment (for manipulated area)
3.  Limit edema formation
4.  Decrease joint effusion
5.  Establish environment for new collagen formation
6.  Reassure patient and stabilize doubts and fears about MUA

In the acute and subacute stage the patient's main concern will be doubt and fear with respect to the latent pain residual post-MUA. Analgesia and control of inflammation, local to the affected area, is a must to help ease their fears. Ice/cold packs and IFC are used to accomplish this goal.

The results of cryotherapy have long been documented as a benefit in controlling the inflammatory process. Some of the physiologic responses to cryotherapy that are important with respect to the post-MUA patient are as follows:[2,3]

*   Vasoconstriction of vasculature
*   Decreased nerve conduction velocity
*   Decreased metabolism
*   Enkephalin production

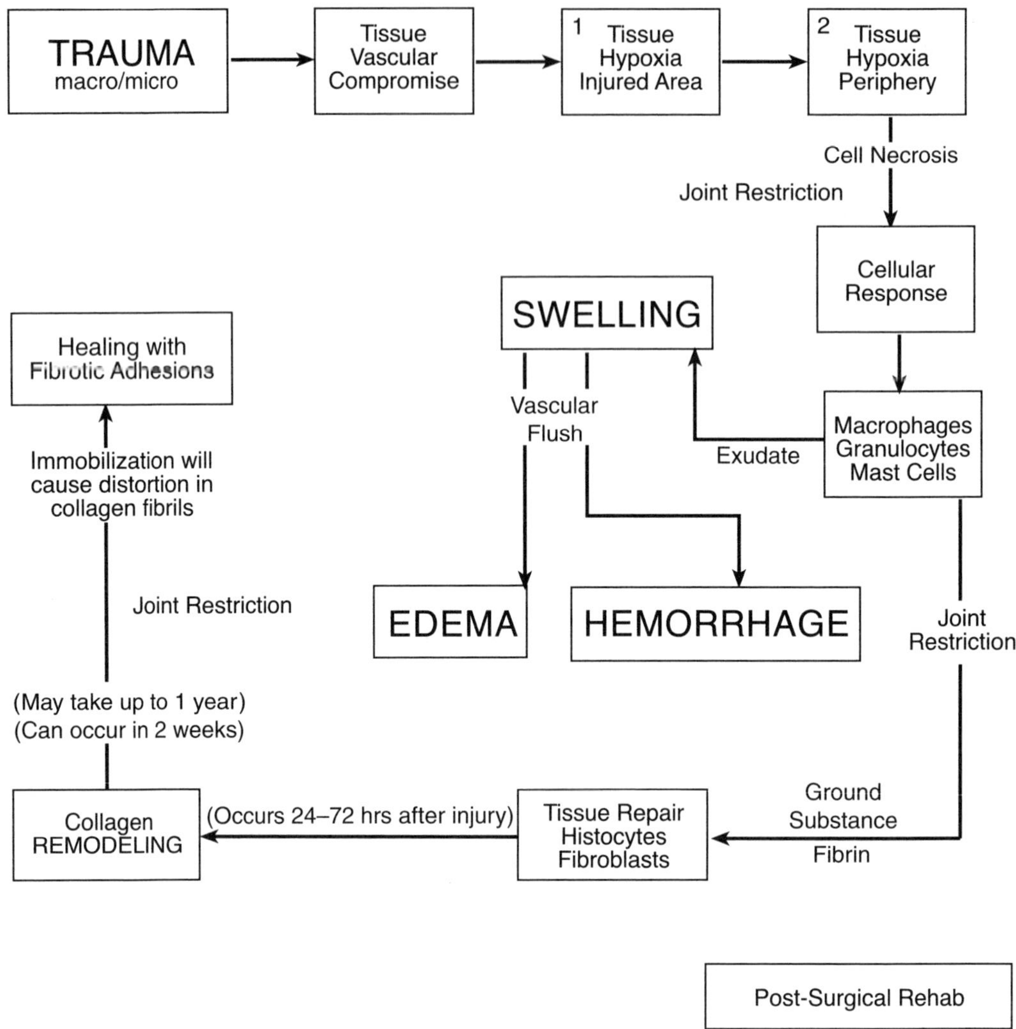



**FIGURE 13.1** The inflammatory cycle — the core of MUA.

It is the opinion of this author that cryotherapy, initiated as early as possible (post-MUA), has the most beneficial effect in immediate care of acute musculoskeletal injuries. Studies show that patients are rehabilitated nearly twice as fast with early cryotherapy (treatment initiated within 36 h post-injury) than with late cryotherapy (treatment initiated after 36 h).[1]

Many authorities are in agreement that cold application decreases blood flow via local and reflex vasoconstriction, thereby diminishing the amount of hemorrhage into traumatized tissue. Application of cold also decreases the local metabolism that serves to protect against secondary hypoxic injury to the tissue cells on the periphery of the primary injury.[1,3] (See Figure 13.1.)

Trauma is induced to an area, resulting in compromise of tissue microvasculature and macrovasculature. This causes primary tissue hypoxia in the traumatized area, for which cold has no overt beneficial effect, as well as secondary tissue hypoxia, which affects the tissue surrounding but not including the primary trauma area. By decreasing the metabolism for the cells at the periphery of the traumatized area by application of cold, these cells can then survive the initial compromise of the injured vasculature. This will result in less total damaged tissue, will produce a smaller cellular response, and will allow for quicker repair on a smaller injury site. Although cold application may not have any profound effect on primary tissue hypoxia, it does appear to have a profound effect on the inflammatory reaction of these tissues at the primary injury site.[3]

In response to tissue injury, the body reacts by sending macrophages, granulocytes, and mast cells to the site. These cells can survive under anaerobic conditions and serve as primary mediators in tissue cleanup and repair. Macrophages eat up cellular debris, which is carried out of the injured area by the local vasodilatory effect on the surrounding vasculature via bradykinin and the mast cells as they secrete histamine and serotonin. If cryotherapy is applied as soon as possible (less than 2 hours) post-injury, the inflammatory response by the body can be greatly diminished. Swelling is a symptom that results from the inflammatory response. It can be due to:

- Direct hemorrhage into traumatized area
- Edema formation
- Local tissue reaction to increased vasodilation from chemical mediators and the repair process

Under normal conditions, the capillary filtration pressure may be slightly positive, causing a flow of fluid from the vascular system into the tissues. This results in the gradual buildup of fluid, which is carried away by the lymphatic system and returned to the vasculature system. "Edema results from an increase in tissue osmotic pressure, which is caused by increased free proteins which attract fluid."[3] Therefore, as the damaged tissue is being broken down by macrophages, increased amounts of free protein are liberated, causing increased edema. The greater the extent of tissue damage, the greater the edema accumulation. This process can account for the delayed onset of most swelling. By utilizing cryotherapy, there will be decreased secondary hypoxic injury response and decreased tissue debris. This will result in less free protein, lower tissue osmotic pressure and, therefore, less edema.[3,4]

As inflammation and cellular debris are controlled, cellular regeneration can begin. This starts by endothelial cell proliferation, resulting in capillary bud formation. These eventually connect to reform the injured vasculature, which allows for transport of oxygen and important nutrients (vitamins, amino acids, enzymes) to the damaged area. Once oxygen presence is reestablished (terminating the cell destructive anaerobic environment), fibroblasts can then become active, which will add to collagen production. As collagen is produced, an enyme collagenase is being released by the continued cleanup efforts of the macrophages and granulocytes, which results in dissolution of a portion of the collagen laid down. This occurs primarily during the first 2 weeks post-injury. Therefore, during these first 2 weeks, the collagen that is produced will be of decreased tensile strength. These healing tissues are then reinforced by ground substance, which adds strength and defines the character of the collagen that will eventually develop.[1]

It is the author's belief that the crucial period in the patient's rehabilitation post-MUA is at this point. As the old fibrotic adhesions are broken, new ones can and will form identical to the ones that the procedure was designed to eliminate. This is why the initial phase of the rehabilitation process (i.e., cryotherapy) is vital, along with the reestablishment and preservation of full range of motion to the affected area. As the collagen is newly formed and is of decreased tensile strength, the initiation of passive range of motion (PROM) exercise is imperative so that, as the ground substance reinforces the healing areas, flexibility is maintained.[1] This will result in flexible adhesion formation that will promote spinal stability yet maintain full active range of motion (AROM). It should also be noted that full collagen maturation may take up to one year.[1,5,6]

Now that local metabolism and the inflammatory response are under control, the patient's sensory perception of pain can now be addressed as cryotherapy and electrotherapy are combined.

It is beyond the scope of this section to explain the neurophysiology of the body's response to the perception and transmission of pain. (Refer to Chapter 3.)

By the application of cryotherapy, both sensory and motor nerve conduction velocities are similarly affected. As the temperature (both on the skin and eventually intramuscular) drops, so does the sensory and motor nerve conduction velocity. Numerous studies corroborate this finding.[7–10] Several factors are involved in considering the varied rate of decrease noted:

- Temperature range of cooling modality selected
- Overlying tissue density
- Depth of nerve from cryotherapy application
- Length of application

These studies are important due to the areas of the body affected by the MUA procedure, namely the cervical (C-spine), upper thoracic (T-spine), and lumbar spine (L-spine.)

The C-spine region and the paracervical musculature are, on most patients, the thinnest areas in relation to tissue density and depth of nerve roots. It should, therefore, follow that sensory and motor nerve conduction velocities should be decreased quickly with respect to time needed to achieve analgesia via cryotherapy. Subsequently, increased times should be necessary for the T-spine and L-spine regions, respectively, due to the increased tissue density related to the overlying subcutaneous tissue and musculature. This is, however, not absolute, as patient size, weight, and musculature will vary individually. In the C-spine, we apply cryotherapy in the form of cold packs for 10–15 min vs. 15–30 min in the L-spine for at least the initial 3 d of post-MUA physical therapy. The continuation of cryotherapy utilization beyond day 3 depends on the patient's tolerance. If severe pain persists, the doctor may choose to extend the duration to help manage the pain cycle. Like any modality, cryotherapy is not without contraindications, which are as follows:[2,3,11]

- Primary and secondary Raynaud's disease
- Hypersensitivity to cold
- Previous frostbite
- Desensitized skin area
- Vasospastic disorders and cardiac conditions

Do not apply cryotherapy directly to exposed skin. Always place at least one layer of toweling down between the cryotherapy of choice and the patient's skin. It is useful to wet the toweling layer in warm water to help ease the patient's initial response to the cold application.

In addition to the analgesic effect that cryotherapy alone will produce, electrotherapy is a welcomed adjunct in helping to disrupt the pain cycle. (See the flowchart in Figure 13.2.) The general goals of electrotherapy are to:[2,12,13]

- Relieve pain and promote analgesia
- Decrease muscle spasms
- Stimulate muscle tissue to elicit a contraction
- Stimulate microcirculation
- Decrease edema by promoting lymphatic drainage

All of these goals are achievable with the advent of IFC, as well as many other electrical muscle stimulating modalities, as long as the pulses per second (pps) or cycles per second (Hz) can be preset and changed as desired. Here are some terms to be familiar with:[12,14,15]

1. **Intensity:** Amplitude or volume of current flow expressed to the patient.
    a. **Sensory:** Very light "pins and needles" or "tingling" sensation perceived by patient.
    b. **Light motor:** Increase volume/amplitude to elicit a muscle contraction, then decrease volume just below the point where the muscle contraction was noted.
    c. **Motor:** Amplitude is increased until a visible muscle contraction is elicited.
2. **Frequency:** Repetition rate of a given wave form expressed in pps or Hz.[16]

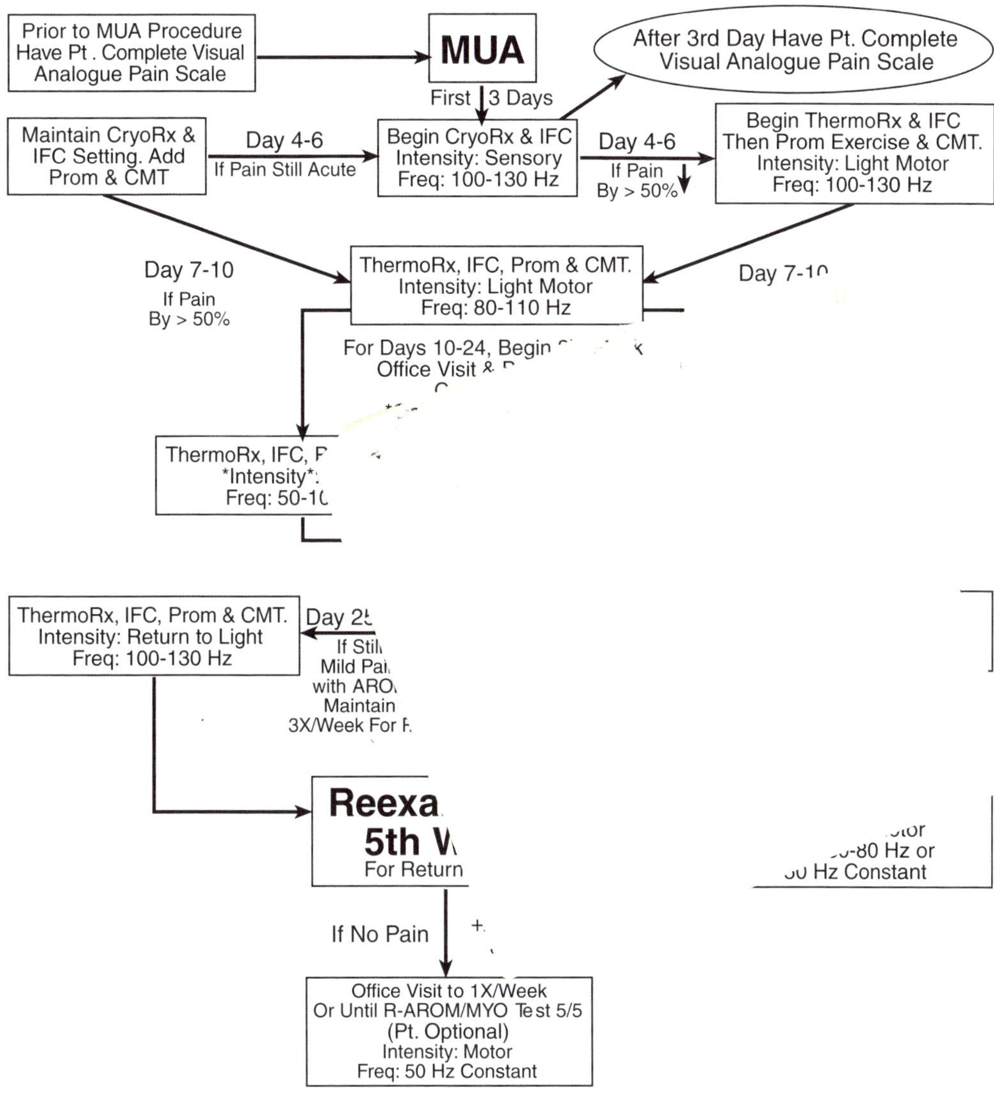


**FIGURE 13.2**

Table 13.1 has been adapted from several sources and is to be used as a guide in selecting the type of physiological response the practitioner or therapist wishes to elicit from the body for a given phase in the rehabilitative scheme.[12–18]

Once the choice of modality is made, electrode placement is to be considered. Important factors in choosing electrode type and configuration are as follows:

- Depth of area to be treated (superficial vs. deep)
- Localization and pain origin or area of discomfort
- Determination of appropriate nerve roots, and dermatomal pattern
- Size of electrodes
- Type of electrodes

When using IFC, the closer the electrodes are to one another, the more superficial the treatment. Therefore, the farther away they are, the deeper the penetration.[12,13,18] The size and composition for

---

**TABLE 13.1**
**Pulse Rate in Hz**

**Clinical Objective**

| | |
|---|---|
| 1–4 or 1–5 | Chronic pain modulation |
| | Beta Endorphin production |
| 1–20 | Muscle fasiculation contraction |
| 10–50 | Stimulate arterial blood flow to muscles |
| 40 | Tetanic muscle contraction without fatigue |
| 20–50 | Reduction of chronic interstitial edema |
| 50 | Tetanic muscle contraction with fatigue |
| 80+ | Tetanic muscle contraction with fatigue |
| | Enkephalin production |
| | Acute pain modulation |
| | Reduction of acute interstitial edema |
| | Stimulate microcirculation |
| 90–110 | Sensory nerve sedation |
| 130+ | Nociceptive system sedation |

---

the electrodes also play an important role. The two types of electrodes discussed are the basic carbon-backed and the adhesive gel-backed, although many other similar models and types are commercially available. The carbon-backed are 3" round and need to be held in close contact to the skin to help decrease tissue resistance via sandbags, hot moist packs (HMP)/cold moist packs (CMP), or velcro strapping. These are fine on flat surfaces of the body where bony contours are not a factor, i.e., the paraspinal musculature of the L-spine region. However, in treating the C-spine region separately, the use of the adhesive gel-backed is more appropriate as they are available in varied sizes and shapes. In addition, the smaller the electrode, the greater the current density per pad. Therefore, mixing different-sized electrodes creates a mixing of current density to a treatment area.

Since the author advocates the use of IFC at our office, these setups will be discussed first. Refer to Figures 13.1, 13.2, and 13.3 for diagrammatic representation.[12,13,18]

1. **Bilateral:** The two pads from one channel are placed on one side of the spine while the two pads from the second channel are placed on the opposite side of the spine (Figure 13.3). This setup can be used when specific dermatomal localization is described by the patient or determined via neurological exam. Bilateral setup is useful for radiating pain referral patterns that affect both extremities.

   **Ex.:** Channel 1: The two pads are placed on the left side of the spine.
   Channel 2: The two pads are placed on the right side of the spine.

2. **Crisscross:** The two pads from one channel line on opposite sides of the spine and form an X with the pads from the second channel, which are placed identically opposite the spine at the same level of channel 1 (Figure 13.4 and Figure 13.5). This setup is used for pain that is diffused in localization or when deeper tissues need to be stimulated.

   **Ex. 1:** To provide analgesia for the C-spine only: Channel 1: One pad is placed on the left side of the C-spine at C-2, and the other pad is placed on the right side of the T-spine at T-2.
   Channel 2: One pad is placed on the right side of the C-spine at C-2 and the other pad is placed on the left side of the T-spine at T-2.

   **Ex. 2:** To treat the entire spine with analgesia:
   Channel 1: One pad is placed on the right side of the C-spine at C-2; C-4 and the other pad is placed on the left side of the L-spine at L-5.

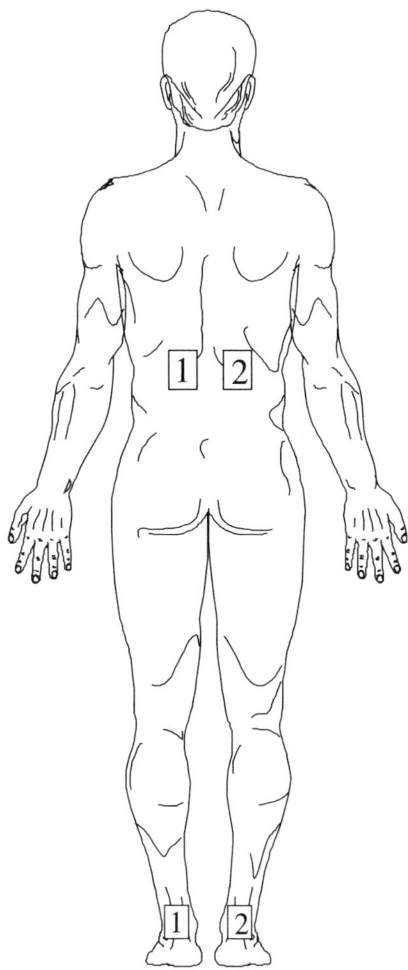

**FIGURE 13.3** Bilateral pad placement for radiating pain affecting both extremities.

  Channel 2: One pad is placed on the left side of the C-spine at C-2; C-4 and the other pad is placed on the right side of the L-spine at L-5.

  Note: The number of C-spine segments covered depends on the size of the adhesive electrode being used. The previous example assumes the use of the smallest-sized pad.

3. **Linear overlapping:** For radiating pain down a single extremity (Figure 13.6).

  **Ex.:** To provide analgesia for right-sided sciatica extending only to the knee: Channel 1: One pad is placed on the left side of the L-5 nerve root, and the other pad is placed at the right sciatic notch in the post gluteal fold.

  Channel 2:One pad is placed on the right side of the L-5 nerve root, and the other pad is placed just superior to the right popliteal fossa.

  Note: If pain extends all the way to the foot, then move the second pad of channel 1 from the sciatic notch to a point 5–6 in. distally at the post-lateral aspect of the thigh, and move the second pad from channel 2 just superior to the medial malleolar fossa.

The above example is just one way to alleviate a radiating pain pattern produced by an inflamed nerve root. Other applications are possible and may change with individual practitioner or therapist variance. Although there are a wide variety of electrical muscle stimulating modalities to choose

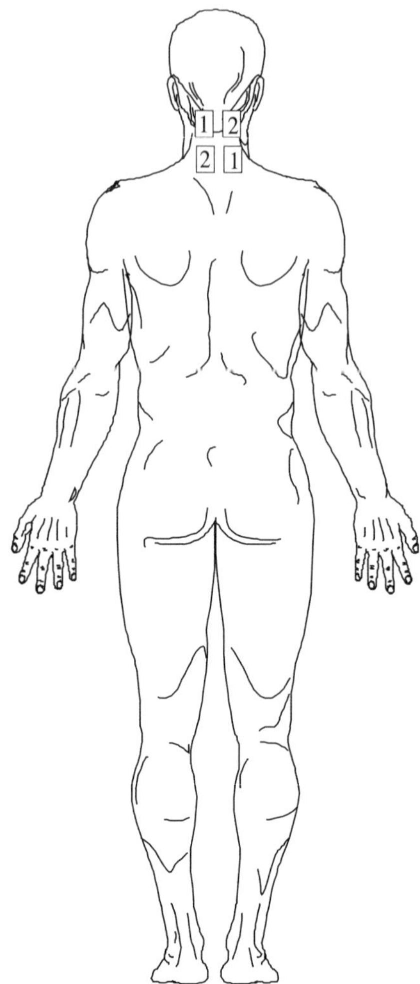

**FIGURE 13.4** Crisscross pad placement for providing analgesia to the cervical spine.

from, it is this author's opinion that IFC provides the broadest range of treatment capacity while minimizing patient discomfort via utilization of a sinusoidal wave form and 4000-Hz carrier frequency to help decrease tissue resistance. Due to the fact that practitioner variance with respect to knowledge, experience, and comfort in utilizing electrotherapy may be wide in range, the semantics of each particular modality and the cause and effect relationship that each has in comparison and contrast to each other will not be discussed.

Other modalities that bear mentioning are transcutaneous electrical nerve stimulator (TENS), low-volt direct current (Galvanism) (LVDC), high-volt pulsed direct current (HVPDC), high-volt alternating current (S 180 Russian Stimulation) (HVAC), low-volt alternating current (VMS, Med-collator) (LVAC), ultrasound (US), and diathermy.

Of the above mentioned, HVPDC is probably the most common modality found in a chiropractic office. Each modality has its own tenets and limitations; therefore, it is up to the individual practitioner to decide which one will have the most beneficial effect.

According to Savage, there are relatively few contraindications to IFC. These include the following:[18]

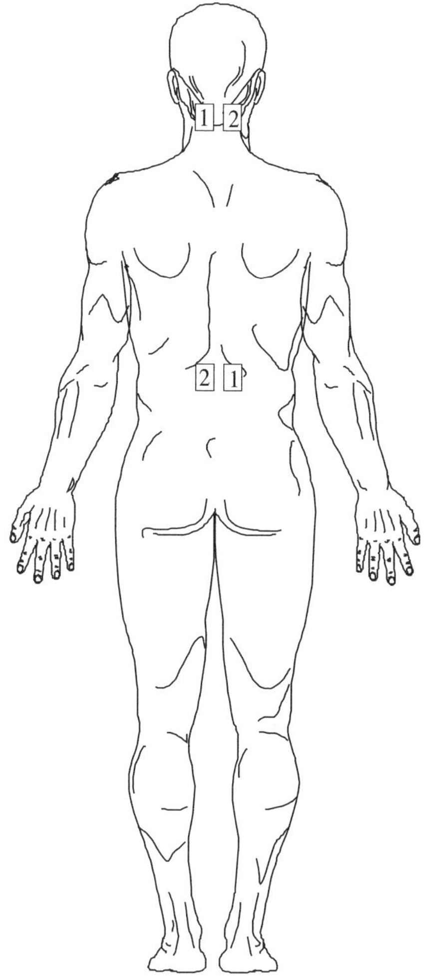

**FIGURE 13.5** Crisscross pad placement for treating the entire spine with analgesia.

- Patients with pacemakers
- Avoidance of stellate ganglion and of the heart itself
- Patients on anticoagulant medication for a thrombotic condition
- Patients with Miliary disease (TB) or any bacterial infections
- Shortwave diathermy (SWD) (IFC must be at least 20 ft. away or patient may experience current surge when SWD is turned off)
- Over the carotid sinus
- Avoidance of pregnant uterus or pelvic organs during menstruation

One distinct advantage that IFC offers over all the other electrical muscle stimulating modalities is that there is no contraindication to metallic implants or heat production in the tissues.[18]

It is generally recognized that some of the therapeutic effects of heat are as follows:[2,11]

- Analgesia
- Decreased muscle spasm
- Increased blood flow
- Increased extensibility in collagen tissues

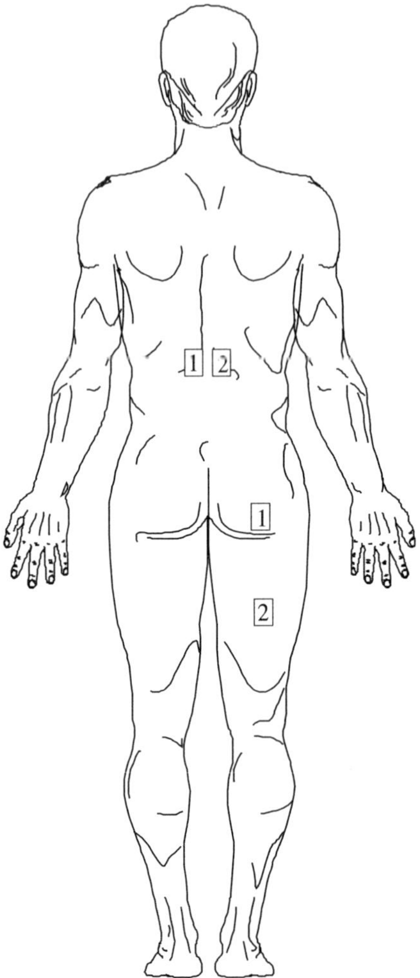

**FIGURE 13.6** Linear overlapping pad placement for radiating pain down a single extremity.

- Decreased joint stiffness
- Increased metabolic rate

These six effects were chosen due to their immediate relationship in the switch from cryotherapy to thermotherapy. "In any deep heating modality, heat results from the conversion of energy into heat as it penetrates into the tissues of the body."[11] Therefore, indications for choice of modality will depend on tissue density and composition of the involved area as noted previously. "If the temperature elevation in some parts of the exposed tissue reaches a point where increase in blood flow is triggered, cooling occurs selectively in that area, since blood rushing into this area is of a lower temperature than the temperature of the tissue heated."[11] This is important in discussing superficial versus deep heating. HMP and infrared are examples of superficial heaters that will raise the temperature at the skin level and possibly into the most superficial layer of subcutaneous fat (3–5 mm). They, however, are subject to the rapid cooling associated with the influx of blood to the skin level, due to the blood being at a significantly lower temperature than that of the tissues heated. HMP are made of silica gel contained in a cotton bag which is immersed in a water bath at 160°F–175°F. These are applied to the patient for 20–30 min with a minimum of six–eight towel layers between the HMP and the patient.

                                                  

The highest temperature is obtained in the skin after approximately 8 min at 42°C with a subsequent decrease in tissue temperature thereafter.[11] Tissues below the subcutaneous fat layer are not affected because the fat layer acts as a thermal insulator. Superficial heat (HMP) has been shown to help alleviate pain in a variety of musculoskeletal conditions. As Lehman and DeLateur noted,[11] with heat-induced increase of blood flow to musculature, pain that could be due to ischemia would be naturally decreased from the hyperemic effect.

Superficial application of heat does have its limitations, however. Many studies agree that tissue temperature elevations needs to be in the 40°C–45°C (104°F-113°F) range for therapy to be effective.[19–22] This is why deep-heating modalities are a better selection. Studies by Lehmann et al.[20] have shown that, although the therapeutic range can be achieved via superficial heaters, maintaining the optimal range over the course of the treatment cannot be accomplished because of the increased vasculature at the skin's surface. Also with HMP, over a period of 20 min, the temperature 1.0 cm below the skin's surface was only raised 3°C (from 34°C resting body temperature at skin surface to 37°C at 1 cm below surface). The skin surface temperature, however, was raised 10°C (from 32° to 42°C) over that same period.[11]

With deep heaters (SWD, US), limitations are not a problem. Both SWD and US have the capacity to raise tissue temperature to the desired therapeutic range and maintain it over the extended time period necessary for effective treatment. Deep-heating modalities may not always be indicated due to individual morphological variance or other physical contraindications. For example, in the C-spine region on a small-framed female, the tissue density may only be 1–2 cm in density, with the C-spine and associated nerve roots located very closely to that range. However, in an obese, large-framed male, a superficial heater would definitely not be indicated due to the limited penetrating power of HMP. Therefore, patient morphological structure and desired therapeutic physiologic response (elicited from the body by the chosen modality) must be carefully examined before treatment is initiated.

In the example of the large-framed male patient, if the desired effect is to be increased blood flow, then the deeper penetrating modalities are warranted. This reasoning is illustrated via studies by Siems et al.[22] and Guy et al.[16] Studies by Johns and Wright,[23] later confirmed by Baklund and Tiselius,[24] showed that elastic stiffness was significantly decreased by warming the joint. They found a "20% decrease in stiffness at 45°C as compared to 33°C when a selective joint was treated with superficial heat."[25]

Lehman[26] suggests a relationship between the percentage of hyperemia and temperature. His results indicated that the tissue temperature must be raised above 41°C to produce any significant reaction, and that a temperature nearer 45°C was needed to obtain a maximal response. They also showed that, "with a initial tissue temperature of 34°C, an increase in temperature to 40°C would produce a 77% increase in metabolic rate."[26]

The author's approach to the rehabilitation process (post-MUA) relates directly to the deposition and realignment of the collagen formation. "Most joint contractures are due to limitations in the range of motion resulting from shortened structures which cross the joint. In most of these cases, the tightness of the offending structure is the result of deposition of fibrous, that is, collagenous tissue."[11]

Kottke states that "after injury collagen fibrils can be detected as early as the second day (via electron microscope) by biochemical means by the third day, and by use of light microscope only a day or two later."[5]

Within 4–5 days, collagenous adhesions begin to form and histologic evidence of fibrosis may occur as early as 4 days. "Gross evidence of restriction of motion begins to occur in approximately 4 days and develops progressively from that time. Immobilizations of a normal joint for 4 weeks results in diminutions or loss of motion because of formation of dense connective tissue. Immobilization of an injured joint for 2 weeks results in connective fiber fusion and loss of motion at that joint."[5]

It therefore stands to reason that, if physical therapy, PROM, and manipulative therapy (CMT, OMT) are not initiated immediately, then the body will repair the injury site as it sees fit. The author refers the reader to the collagen deposition, repair, and realignment section in Chapters 2 and 4 for a more detailed description of the repair process.

It is imperative that the patient's progress be monitored very closely with respect to the range of motion increasing and the amount of pain present daily. This can be accomplished by thorough questioning (before beginning therapy) pertaining to the quality, location, duration, onset, and consistency of the pain. If the rehabilitation process does not proceed along the guidelines as indicated, the patient could possibly expect a return to abnormal function/dysfunctional state.

Three types of connective tissue can form: organized, loose (areolar), and dense. Organized connective tissue is the type that forms tendons and ligaments where collagen fibers and fibrocytes form linear columns along the long axis of the tendon or ligament to be repaired. Loose (or areolar) and dense are the types that the rehabilitative approach focuses on. Loose connective tissue is the type that forms between organs, fascia, capsules, intramuscular layers, and subcutaneous tissue, where movement can occur repeatedly.

"Histologically, networks of collagen and reticular fibers run in all directions without a regular pattern. When these fibers are laid down or replaced, their length and mobility between attachments depend on the motion of the part during the period of formation."[5] Therefore, the less movement allowed as the new network of collagen is forming, the greater the potential for restricted movement (in that same area pre-MUA) to return. This course of action will lead to the formation of dense connective tissue, most commonly found in scars.

"In areas where motion does not occur, such as fascial planes, and capsules of muscle or organs, collagen is laid down as dense meshworks, sheets or bands. In areas immobilized by edema, dense connective tissue will develop. If the part is externally immobilized, a dense contracted scar will form. But if motion is maintained during healing of a wound, loose connective tissue will form."[5]

It is for this reason that the early advent (days 4–6) of the stretching and PROM are imperative. The physician or therapist has direct control over the type of connective tissue that is allowed to form and the range of motion of that particular area affected. With the addition of the continued manipulations over the remainder of the rehabilitation (days 4–35), normal joint range of motion and biomechanics can also be reestablished for that previously affected area.

This concludes the discussion on the pertinent theories behind the physical therapy modalities and their application. The reader is now referred to the flowchart in Figure 13.2 for the remainder of this chapter.

In order to establish a firm baseline on the patient's subjective pain response and progress, this author suggests utilizing a visual analogue pain scale (Figure 13.7).

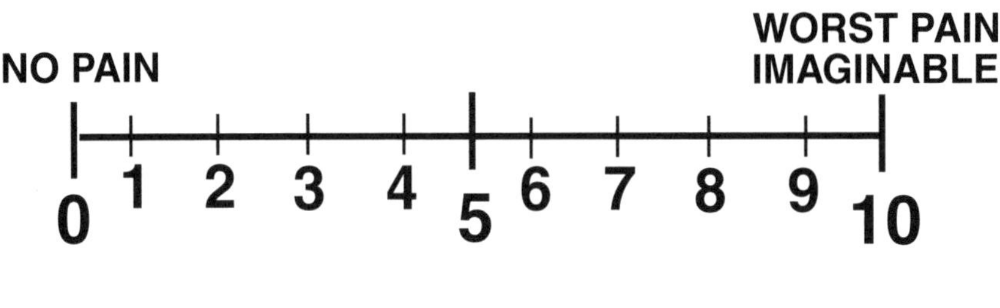


**FIGURE 13.7** Visual analog scale.

The patient must fill out a pain scale prior to undergoing the MUA procedure, after the third MUA procedure, and prior to initiating therapy on day 7 as well as after the final reexam. This scale will be utilized as a prognostic indicator to monitor when the switch over to thermotherapy will be indicated.

For the patient's first 3 days of MUA, the patient should receive cryotherapy on the manipulated area of the spine as soon as possible post-manipulation. This can be provided by the outpatient facility or by the patient bringing in ice in a small cooler.

If the patient is to receive physical therapy at the hospital, the intensity should be set at "sensory" and the frequency at 130 Hz "constant" or a sweep of 100–140 Hz. These settings are also utilized in the private office.

If the patient has to travel an appreciable distance back to his or her practitioner's office, proper instruction on the application of cryotherapy should be thoroughly explained.

On days 4–6, if the pain on the visual analog pain scale (Figure 13.7) is decreased by 50%, thermotherapy is initiated by either using HMP placed on top of the IFC setups or by preheating the affected areas with SWD or US and then utilizing the IFC therapy. In either case, the intensity should be a "light motor" muscle contraction, with a small sweep of 100—130 Hz or a "constant" setting of 130 Hz.

If thermotherapy is initiated (days 4–6), PROM exercise is also added. It is recommended that the stretching techniques be implemented as outlined in the MUA protocol prior to instituting the PROM exercises. Utilize passive movement throughout only the "pain-free" range of the appropriate spinal area involved. Examples of standard PROM and AROM exercises can be found in most physical therapy texts. This author's reference came from *Therapeutic Exercise — Foundation and Technique*, by Kisner and Colby.[27] This exercise should be followed by manipulation to the appropriately involved area.

After day 3 of post-MUA, if the pain is not decreased by 50% the practitioner/therapist should maintain the use of cryotherapy applied over to the IFC setup. The intensity should be retained at "sensory" level and the frequency at 130 Hz constant. PROM and chiropractic or osteopathic manipulative therapy (CMT, OMT) should still be continued even if pain is not decreased by the required 50%. Prior to initiating therapy on day 7, the patient should be given another visual analogue pain scale. By this time, the patient pain intensity should be decreased by 50%. If so, then proceed to the settings for days 7–10. If not, then maintain the use of ice and IFC, using the frequency noted above for days 7–10, while again also instituting PROM and manipulation.

If the therapy for days 4–6 is progressing favorably, (i.e., pain at approximately "3" on the visual analogue pain scale), then for days 7–10, the only difference from days 4–6 is the changing of the IFC frequency from the 100—130 Hz sweep to 80–110 Hz sweep.[13,17] This will begin to elicit a muscle contraction for a portion of the sweep (at 80 Hz)[18] while still sedating the sensory nerves at 110 Hz.[18]

This now concludes daily care for days 11–24; at this point, the office visits are reduced to three times a week. If the PROM exercise is pain free, the patient may begin to experience muscle contractions in the physical therapy sessions and begin AROM exercises two times a day at home. Thermotherapy and IFC are continued, but now the frequency and intensity are changed to promote more muscle involvement. The frequency sweep is broad, with the baseline at 50 Hz (for muscle strengthening)[13,17] contraction to 100 Hz, which will still provide some sedation of the sensory nerves.[18] Keep in mind, the more broad the frequency sweep, the less amount of time the current spends on a given frequency within that sweep. Therefore, a more "narrow" or even "constant" setting should be preferred when an analgesic environment is desired, versus a "broad" sweep for working the muscles. The intensity for this 2-week period should be "motor" (i.e., a visible muscle contraction) with manipulation to follow the physical therapy.

This is now the prerehabilitation phase of post-MUA therapy.[28] During these two weeks, the patient is to be given AROM exercise to be done at least two times a day at home. These exercises are to be absent of any resistance and should be taught to the patient while in the office setting initially, to ensure that the patient understands and can perform the exercises correctly.

After the second week of AROM exercise, the patient is to receive a reexamination. Active range of motion should be measured and recorded, and the appropriate orthopedic/neurological test (if any) should be performed. Another analogue pain scale should also be filled out for progress assessment and records.

For days 25–35 (post-reexam) the patient office visit frequency is again reduced, now to two times a week. The patient is now instructed on how to add resistance to the AROM exercises still to be performed two times a day, while the physical therapy is optional from this period onward. If instituted, the intensity should still be "motor" with the frequency sweep at the 30–80 Hz range. This will provide muscle stimulation throughout the frequency sweep range.[13,15,17]

Following the fifth week of therapy, the patient should be given a final examination to determine whether a return to activities of daily living is permissible. Range of motion measurement should again be recorded and a muscle strength assessment/grade be evaluated for the appropriate area muscles. The orthopedic and neurological evaluation should be unremarkable at this point, and maximum medical improvement (MMI) should be approaching.

The following constitutes formal rehabilitation.[28] For days 35 and on, office visits are reduced to one time per week (note: there may be clinical exceptions) until the resisted ROM and/or the muscle testing of the involved area muscles are 5 out of 5. Physical therapy is again optional, with the intensity at "motor" and the frequency at 50 Hz constant for an optimal muscle strengthening contraction.[13,15]

Once the patient has reached MMI, the patient should be counseled with respect to the fears and expectations of returning to a lifestyle that is free of pain with no restriction of range of motion. It is also important to discuss a program designed to maintain and monitor the strength and flexibility of the affected areas because as was noted previously, collagen repair and maturation may take up to one year to complete.

This is a point where individual practitioner variance will be subject to further study and debate as to the frequency and efficacy of future patient visits.

In conclusion, this author maintains that the post-MUA physical therapy and rehabilitation program is of utmost importance in facilitating the proper environment needed for functions realignment of the collagen network. If the guidelines contained in this chapter are not adhered to, it is this author's belief that certain functional disabilities are sure to return to the patient. Rehabilitation is a specific and time-consuming venture. If the clinic/office is not adequately oriented to achieve maximum results, the patient should be referred out to an appropriate facility.

## REFERENCES


1. Roy, S., Irvin, R., Sports Medicine, *Prevention, Evaluation, Management, and Rehabilitation*, Prentice-Hall, Englewood Cliffs, NJ, 1983: 125–28.
2. Jaskoviak, P.H., Schafer, R.C., *Applied Physiotherapy,* Arlington, VA: American Chiropractic Association, 1986.
3. Knight, K., *Cryotherapy: Theory Technique and Physiology*, 1st ed., Chattanooga, TN: Chattanooga Corp., 1985.
4. Guyton, A.C., *Textbook of Medical Physiology*, 7th ed, WB Saunders, Philadelphia, 113–16, 1986.
5. Kottke, F.J., Therapeutic exercise to maintain mobility, in *Handbook of Physical Medicine and Rehabilitation*, Kruser, Kotlke, Elwood, eds., WB Saunders, Philadelphia, 389–401, 1971.
6. Robbins, S., *Pathology*, 3rd ed., WB Saunders, Philadelphia, London, 63–67, 1967.
7. Abramson, D.I. et al., Effect of tissue temperature and blood flow on motor nerve conduction velocity, *J. Am. Med. Assoc.* 198 (10), 1082–88, 1966.
8. Halar, E.M. et al., Nerve conduction velocity: relationship of skin subcutaneous and intramuscular temperatures, *Arch. Phys. Med. Rehab.*, 61, 199–203, May 1980.

9. Lee, J.M. et al., Effects of ice on nerve conduction velocity, *Physiotherapy*, 64, 1–6, 1978.

10. Olsen, J.J., Johnson, E.W., Clinical value of motor nerve conduction velocity determination, *J. Am. Med. Assoc.* 172, 2030–35, 1960.

11. Lehman, J.F., DeLateur, B.J., *Therapeutic Heat in Therapeutic Heat and Cold*, 3rd ed., Lehman, J.F., ed., Williams & Wilkins, Baltimore, Maryland, 1982.

12. DeDominico, G., *New Dimensions in Interferential Therapy — A Theoretical and Clinical Guide*, Linfield, Australia, Reid Medical Books, 1987.

13. Nelson, R.M., Currier, D.P., *Clinical Electrotherapy*, Appleton & Lange, Norwalk, CT, 1987.

14. Alon, G., DeDominico, G., *High Volt Stimulation: An Integrated Approach to Clinical Electrotherapy*, Chattanooga, TN, Chattanooga Corp., 1987.

15. Snyder-Mackler, L., Robinson, A.J., *Clinical Electrophysiology*, Williams & Wilkins, Baltimore, MD, 1989.

16. Guy, A.W., Biophysics of high frequency currents and electromagnetic radiation, in *Handbook of Physical Medicine and Rehabilitation*, Krusen, Kotlke, Elwood, Eds., WB Saunders, Philadelphia, 1971, 213–17.

17. Kahn, J, *Principles and Practices of Electrotherapy*, Churchill Livingstone, New York, 1987.

18. Savage, B, *Interferential Therapy*, Faber & Faber, Ltd, Great Britain, Richard Clay, Ltd, Bungay Suffolk, 1984.

19. Gersten, J.W., Effect of ultrasound on tendon extensibility, *Am. J. Phys. Med.*, 1955, 34, 362–69.

20. Lehman, J.F. et al., Effect of therapeutic temperatures on tendon extensibility, *Arch. Phys. Med. Rehab*, 51, 481–87, 1970.

21. Mason, R., Rigby, B.J., Thermal transitions in collagen, *Biochem. Biophys. Acta.* 66, 448–50, 1946.

22. Siems, L. et al., A comparative study of shortwave and microwave diathermy on blood flow, *Arch. Phys. Med.* 29, 259, 1948.

23. Johns, R.J., Wright, V., Relative importance of various tissues in joint stiffness in rheumatoid arthritis, *Acta. Rheum. Scand.* 13, 275–88, 1967.

24. Bakund, L., Tiselius, P., Objective measurement of joint stiffness in rheumatoid arthritis, *Acta. Rheum. Scand.*, 13, 275–8, 1967.

25. Lehman, J.F. et al., Heat and cold, *Clin. Orthop. Rel. Res.*, 99, 207–45, 1974.

26. Lehman, J.F., Therapeutic heat, in *Handbook of Physical Medicine and Rehabilitation*, Krusen, Kotlke, Elwood, eds., WB Saunders, Philadelphia, 273–345, 1971.

27. Kisner, C., Colby, L.A. Stretching, from *Therapeutic Exercise Foundations and Techniques*, 2nd ed., F.A. Davis, Philadelphia, 109–20, 1990.

28. Gordon, R. with contribution from Furno, P., from syllabus copyright, Cornerstone Professional Education, Inc. MUA syllabus currently sponsored by the National University of Health Sciences, 5th ed., August 1998.

*Part II*

# 14 Hospital Staff Privileges and Ambulatory Surgical Center Protocols (For the Chiropractic Physician)

*Robert C. Gordon*

## CONTENTS

Although this text is written from a multidisciplinary perspective, it is important to address information for the practitioners who are usually not involved in the hospital or the ambulatory surgical setting. The chiropractic professional, although very skilled in the techniques of manual therapy, has not been exposed to the hospital setting. This chapter is written specifically to address the hospital environment.

Hospital staff privileges carry a considerable responsibility. Medical staff membership privileges are a multidimensional integration of many different disciplines. The desired outcome is to provide the highest quality of care to the patient.

As chiropractic physicians, we are not the "favored son" in this arena. As health care changes and more providers are looking for a holistic approach, we should be involved from now on. The MUA procedure is one of the best avenues to propel chiropractic into the hospital environment, and it carries with it the credibility that we have long sought to achieve.

There is always going to be opposition in the ranks of our profession and the medical profession. If you choose to be among the pioneers in this endeavor you can expect to take the heat from many in both professions who feel that you are overstepping your boundaries. This could not be further from the truth, but you can expect a somewhat adversarial position.

But once again we must negate the negative to propel the positive outcome of our profession.[1,2]

Those of us who are involved in the MUA program and, as such, the hospital setting, are finding new dimensions in interdisciplinary relations, and although there still remains opposition from the medical community, the benefits outweigh the controversy.

Consider cross-examination in the courtroom scenario, where in the past it was commonly asked "Doctor, you are not associated with a hospital as a chiropractor, are you?" The question always held the connotation of inferiority; but now with the affirmative answer it only lends credibility to those doctors who are involved in hospital environments.

One of the most significant benefits of hospital staff privileges concerns the fact that now we are able to follow our patients who are referred for hospital stays without losing the patient to the medical establishment without any further contact. As a co-admit staff physician, you become involved in referring the patient to your co-admit MD or DO, and have hospital privileges to seek justification for much of the testing that goes on, especially those tests that revolve around your customary scope of practice.

This not only benefits the patient, but now also gives you the credibility you deserve in the eyes of the patient and the respect of the referring medical staff members who look upon you as an integrating member of their medical community. This is done without losing your chiropractic identity, but, more important, provides a means for intraprofessional discourse.

Hospitals are not eager to admit chiropractors to their staffs and are looking to allow only those physicians who show a willingness to adapt to the hospital environment, and who also are willing to demonstrate intellectual and academic substantiation for the care being provided to their patients.

## DEVELOPING CHIROPRACTIC–HOSPITAL RELATIONSHIPS

The MUA procedure is one of our greatest avenues for admission into the hospital medical staff. In the past, the chiropractor was limited to the number of patients who might be referred to the hospital simply by the nature of conservative chiropractic care. As we become involved in the MUA procedure, we are now adding a new dimension to this referral base. We now have another step in the referral cycle for chronic recurrent neuromusculoskeletal and specifically spinal-related problems, which in the past have had conservative care to include chiropractic care and possible drug therapy or surgery. We now have the MUA procedure as an alternative between exhausted conservative care and surgery. With that in mind, we now approach hospitals that are receptive to having chiropractic care on staff.

## INITIAL CONTACTS

Individuals most likely to be interested in the MUA procedure and also in establishing co-admit privileges are those who play a significant part in the team approach to manipulation under anesthesia and wish to see the procedure become part of the treatment protocols in their facilities.

### CHIEF OF ANESTHESIOLOGY

This is the physician who plays the most important role in advising the medical staff of your intentions to bring a viable procedure to the facility. The anesthesiologist's responsibility is to provide the anesthesia portion of the procedure. Before most CEOs respond to your request to be on staff, this physician will most likely review the opinions of the anesthesiology staff.

### HOSPITAL ADMINISTRATOR

The hospital administrator is the next most important person who you will want to meet. This person is responsible for running the hospital, and if the facility is corporate owned, this person is responsible to the corporation for any decisions that are made on behalf of the hospital. This individual will make the decision to move forward with the MUA project, and will hold the key to determining who will be the right people in the hospital to initially contact for support. I place this person at the position of second in your initial contact because of the importance that they place on the anesthesiologist's decision as to how the anesthesia will be provided and whether the anesthesiology group is willing to provide the service to bring MUA into the mainstream of their facility. It is much easier for the CEO/hospital administrator to make a case for having MUA performed in their facility to the medical staff if they have the support of the anesthesiology group.

### PHYSICAL MEDICINE RELATIONSHIP

If you have developed a relationship with a physiatrist, this person is usually a good referral source to help you establish your program.

## PODIATRIST

A staff podiatrist is a good source for helping you establish your program because podiatrists have the same types of problems getting on staff as you are trying to overcome.

## ORTHOPEDIST

If you have established a good working relationship with an orthopedist who is interested in becoming involved in your program, they might be willing to help you get established in the facility.

## NEUROLOGIST

A neurologist who develops an interest in providing second opinions for your program may be a good referral for establishing your program.

## INTERNIST/GENERAL PRACTITIONER

Staff physicians make excellent co-admit physicians because they are readily available to help admit your patients and perform any required invasive testing you may agree on as well as any drug therapy needed. Because they feel less experienced with neuromusculoskeletal conditions, they will usually allow more latitude than some of the other physicians. These are good physicians to seek for medical clearance.

# INTERHOSPITAL POLITICS

The next step to overcome in establishing hospital privileges is the interhospital politics. A hospital is run like a large corporation, with a CEO or administrator as the corporate representative.

The CEO will have an executive committee, which is formed from various staff members and, in some instances, community laypeople who act as an advisory body to the hospital in community affairs.

If the hospital is corporate owned, the CEO is also responsible to the corporation for any decisions that are made for the hospital.

Because of the last group, the CEO will be very careful to recognize the corporate opinions with regard to chiropractic involvement, and to having the MUA procedure.

It is best to form a good relationship with the CEO in establishing the chiropractic program whether MUA is at the forefront or not, by having one or more of the physician specialists act as intermediaries or even mentors in your initial contact.

The executive committee usually, but not always, has the final vote for the decision to have a chiropractic department. This decision is usually based on several factors:

1. Current hospital bylaws.
2. Department(s) ratification.
3. Three-fourths vote of approval.
4. Joint Commission on Accreditation of Healthcare Organizations (JCAHO) standards for the hospital.
5. Quality assurance standardization: What standards of care will be used to monitor the procedures being used by the chiropractors, etc.
6. Choice of department that the chiropractic procedures will fall under, including the MUA procedure (many times it's the department of surgery) It is recommended that either "general medicine," "physical medicine," or "pain management" be the department of choice to include the department of chiropractic. The department of "surgery" sometimes causes irritation in the medical and chiropractic communities with the connotation that "surgery implies cutting."

Personnel who will have direct effect on establishing a chiropractic department include:

1. CEO/administrator (corporate owner)
2. Administrative chief operating officer
3. Anesthesiology
4. Nursing staff — recovery, operating room (for MUA)
5. Neurology/orthopedics (if they control the referral base)
6. Radiology (CTs, MRIs, etc.)
7. General family practitioners/internists (if they become involved)
8. Billing (if the hospital does the billing for the chiropractors)
9. Medical credentialing
10. Medical records

## INTERRELATING WITH HOSPITAL EMPLOYEES, ADMINISTRATION, STAFF, AND OTHER PROFESSIONALS

The team approach involves working with the following groups:

Nursing Staff
- Director of Nursing (DON)
- OR Supervisor (ORS)
- Surgical techs
- RNs and LPNs

Administration
- Hospital administrator
- CEO
- Attorney
- Medical records
- Clerks and other personnel

Staff physicians
- Chief of Staff
- Radiology
- Anesthesiology
- MD and DO
- Paraprofessionals, i.e., psychologists, optometrists, pharmacists
- Other

## EXECUTIVE BOARD OF DIRECTORS

The executive board of directors of a hospital has the final word in the decision-making process of the hospital. In many cases, they are governed by an outside owner.

The executive board has the following pertinent responsibilities:

1. The CEO of the hospital and the administrative staff control hospital function on direct command from the owners.
2. The CEO controls the business end of the hospital.
3. The positions held with the executive board are appointed by the CEO/administration.
4. The executive board hires staff who are pertinent members of the hospital.
5. Responsible for establishing the hospital bylaws.

6. Has the final word in deciding what delineation of privileges will be allowed by each practitioner.
7. Makes the final decisions and reviews all reports submitted by the various hospital departments.
8. Decides whether you will be on staff, and has complete autonomy for deciding whether your particular specialty is a desired addition to the hospital.
9. Considers all applications presented by the credentials committee, but do not have to act on all applications submitted. (i.e., your application could be tabled for an indefinite period of time).
10. Expects the highest quality of care and professionalism from its doctors and will not allow physicians to practice in a haphazard manner. The members are directly responsive to the guidelines of established standards set by quality assurance.

## Sample Cover Letter Presenting MUA Technique to a Hospital

Dear Administrator (CEO):

I am currently a practicing chiropractic physician in the area and have completed certification to perform a procedure called manipulation under anesthesia.

This is not a new procedure. In fact, it has been in existence since the late 1930s and was performed originally by the osteopathic profession.

Our new approach requires hospital involvement in an environment where rapidly acting anesthetics allow the procedure to be completed in 15–30 min with 30- to 45-min recovery time, many times requiring a 3-d series of procedures to accomplish the desired outcome.

The addition of a chiropractic department to your hospital would certainly broaden your present patient base as you would be establishing a very favorable relationship with the chiropractic physicians in the area who are certified to perform MUA.

In addition to having this very valuable procedure performed in your facility, the establishment of a chiropractic department is an ideal way to increase the number of referrals to other medical specialists in the facility primarily because most chiropractic clinics see anywhere from 150 to 300 patient visits per week for conservative care for various neuromusculoskeletal problems within our scope of practice.

The MUA procedure is usually an outpatient procedure, but has required inpatient observation as well. The hospital would not only increase its patient base by having certified chiropractic MUA physicians on staff, but would be looking at considerable ancillary diagnostic testing, pre-op testing, post-MUA rehabilitation and/or physical therapy, plus pre- and post-documentation diagnostics for research purposes.

We would consider it a great pleasure to present this concept to you and your staff at your earliest convenience and look forward to working with you on this project in the near future.

Sincerely,

## SAMPLES OF CHIROPRACTIC DEPARTMENT BYLAWS FROM DIFFERENT HOSPITALS

Application

I fully understand that any significant misstatements in or omissions from this application constitute cause for denial of appointment or cause for summary dismissal from the medical staff. All information submitted by me in this application is true to the best of my knowledge and belief.

In making this application for appointment to the medical staff of the facility, I acknowledge that I have received and read the bylaws of the facility, and that I am familiar with the principles, standards of the Joint Commission on Accreditation of Healthcare Organizations (JCAHO) (if applicable), on the ethics of the national, state, and local associations that apply to and govern my specialty and/or profession, and I agree to be bound by the terms thereof if I am granted membership or clinical privileges. I further agree to be bound by the terms thereof without regard to whether or not I am granted membership or clinical privileges in all matters relating to the consideration of my application for appointment to the medical staff, and I further agree to abide by such center and staff rules and regulations as may be from time to time enacted.

By applying for appointment to the medical staff, I hereby signify my willingness to appear for the interviews in regard to my application, and authorize the center, its medical staff, and their representatives to consult with administrators and members of medical staffs of other hospitals or institutions with which I have been associated and with others, including past and present malpractice carriers, who may have information bearing on my professional competence, character, and ethical qualifications. I hereby further consent to the inspection by the facility, its medical staff, and its representatives of all records and documents, including medical records at other hospitals that may be material to an evaluation of my professional qualifications and competence to carry out the clinical privileges requested, as well as my moral and ethical qualifications for staff membership. I hereby release from liability all representatives of the facility and its medical staff for their acts performed in good faith and without malice in connection with evaluating my application and my credentials and qualifications, and I hereby release from any liability any and all individuals and organizations who provide information to the facility, or its medical staff, in good faith and without malice concerning my professional competence, ethics, character, and other qualifications for staff appointment and clinical privileges, and I hereby consent to the release of such information.

I hereby further authorize and consent to the release of information by this facility, or its medical staff, to other hospitals, medical associations, and other interested persons on request regarding any information they may have concerning my professional expertise and this information is given in good faith and without malice. I hereby release from liability this facility and its staff for investigating me in this manner.

I understand and agree that I, as an applicant for medical staff membership, have the burden of producing adequate information for proper evaluation of my professional competence, character, ethics, and other qualifications and for resolving any doubts about such qualifications.

I will not participate in any such form of fee-splitting. Moreover, I pledge myself to shun unwarranted publicity, dishonest money-seeking, and commercialism, to refuse money trades with consultants, practitioners, makers of surgical appliances and optical instruments, or others, to teach the patient his or her financial duty to the physician and to expect the practitioner to obtain his or her compensation directly from the patient, to make my fees commensurate with the services rendered and with the patient's rights, and to avoid discrediting my associates by taking unwarranted compensation.

I have not requested privileges for any procedures for which I am not certified. Furthermore, I realize that certification by a board does not necessarily qualify me to perform certain procedures. However, I believe that I am qualified to perform all procedures for which I have requested privileges.

Signature of Applicant _______________________________________________________

☐ Appointment Recommended        ☐ Appointment Not Recommended

☐ Appointment Deferred

Date ______________________        Chairman, Advisory Committee

☐ Appointment Recommended        ☐ Appointment Not Recommended

☐ Appointment Deferred

Date ______________________        Chairman Board of Directors______________________

## DELINEATION OF PRIVILEGES FOR THE CHIROPRACTIC SERVICES PROGRAM: MANIPULATION UNDER ANESTHESIA SPECIFIC

The following services provided by the chiropractic physicians involved in providing patient care for the procedure of manipulation under anesthesia (MUA) shall be recognized at ______________ hospital.

- Evaluation of and patient selection for MUA procedure.
- Diagnostic referral for further evaluation.
- Referral for medical clearance and co-admittance for the MUA procedures
- In-hospital evaluation of MUA patients before and after MUA procedures
- Orders for daily discharge written by the chiropractic physician for daily aftercare
- Recognition and responsibility for dictating OP reports and discharge summaries on each patient undergoing the MUA procedure

Procedures

- Passive stretch as outlined by the MUA procedure as taught by CCE-accredited chiropractic colleges that teach the MUA procedure
- Patient mobilization (fibrosis release procedures) as outlined by the MUA procedure as taught by CCE-accredited chiropractic colleges that teach the MUA procedure
- Specific chiropractic adjustive, mobilization and manipulative procedures for the
    - Cervico/occipital cranial region
    - Cervical spinal area
    - Cervical thoracic spinal area
- Shoulder stretching and mobilization techniques

- Thoracic spinal area
- Rib articulation
- Thoracolumbar spinal area
- Lumbar spinal area
- Lumbosacral spinal area
- Hip and pelvic area
- Shoulder articulation
- Extremities to include knees, ankles, elbows, wrists

## BYLAWS FOR CHIROPRACTIC DEPARTMENTS IN AMBULATORY SURGICAL CENTERS AND HOSPITALS

The bylaws that your particular facility establishes will come under close scrutiny in the initial setup phase. How well this is done and to what depth will depend a great deal on the success of your initial contacts. The willingness of the administration of your facility to accept you at the fullest limit of your licensure will depend on how well you conduct yourself through those initial phases.

There are multiple levels in which this process of creating department bylaws can progress depending on what is desired by the facility. These same bylaws can be established in ambulatory surgical centers once multiple doctors providing the MUA procedure are hired. Some of the options are as follows:

- A separate chiropractic department
- A department of chiropractic under the general medical department
- A division of chiropractic under an already established major department, such as pain management

It may be suggested that you take a position as an allied health care professional. This is not a bad way to get started in the hospital, but the CEO needs to be made aware that full staff privileges with co-admit status are desired as you progressively show the value of having your skills involved in treating patients at the facility. Not all of my colleagues agree with this because it has a tendency to give the impression that we are somehow on the same level as the nursing staff or the PTs. This is not the case, and getting started in this capacity sometimes helps bring you on staff, lets you get started providing the MUA procedure to your patients, and gives the medical staff a chance to see the value of having you as part of the staff. Remember, you have not received the training in hospital protocols that the other physicians were exposed to during their medical training, and you need to become acclimated to this new environment as you provide the MUA procedure. Historically once you are involved in the daily function of the hospital, the CEO and medical staff will offer you a more significant staff position under co-admit status.

## MEDICAL STAFF

### Section A — Division of Medical Staff

Consulting staff consists of physicians, dentists, and podiatrists eligible for staff membership who may attend private patients in the facility. The members of the consulting staff may perform those procedures as recommended by the medical advisory committee and approved by the board of directors. A member of the consulting staff will not be eligible to vote or hold office.

1. Active staff will consist of physicians, dentists, and podiatrists who have qualified for active staff appointments and have indicated a desire to participate in the facility. They

may be appointed by the board of directors, upon recommendation of the medical advisory committee. All active staff members are subject to periodic review by the medical advisory committee and the board of directors. Members of the active staff will be entitled to vote and hold office except those active staff members on provisional or temporary status.

2. The provisional staff will consist of physicians, dentists, and podiatrists eligible for staff membership, who are awaiting approval of privileges and who may attend private patients in the facility. Members of the provisional staff will not vote or hold office and are subject to 6-month probation. Sometimes, the CEO will place the chiropractic physician in this position so that the medical staff can become familiar with the services provided. This is sometimes more palatable to the chiropractic physician rather than allied staff privileges, and sometime the medical staff will accept this status for the chiropractic physician in order to help with the process of obtaining full staff co-admit status. Under special circumstances, a physician may be immediately appointed to the active staff by the board of directors upon the recommendation of the medical advisory committee for one-year temporary status. All provisional staff members are subject to review by the medical advisory committee, and upon its recommendation may be appointed to the active staff by the board of directors.

3. The members of the courtesy staff must hold the rank of courtesy for at least 6 months before they may be promoted to active staff. All promotions from provisional staff to active staff will be on a provisional basis for a period of at least 6 months. During this time, a member's privileges may be reduced, or in the case of provisional appointments, withdrawn upon recommendation of the medical advisory committee of the medical staff and the approval of the action by the board of directors.

4. The courtesy staff will consist of those physicians providing continued medical care for patients served in the facility. Practitioners on the courtesy staff will be privileged to take medical histories, perform physical examinations, and treat medical problems associated with the treatment rendered all patients in the center. Members of the courtesy staff will not be eligible to vote, hold medical staff office, or serve as chairman of any medical staff committees; e.g., internists or cardiologists.

5. Paramedical personnel or physician's assistants' staff privileges will be granted to nonmedical, dental, or podiatric personnel such as certified registered nurse anesthetists who are qualified to be, and are, credentialed by the board of directors. These persons will not have independent authority for the care of patients but will practice under the supervision or direction of a member of the medical staff.

6. The allied health professional staff will consist of persons trained and qualified in allied health disciplines who exercise independent judgment and provide special professional advice or specified services to patients or the medical or administrative staffs. Allied health persons will be qualified by training, education, and licensure appropriate for their special services and will serve within the scope of their recognized professional qualifications and skills. Allied health persons will be appointed or reappointed and granted privileges according to the procedures provided in Articles IV and V of these bylaws. They will be subject to the provisions of these bylaws pertaining to privileges, duties, and ethical practice of the professions. Allied health persons will be assigned to a service of the medical staff by the governing board and will be responsible to the medical director. Allied health persons may not admit or discharge patients. When requested by a patient's attending physician, they may, within the scope of their privileges and these bylaws and rules and regulations, attend that patient in the hospital. The extent of the service will be determined by the staff and the attending physician who has thc final responsibility for the welfare of the patient. Allied health professionals will not be considered members of the medical staff, and as such will not be expected to attend medical staff meetings

or to have committee duties. They will be required to provide appropriate documentation on the medical records, including notes.

## SECTION B — CLINICAL DEPARTMENT

There will be clinical departments consisting of the following:

1. Surgery — Monitors surgical procedures performed in the facility and will keep, or cause to be kept, careful supervision over all surgical procedures performed in the facility. This department will consist of the subspecialties of general surgery, plastic surgery, otolaryngology, orthopedic surgery, gynecology, urology, podiatry, and such subspecialties as recommended by the medical advisory committee and approved by the board of directors.
2. Anesthesiology — Responsible for the administration of anesthesia, relief of pain, and all the fields of analgesia. Anesthesiology determines the acceptability of patients for ambulatory care, in accordance with the bylaws, rules, and regulations.
3. Dentistry and podiatry — Responsible for the clinical procedures performed in the facility and will keep, or cause to be kept, careful supervision over all clinical work performed in the facility.
4. Medicine — Responsible for procedures in the field of medicine and will be concerned with the supervision of all nonsurgical procedures performed in the facility.
5. Radiology — Responsible for procedures in the field of radiology and will be concerned with the supervision of all radiological procedures performed in and/or for the facility.
6. Pathology — Responsible for the supervision of all pathological procedures performed in and/or for the facility. Membership on the medical staff of the center will be a privilege restricted only to those professionally competent practitioners within the facility's primary service area who consistently meet the qualifications, standards, and requirements set forth in these bylaws.
7. Chiropractic — Responsible for the procedures in the field of chiropractic medicine and will be concerned with the supervision of manipulation under anesthesia by the chiropractic staff and all other chiropractic procedures performed in the facility.

## SECTION C — MEMBERSHIP QUALIFICATIONS

1. Appointment to the medical staff will be made by the board of directors upon recommendation by the medical advisory committee of the medical staff. Initial appointment will be for a probationary period of 6 months. Upon review, if subsequent appointment is allowed, such appointment will be made for a 2-year period, subject to the bylaws of the medical staff. For the purpose of these bylaws, the medical staff year commences on the first day of January and ends the thirty-first day of December of each year.
2. An applicant for staff membership will be registered and legally licensed to practice in the state of __________. All applicants requesting surgical admitting privileges who must have hospital co-admitting privileges, must have admitting privileges in a local accredited hospital and must be either board certified, board eligible, or board qualified, according to the requirements of each board and recommended by a majority of the medical advisory committee as qualified to serve on the medical staff by virtue of their qualifications and experience. Those physicians who are not board certified and recommended for staff membership by a majority of the medical advisory committee may be given temporary privileges for one year or longer, relative to the eligibility requirements of their specialty and duration as a staff member. Board certification is at the discretion of the medical advisory board and may or may not be a requirement for staff privileges. Those who are

board eligible will be given temporary privileges for three years or longer, relative to the eligibility requirements of the specialty at the time of completion of specialty training. The codes of ethics as adopted or amended by the American Medical Association, the American College of Surgeons, the American Chiropractic Association, and the National Academy of MUA Physicians, respectively, will govern the professional conduct of the members of the staff.

3. Podiatrists will be given certain privileges in accordance with the rules and regulations of the medical staff, Section H.3 (Staff Privileges).

4. Chiropractic physicians will be given certain privileges in accordance with the rules and regulations of the medical staff, H.3 (Staff Privileges). Chiropractic physicians desiring to perform manipulation under anesthesia at the facility must have been in private chiropractic practice for a minimum of ________ years and be observed in the procedure of manipulation under anesthesia in a minimum of five procedures by one of the on staff chiropractic physicians (proctors) certified in manipulation under anesthesia.

5. An applicant for the medical staff of the facility will present his written application for appointment and privileges for specific procedures to the medical director utilizing the form prescribed by the board of directors of the facility. Upon making application, the applicant will also signify agreement to abide by the bylaws, rules, and regulations of the medical staff and the facility in accordance with subsection 5 hereof. Application will include detailed information concerning the applicant's education, training, and experience, and give information as to whether the applicant's clinical privileges have ever been revoked, suspended, reduced, or not renewed at any hospital or institution, or whether his or her license to practice his or her profession in any jurisdiction has ever been suspended or terminated.

The applicant will have the burden of producing adequate information for a proper evaluation of their competence, character, ethics, and other qualifications, and for resolving any doubts about such qualification.

As a condition for membership, the applicant must provide evidence of current professional liability coverage with minimum requirements as the Surgery Center's board may from time to time be determined, but at least $1 million individual/$3 million per occurrence for chiropractors who perform non-invasive MUA.

Furthermore, the applicant will

- Appear for interviews in regard to his or her application.
- Authorize consultation with members of the medical staffs of facilities with which the applicant has been associated and with others who may have information on his or her competence, character, and ethical qualifications.
- Consent to inspection of all records and documents that may be material to an evaluation of his or her professional qualifications and competency to carry out the privileges he or she requests, as well as his or her moral and ethical qualifications for medical staff membership.
- Release any liability for all representatives of the facility and its medical staff for their acts performed in good faith and without malice in connection with evaluating the applicant and his or her credentials.
- Release from any liability all individuals and organizations who provide information in good faith and without malice concerning the applicant's competence, ethics, character, and other qualifications for medical staff appointment and privileges.
- Upon receiving the application, the medical director of the designee will make all necessary checks on references, licensure, and other information, which would indicate

the applicant's qualifications for staff privileges sought. The medical director will then transmit the application to the medical advisory committee for evaluation.

- The medical advisory committee will review the character, qualifications, and professional standing and will submit a written recommendation to the board of directors. Failure to complete the review process within ninety (90) days, unless extended by mutual agreement of applicant and the administrator, will be considered to be a denial of the application. All applicants, as well as members of the medical staff, consent to the release of pertinent information for any purpose set forth in these bylaws and release from liability and agree to hold harmless any person or entity furnishing or releasing such information concerning application for medical staff status. The recommendations of the medical advisory committee will be transmitted to the board of directors through the administrator and upon receipt of the reports, the board of directors will review the medical advisory committee's recommendations. When determining qualifications, the medical advisory committee will recommend privileges for specific procedures to be granted, commensurate with physician's education, training, and experience as provided in these bylaws. Each applicant must indicate in writing the specific procedures which he requests to perform at the facility. The board of directors will either accept or reject the recommendations of the medical advisory committee, or refer them back for further consideration, stating the reasons for such action. This will be done by the next regular scheduled meeting of the board of directors or not longer than ninety (90) days after receipt by the board of directors of the report of the medical advisory committee and failure of the board to act within ninety (90) days of receipt, unless extended by the mutual agreement of the applicant and the administrator, will be considered to be a denial. In the event the application is deferred by the board of directors, in no instance will the report be delayed more than ninety (90) days from the date of review of the application by the medical advisory committee and the applicant will be notified. Failure to take action by the board of directors within ninety (90) days of the review by the medical advisory committee, unless extended by mutual agreement of the applicant and the administrator, will be considered to be a denial. When final action has been taken by the board of directors, the administrator will transmit the information to the candidate, and if accepted, secure a signed agreement to be governed by the bylaws, rules, and regulations. This agreement is to be signed and returned to the administrator within one week of notification by the administrator.

- During the time the staff application of a physician, dentist or podiatrist is pending, temporary privileges may be granted by the concurrence of the chairperson of the medical advisory committee and the administrator. This request will be made in writing by the applicant concerned and directed to the chairperson of the medical advisory committee. Approval of temporary privileges will be confirmed in writing. These privileges may be granted for a period of thirty to ninety days subject to renewal of request and reviewed at the time of expiration of the special privileges.

6. Upon becoming a member of the staff, each physician will agree not to engage in the practice of the division of fees under any guise whatsoever. Specifically, each member of the staff will sign the following pledge, an original executed copy of which will be maintained by the facility during staff membership:

"I agree to abide by the bylaws, rules, and regulations of the medical staff and by such bylaws, rules, and regulations as may be, from time to time, enacted of the

_______________________________.

"Moreover, I hereby declare that I will not engage in the practice of the division of fees under guise whatsoever. In complying with this principle, I understand that I am not to collect fees for others to collect fees for me, nor make joint fees with physicians referring patients to me for operation or consultation, nor permit any agent or associate of mine to do so. Further, I agree to comply with the principle that all physicians participating in the care of a patient will render separate bills and receipts."

7. Staff appointments are for 6 months temporary probation and thereafter for 2 years. All appointments and privileges will be reviewed for reappointment at the appropriate time. Each applicant for reappointment to the medical staff will submit to the medical advisory committee and the administrative director all information necessary to update the medical staff file on the staff member's health care–related activities, which will include, but not be limited to, a specific request for privileges; the staff member's continuing training, education, and experience since the previous appointment; the staff member's current health status; sanctions of any kind imposed or pending by any other health care institution, professional health care organization, or licensing authority with respect to the staff member; and a complete summary of the staff member's malpractice insurance coverage and any malpractice claim, suits, and settlements involving the staff member. No staff member will be reappointed without specific review of the individual's performance and qualifications by the medical advisory committee, which will make specific recommendations to the board of directors, setting forth its recommendations for renewal of staff privileges for each physician. The board of directors will either accept or reject the recommendations of the medical advisory committee or refer them back to the medical advisory committee for further consideration, stating the reasons for such action. This will be done by the next regular meeting of the board of directors. When final action has been taken by the board of directors, the administrator will transmit the information to the candidate for reappointment.
8. If the board's action with respect to an application for appointment to the medical staff is adverse to the applicant or staff member, as the case may be, defined in Article III, Section E hereof, the administrative director will promptly so inform the applicant or staff member by certified mail, return receipt requested, and the applicant or staff member will be entitled to the procedural rights as provided in Article III, Section E.

No physician, dentist or podiatrist will be entitled to membership on the medical staff or to the exercise of particular privileges merely by virtue of the fact that he or she is a member or any professional organization, or that he or she had in the past, or presently has, such privileges at another hospital or similar facility.

## HOSPITAL DEPARTMENT OF CHIROPRACTIC — RULES AND REGULATIONS

### PREAMBLE

Recognizing that the Department of Chiropractic is responsible for the quality of chiropractic care in the hospital and that the chiropractic staff, being a department of the medical staff, must function within the overall guidelines of the medical staff bylaws of _______________ Hospital.

The chiropractors practicing in this hospital hereby organize themselves paralleling and in conformity with the general medical staff bylaws and rules and regulations as hereinafter stated.

### ARTICLE I — PURPOSE

The purpose of the department will be

1. To ensure that all patients admitted or cared for by a chiropractor receive the best possible quality care
2. To monitor and evaluate patient care according to the 10-Step Quality Assurance Program outlined by JCAHO
3. To perform other staff functions so described in the medical staff bylaws
4. To provide a means whereby problems of a chiropractic administrative nature may be discussed by the chiropractic staff with appropriate recommendations to the medical executive committee
5. To initiate, recommend, and maintain rules and regulations for governing of the chiropractic staff

## ARTICLE II — MEMBERSHIP

### Section 1. Qualifications

A. Applicants for membership will be qualified legally, professionally, and ethically for the categories of membership and for privileges that they are granted.
B. Privileges of all members will be based on professional qualifications and demonstrated professional ability.
C  Applicants will be licensed by the state of ______________.
D. Applicant has been a practicing chiropractor for at least _____ years.
E. All should be members of their national, divisional, and local associations.

### Section 2. Ethics and Ethical Relationships

A. The professional conduct of members of the chiropractic staff will be governed by principles and ethics outlined in the medical staff bylaws. Specifically, all members of the chiropractic staff will pledge themselves that they will not receive from, or pay to, another physician, either directly or indirectly, any part of a fee received for professional services.
B. In addition, all staff members of the (State) Chiropractic Association, Inc., will comply with all provisions of the code of ethics of the (State) Chiropractic Association, and all other members of the chiropractic staff will comply with codes of ethics of their respective associations or societies.

### Section 3. Terms of Appointments

A. Appointments will be made by the governing board of the hospital after recommendation of the chiropractic staff with concurrence of the medical executive committee and will be for a provisional period.
B. In no case will the governing board take action on an application, refuse to renew an appointment, or cancel an appointment previously made without conference with the chiropractic staff.
C. Appointment to the chiropractic staff will confer on the appointee only such privileges as may hereinafter be provided.

### Section 4. Procedure of Appointment

A. Application for membership on the chiropractic staff will be presented in writing and will state the qualifications and references of the applicant and will so signify his or her agreement to abide by the bylaws, rules, and regulations of the medical staff. The application for membership on the chiropractic staff will be presented to the administrator of the hospital, or his or her designee, who will transmit it to the chiropractic staff.

B. At the first regular meeting thereafter, the application, with appropriate credentials and letters of reference, will be presented at the chiropractic meeting.

C. The chiropractic staff will then vote on the applicant and forward their recommendation to the medical executive committee for their recommendation to the governing board, which will make the ultimate decision.

## ARTICLE III — DEPARTMENT

The chiropractic staff is organized as a department of the medical staff.

## ARTICLE IV — OFFICERS AND COMMITTEES

### Section 1. Officers

The officer of the chiropractic staff will be the chairman of the department. This will be an elected position by 2/3 vote of the chiropractic department. The election will be open and/or by secret ballot. Term of office will be for one year, January 1st to December 31st. However, a chairperson can serve two (2) consecutive terms. The chairperson is responsible for the organization and administration of the chiropractic staff. Responsibilities of the department chair include, but need not be limited to, the following:

1. Being accountable for all professional and administrative activities within the department
2. Continuing surveillance of the professional performance of all individuals who have delineated clinical privileges in the department
3. Recommending to the Department of Chiropractic the criteria for clinical privileges in the department
4. Recommending clinical privileges for each member of the department
5. Assuring that the quality and appropriateness of patient care provided within the department are monitored and evaluated

Accurate and complete minutes of all meetings will be kept.

### Section 2. Sponsorship

1. The chairperson of the department, or his or her qualified designee, is to be the sponsor.
2. The physician to be sponsored must observe at least one (1) MUA being performed before performing one himself or herself.
3. The physician being sponsored must perform a minimum of ____MUAs while being proctored.
4. After the performance of five (5) observed MUAs by the chairperson of the Chiropractic Services Department, the report and accompanying charts will go to the Department of Chiropractic Quality Assurance and then on to the medical executive committee.
5. If a physician has never manipulated a frozen joint (i.e., shoulder), he or she must observe a minimum of_____ manipulation(s) being performed before being allowed to participate in this maneuver.

Note: When a physician will be manipulating a frozen joint or performing on any type of unusual case, invitation should be made to other members of the chiropractic staff to observe such procedure.

## ARTICLE V — MEETINGS

### Section 1. Regular Meetings

The chiropractic staff will meet monthly on the _______of the month to conduct business of the chiropractic staff, to hear the reports of the assigned committees, and to present educational programs when possible. This will also be the meeting to present the MUA procedures that will be performed for that month.

### Section 2. Special Meetings

Special meetings of the chiropractic staff may be called at any time by the chairperson at the request of the governing board, the executive committee, or any five members of the active chiropractic staff. At any special meeting, no business will be transacted except that stated in the notice calling the meeting. Written notice of such meetings will be postmarked at least 7 days in advance of the said meeting.

### Section 3. Attendance at Meetings

A.  Active staff members and courtesy staff members will attend at least 50% of the meetings unless excused for just cause, such as sickness or absence from the community. Non-compliance will be considered as a resignation from the chiropractic staff.
B.  Reinstatement of members of the active staff to positions rendered vacant because of absences from meetings may be made upon written application to the chairperson of the chiropractic section. This application must then be brought to the next chiropractic staff meeting for action.
C.  Members of the honorary or consulting categories of the chiropractic staff will not be required to attend meetings, but it is expected that they will attend and participate in these meetings unless unavoidably prevented from doing so.

### Section 4. Quorum

Fifty percent of the total membership of the active chiropractic staff will constitute a quorum.

### Section 5. Agenda

The agenda at any regular meeting will be (1) call to order, business meeting; (2) acceptance of the minutes of the last regular and of all special meetings; (3) communications, quality assurance; (4) committee reports; (5) unfinished business; (6) new business; presentation of grand round cases and the new cases for the month for MUA. In the event there is a continuing education program, this will follow the new business and the closing of the regular business meeting. At the discretion of the chairperson, the continuing education session may, with the approval of the members of the chiropractic staff, be placed as the first order of business.

## APPLICATION FOR CHIROPRACTIC STAFF PRIVILEGES
## (HOSPITAL OR AMBULATORY SURGICAL CENTER)

1.  This application is for membership as an active health practitioner on the medical staff of the chiropractic department.
2.  The application for medical staff privileges must be completed and returned to the hospital executive offices.

3. By applying for medical staff appointment, you are willing to appear for an interview in regard to your application.
4. If you choose to make application, you will be responsible to read and agree with the parameters established for medical membership as established in the bylaws for your department and the hospital.
5. A dossier of your application will be referred to the credentials committee after being received by the chief of chiropractic services.
6. You will be required to appear for interview with the board of chiropractic at one of the regularly scheduled monthly meetings.
7. When the credentials committee has completed its investigation, a report will be submitted to the executive board with a recommendation for acceptance, deferment, or rejection of the application.
8. I hereby certify that I have read and am familiar with the above instructions and the bylaws of the Department of Chiropractic Services, and will abide by such laws and hospital rules and regulations as will apply to the Department of Chiropractic Services.

Signature_________________________________________ Date _____________________________

Professional affiliations ______________________________________________

_______________________________________________

_______________________________________________

_______________________________________________

If answers to any of the following questions are "Yes," please give full details on a separate sheet of paper.

1. Has your license to practice chiropractic ever been limited, suspended, revoked, or voluntarily surrendered? yes _________no_________
2. Have you ever been refused membership on a hospital staff when other chiropractors have been admitted? yes_____ no _________
3. Have you ever been denied membership or renewal thereof, or been subject to disciplinary action in any chiropractic organization? yes_____ no_____
4. Have you ever failed to complete any basic chiropractic training? yes_______ no_________
5. Is your license currently under investigation by any state, government, or chiropractic organization? yes ______ no _________

## THE SCIENTIFIC BASIS OF CHIROPRACTIC AS PERTAINING TO CHIROPRACTIC PHILOSOPHY FOR THE CHIROPRACTIC PHYSICIAN

This is required in most department bylaws to clarify the type of health-care practitioner involved in a particular department. This is not just required of the chiropractic department, but of all of the departments.

"Chiropractic is the study of problems of health and disease from a structural point of view with special consideration given to spinal mechanics and neurological relations."[3]

The chiropractic physician bases his or her philosophy on several basic scientific principles:

• Disturbances in the body structural systems are also disturbances in function of the body called disease.

- Disease may be caused by disturbances in the nervous system.
- "In the complex multicellular organism, the nervous system resides preeminent in controlling, coordinating and synergizing the functions of the body."[3]
- The spinal vertebrae may become misaligned, and these "off centerings"[3] are called subluxations, which is a common biomechanical pathology.
- Chiropractic philosophy relates to the relationship of mechanically produced disturbances of the nervous system by the biodynamic misalignment of the vertebrae, which interferes and impairs bodily function.
- "Mechanically produced disturbances of the nervous system may cause or aggravate disease processes in various parts and functions of the body."[3]
- The basic premise in the chiropractic philosophy is that correction of the dysrelationship of the articulations which we term "subluxation" will restore biomechanical function to the source of dysrelation and provide improved function.
- "The philosophy of Chiropractic is based on the relationship of biomechanics to biodynamics. Biomechanics is the science of mechanical forces as they are applied to a living organism while biodynamics refers to the study of the nature and determinants of an organism's behavior during motion."[3]
- The correction of the dysrelationship is accomplished by the specific chiropractic adjustment.
- "Reduction of the subluxated spinal segments and extra spinal articulations by application of a specific chiropractic adjustment for the purpose of normalizing the relationship of the segment within its motor articular bed, serves to relieve the attending neurological disturbance, reduce the symptom expressions and mitigates the possible attending disease process."[3]

The chiropractic physicians who are granted staff privileges endorse the following overview of the practice responsibilities of a chiropractor as provided in the practice act of the Board of Chiropractic Examiners:

1. The chiropractor will be responsible for taking a comprehensive history while initially interviewing the patient.
2. The chiropractor will conduct systematic physical, orthopedic, neurological, and chiropractic examinations, which will identify the patient's chief complaint, but will also identify those abnormalities that may also alter the normal health status of the patient and inform the patient of same.
3. The chiropractor will identify any underlying health-related problems in the course of an examination for a specific complaint, and will recommend further investigation of any abnormal findings by follow-up diagnostic testing and/or referral to appropriate allied health practitioner.
4. The chiropractor practices those techniques that are within the scope of his or her practice act to assist the patient with the recovery of the patient's chief complaint.
5. The chiropractor may incorporate one or more of the following as the scope of his or her license permits:
   a. Adjust specific spinal vertebrae.
   b. Prescribe and administer physical therapy to the involved area.
   c. Prescribe nutritional advice and dietary instruction to enhance the care and well-being of a patient.
   d. Make use of first aid, strapping, and taping in course of therapy to the area of chief complaint.
   e. Counsel the patient on daily living standards, which help with the care and treatment of the patient's chief complaint.

6. The use of the following is adjunctive physiological therapeutics to the specific adjustment: ultrasound; interferential therapy; electrical muscle stimulation; diathermy; moist hot packs; cryotherapy; cold packs; acupressure and acustimulation acupressure (if certified); exercise therapy; traction (mechanical and manual); and other modes of physiological modalities that have been found to promote the healing process, such as massage.

7. The chiropractor evaluates the progression of the patient at periodic intervals and devises further progressive plans of action, or referral plans for secondary opinions.

8. Manipulation under anesthesia or medication-assisted manipulation with fibrosis release procedures are within the scope of practice for chiropractic physicians by the fact that the program for certification is sponsored by CCE-accredited chiropractic colleges and universities. Manipulation under anesthesia requires additional postgraduate classroom instruction and completion of actual procedures as part of a proctorship for certification.

The chiropractic physicians also embrace the bylaws and rules and regulations of the medical staff and of the Department of Chiropractic Services and agree to adhere to same. The chiropractic staff recognizes that these bylaws and rules and regulations are in accordance with federal, state, and local laws as well as Joint Commission and Medicare regulations.

Chiropractic staff membership is granted only to those chiropractic physicians who accept the above stated philosophy and principles of chiropractic and who abide by the bylaws and rules and regulations. Any violation of these is grounds for rescinding of privileges by the medical executive staff and governing board.

---

Signature of Applicant                                                                                   Date

## DEPARTMENT OF CHIROPRACTIC SERVICES

### PREAMBLE

The Department of Chiropractic Services of _______ will function under a division of the department of _______________. The Department of Chiropractic Services will provide comprehensive chiropractic patient care in a limited area of specialty that will be called manipulation under anesthesia and will function only within the scope of the Chiropractic Practice Act of the state of

_______________.

### OBJECTIVES OF THE DEPARTMENT OF CHIROPRACTIC SERVICES

### (For Manipulation under Anesthesia)

1. The Department of Chiropractic Services (DCS) will provide high-quality chiropractic care on patients referred into the manipulation under anesthesia program. Chiropractic physicians credentialed into the DCS will always endeavor to maintain the highest standards of chiropractic care consistent with the dictates of the ___________ state law on chiropractic and of the chiropractic code of ethics, which this department recognizes as that code of ethics developed by the state Chiropractic Association.

2. The DCS will encourage continuing education programs for the chiropractic physicians involved in the MUA program, and incorporate an adjunct medical education program so that the medical staff will have access to research and development in the chiropractic field.

3. The DCS will provide a forum, by means of staff and committee meetings, wherein problems of mutual concerns to the committee, hospital, administration, medical staff, and chiropractic staff may be discussed and resolved.
4. The DCS will provide high-quality care by participation in the hospital-wide quality assurance program.

## CHIROPRACTIC PROTOCOL AND PROCEDURES

### Section 1. Normal Office Patient Procedures

- Perform systematic physical, neurological, and orthopedic examinations.
- Perform postural and spinal analysis unique to chiropractic diagnoses
- Evaluate and update records to determine case progress and required treatment.
- Improve, correct, or prevent any and/or all components of a subluxation complex of any articulation of the musculoskeletal system.
- Improve any or all components of any abnormal biomechanical condition of the spine or musculoskeletal system.
- Instruct in dietary regimens, nutritional supplements, and physical and mental attitudes that affect health and personal sanitation.
- Instruct in occupational safety, posture, rest, work, rehabilitative exercises, recreational activities, health habits, adaptive lifestyles, and the many other activities of daily living that would enhance the effects of chiropractic health care.
- Physical therapy to include, but not limited to, ultrasound, electrical muscle stimulation, interferential therapy, acupuncture therapy, traction, flexion distraction, diathermy, paraffin bath, galvanic therapy, heat packs, cryotherapy, and soft tissue massage therapy.
- Specific spinal adjustive techniques that are used to mobilize the articulations that help restore spinal or extremity joint flexibility and the subluxation syndrome.

### Section 2. Procedures Required for MUA

- The patient may be required to obtain pre-operative testing. which may include CBC, SMA 6, chest x-ray, or EKG for patients over 50 years of age and pregnancy testing for women of child-bearing age.
- Manipulation under anesthesia is performed in a special operative area equipped with the proper anesthetic and vital sign–monitoring devices, as well as crash cart and ventilation equipment for emergency procedures.
- The number of MUAs is left to the discretion of the doctor of chiropractic and is based on the severity of the problem and the desired outcome. (Follow standards and protocols as established by the National Academy of MUA Physicians.)
- Physical therapy as prescribed in the text is recommended on the same day of the MUA and on subsequent days of therapy, but is left up to the discretion of the doctor and the results that are to be achieved.
- Protocol for credentialing is left up to the facility where the procedure is performed.

---

Signature of Applicant                                                      Date

# SAMPLE BYLAWS FOR A HOSPITAL-BASED
# CHIROPRACTIC DEPARTMENT

### ARTICLE I

Name
The name of this organization will be the Department of Chiropractic Services (DCS).

### ARTICLE II — DCS MEMBERSHIP SPECIFICATIONS

### Section 1. Membership

Membership in the DCS is a privilege that will be offered only to professionally competent chiropractic physicians who continuously meet the qualifications, standards, and requirements set forth in these articles and the state licensing statutes for chiropractic physicians in the state in which each doctor practices.

### Section 2. Qualifications

Qualifications for membership in the Department of Chiropractic Services:

A. Proof of graduation from a chiropractic college presently holding status with a National Chiropractic accrediting agency by the U.S. Department of Education, as well as CCE accreditation.

B  Licensure to practice chiropractic in the state in which you practice.

C. No violations with the Department of Professional Regulations.

D. No violations with any federal professional regulating agency.

E. No felony or criminal violations.

F. Proof of professional liability insurance in accordance with hospital regulations and bylaws.

G. Documented participation in postgraduate education either presently or within the past year. MUA certification can be used if already taken and within the parameters.

H. Completion of a certification course in manipulation under anesthesia. The individual center will establish its own practical requirement.

### Section 3. Application for Membership

Application for membership to the DCS will be in accordance with the regulations governing the department and the bylaws of the hospital. The application will be presented on the prescribed forms, demonstrating qualifications and references of the applicant. The applicant will have three (3) references from staff physicians, two (2) of which must be from chiropractic physicians on staff. The applicant will sign a statement agreeing to abide by the bylaws and the rules and regulations of the DCS. The applicant will sign a statement of agreement relative to commercial advertising. The applicant will also sign the chiropractic philosophy form agreeing with the statement of philosophy and agreeing to abide by the philosophy.

### Section 4. Appointment to the Department of Chiropractic Services

Appointment to the DCS will be in accordance with the bylaws, rules, and regulations of the hospital, and the DCS. Completed applications will be submitted to the chairperson of the Board of Chiropractic of the DCS. All completed applications will be reviewed by the chiropractic credentials committee within thirty (30) days of their receipt. The DCS credentials committee will forward appropriate recommendations to the medical executive review committee, which will forward its recommendations to the governing board.

Appointment to the DCS will also be based on an interview with the chief of chiropractic services, chiropractic board chair, and DCS board during a regularly scheduled meeting of the board. The applicant will be notified by mail and phone call of the date, time, and place of the scheduled meeting. If two scheduled interviews are missed, the application will be dropped.

## Section 5. Appeals

Applicants denied chiropractic privileges may appeal such a decision in accordance with the provisions for such appeal in the bylaws.

## ARTICLE III — DEPARTMENT OF CHIROPRACTIC SERVICES GOVERNING BODY

### Section 1. Chief of Chiropractic Services

The duties of the chiropractic department head will be established by each facility.

### Section 2. Board of Chiropractic of the Department of Chiropractic Services

The board of chiropractic of the Department of Chiropractic Services will consist of a chairperson, a vice chairperson, and three chiropractic physicians chosen by the chief of chiropractic services and the medical executive committee.

The board will function as the governing body of the chiropractic physicians and will be responsive to the directions of the medical executive committee.

The board will function as the review committee for new applicants for staff privileges in accordance with Article II of this document.

The board will meet once a month to discuss concerns of the body of chiropractic physicians, and at other times when the chief of chiropractic services feels the need for chiropractic board approval.

Members of the chiropractic board may not miss more than two meetings per calendar year unless excused, or a new board member will be appointed by the chief of chiropractic services with approval of the medical executive committee.

### Section 3. Responsibilities of Board Members of the Department of Chiropractic Services

A. The chief of staff will be responsible for fulfilling obligations described in Article III, Section 1, of this document.
B. The chairperson will call and preside over monthly board meetings, and will be responsible for working closely with the chief of chiropractic services to see that quality and appropriateness of care is maintained, to identify and resolve problems, and to follow up on the results of the actions taken as they relate to chiropractic services. The chairperson will also sit on the chiropractic review panel for new applicants. The chairman will serve for one year.
C. The vice chairperson will assume the duties and authority of the chairperson during his or her absence or by special request of the chairperson or chief of chiropractic services. The vice chairperson will sit on the chiropractic review panel for new applicants. The vice chairperson will serve for one year.

D. Board members: Three chiropractic physicians who have been credentialed into the DCS in accordance with Article II will be appointed to the board of chiropractic by the chief of chiropractic services. The board members will serve for one year.

## Section 4. Credentials Committee

The board of chiropractic of the DCS functions as the chiropractic portion of the credentialing of new chiropractic applicants to the hospital.

Chief of Department of Chiropractic Services

_______________________________________________     _______________________________
Signature                                            Date

Chairman of the Board of Chiropractic:

_______________________________________________     _______________________________
Signature                                            Date

Chief of Staff:

_______________________________________________     _______________________________
Signature                                            Date

Governing Board Executive Officer:

_____________________________________________________________________________________

Signature of Applicant _______________________________     Date _______________________

# RESPONSIBILITIES OF THE CHIROPRACTIC PRACTITIONER IN THE HOSPITAL OR OUTPATIENT SURGICAL CENTER

1. Make sure patient has been seen by the pre-op approval doctor.
2. Make sure the patient has appropriate testing.
3. Make sure the patient has been informed about the procedure, including adverse reactions, so he or she can feel comfortable signing the consent forms.
4. Contact and communicate with the billing office to make sure the procedures are covered techniques under the patient's insurance. (Hospital or outpatient surgical facility will take care of most of this.)
5. Work with adjustors in a professional manner to educate them about the MUA procedure.
6. Make the family of the MUA patient comfortable by explaining the procedure.
7. Greet the patient the first day of the procedure and put his or her mind at ease about the procedure.
8. Introduce all doctors involved with the procedure.
9. Make the patient comfortable before and after the procedure.
10. Check with the patient while in recovery and before the patient leaves the facility.
11. Make sure your reports are dictated and signed before leaving each day.
12. Make sure the patient understands post-MUA instructions before leaving the facility.

13. Keep accurate records both in the facility and in the office concerning the MUA procedure.
14. Attend meetings called by the center's board of directors.
15. Participate in subcommittee meetings.
16. Involve yourself in the promotion of the validity of your profession and the MUA technique.
17. If you do not feel comfortable in recommending the use of MUA in the appropriate cases in your practice, you should seriously consider the other alternative treatments available to you in chiropractic.

## MEDICAL CHART SEQUENCE

### CONSENTS

Disclosure and Consent for Rendering of Medical Services
Anesthesia — MAC
General
Photography/Videotaping
Chiropractic History and Physical
Medical Clearance
Consultations
Laboratory Results
Radiology Results
MRI Results
EKG
Progress Notes
Operative Report
Discharge Summary
Pre-operative Anesthesia Orders and Evaluation
Anesthesia Records (in consecutive order)
Pre-operative Instructions
Admission/Pre-op Record
Recovery/Discharge Record (consecutive order)
Follow-up Instructions
Patient Correspondence

### MEDICAL RECORDS/HOSPITAL RECORD KEEPING

1. Authority: The authority for maintaining complete and accurate records must be delegated to the director of medical records in a facility. This person reports to the assistant administrator for professional services. Inter-relationships and intra-relations: The medical records department maintains a close relationship with the medical staff. This department also works closely with the nursing department and other ancillary departments and services of hospital and ambulatory surgical centers. It is an integral part of the day-to-day operations and functions quite differently than the record keeping of our private offices.
2. Standards: All records must be completed, assembled and coded in accordance with the standards established by the American Medical Association, American Osteopathic Association, American Chiropractic Association, the Joint Commission on Accreditation of Healthcare Organizations and each state's licensure (HRS and Department of Professional Regulation). The attending physician is directly responsible for accuracy in the completion of each case record.

Facilities will vary in their time constraints on record completions and being signed. The chiropractic physician must govern himself accordingly.[1]

## MEDICAL RECORDS DEPARTMENT SIGNATURE IDENTIFICATION RECORD

Please sign below in as many ways as you would normally sign a medical record. Example: signature, initials, etc. This is for signature identification only, and is not meant for insurance purposes, although an insurance company might request same.

_____________________________________________________________________________

_____________________________________________________________________________

_____________________________________________________________________________

Date Signed _________________________________________________________________

## RESPONSIBILITIES FOR THE CHIROPRACTIC PRACTITIONER IN RECORDNG A COMPLETE PATIENT CHART

Completion of a patient's chart whether in the office or in the hospital or outpatient surgical setting must contain a concise record of the patient's history of symptoms, record of onset and social history, comprehensive physical examination, diagnostic testing (if required), diagnostic impression from a breakdown of the differential diagnosis, and a working plan of action that has as its cortex the ability to be flexible to the patient's response to treatment.

### History

The purpose of a history is to record all of the pertinent information that the patient relates regarding the primary and secondary symptoms that brought the patient to you. In most instances, it is necessary for the doctor to bring important facts to light by specific questions regarding the patient's feelings both physical and mental since the coordination of both physical and mental entities control the patient's perception of discomfort or what the patient will describe as pain.

A good history should include the following information:

1. Primary patient complaint: What exactly does the patient feel and where is the discomfort principally located? Is there more than one location? Is the sensation the patient feels descriptive or nondescriptive (i.e., pain in my back and burning pain down my leg)?
2. Onset of the primary patient complaint: A description of the way the complaint came on is important in ruling out other entities with similar symptoms.
3. Past history: Has the patient had these same or similar symptoms in the past, and have these symptoms been treated by other physicians? What was the previous diagnosis and what was the outcome?
4. Social history: What familiar history relates to the patient symptoms? What kind of work does the patient do? What kinds of physical activities is the patient engaged in (i.e., exercise program).
5. Personal profile: Should contain age, marital status, number of children, spouse's occupation (may directly relate to how symptoms appeared if wife or husband do the same or similar work, etc.) This would also be an area of the history to inquire about how the patient is able to handle the stress in his or her life. Sleeping habits would fall into this category.

6. Specifics as described by the patient: This is a section of the history in which I let the patient personally describe the sensation he or she is experiencing, point with finger to the exact location, and tell what makes the symptoms better, and what makes them worse. This portion of the history can be redundant, but also may bring out small facts that could lead to significant findings. Here we are specific.

## REPORT OF MUA (OPERATION REPORT)

The operative report is a significant report that describes the daily activities that were accomplished in the operative area.

It is also a section that describes the technique in detail. This portion of the daily report will not usually change a great deal if multiple MUAs are accomplished. The doctor may wish to write any responses that are noted, and then will want to write the patient response in his or her office daily notes when the doctor sees the patient in the office.

The portion on "procedure performed" needs to be written in detail and describes what was actually accomplished with the patient from the time the patient is placed supine on the table until the procedure is completed. (See the sample operative report.) In this report, you will describe the area that is contacted; the procedural stretching that was accomplished; the position the patient's body was in; the specific contact that was made on the patient's vertebrae; what segment or segments were moved; the direction of the movement; and what was accomplished with the movement.

The portion of the report that deals with the physiological description of what was accomplished by the adjustment can vary with the individual MUA instructor you learn the procedure from to describe what happens when an adjustment occurs. Because this is a theoretical consideration and has not as of yet been fully researched, we use general terminology to describe the results of the adjustment so that anyone reading the report would have a descriptive idea of what occurred. The reason for this text is to try to standardize this concept further.

We recommend the phrases –"taking the joint to its full range of motion" and "stretching the ligamentus apparatus to its full elastic barrier." Once this is accomplished, a low-velocity thrust is made toward the rotation of the range and an "audible release" will normally occur. Literature has described this "sound" as "cavitation." Two respected authors, John Triano and Richard Sandoz, refer to this phenomenon as a slight cavity being made by the hyaline cartilage cover of the articulation as the rapid movement is made and the pressure causes a slight indentation, or cupping, which causes release of gases and the suction or "popping" sound. An "audible release" is also an acceptable term and appears to be used more frequently.[4,5]

Each area that is manipulated under anesthesia is described, and then a description of what occurred after the procedure (i.e., the patient was awakened and moved to a gurney for transport to recovery) will follow as the report ends. The report is signed by the primary treating physician and dated. This report needs to be in the patient's file within 24 hours of the procedure.

## DICTATING AN OPERATIVE REPORT

An operative report that is used when the doctor is involved in the MUA program may be new to the doctor of chiropractic. Not that we haven't written reports and narratives in our clinics, but this type of report is specific for a one-day description of a procedure, which we generally are not used to doing. Remember, progress notes are different than operative reports.

In an operative report, the facility, especially a hospital that is governed by quality assurance parameters, must provide justification for doing any procedure that is performed. As such, an operative report is descriptive in nature, concise, and supportive with regard to clinical justification.

Sample operative reports are contained within the text, but the doctor must be cognizant of the fact that a sample is a sample. If you are going to model your report after the sample that we have written, describe your procedure in accordance with the responses you elicit from your patient, and do not in any way make each report sound identical.

I realize that the description of the procedure itself is fairly similar on each day, but maintain unique differences as you describe positions, topography, articular sites, and audible releases or cavitation. These factors will be different in each case, and they should be different on each successive day. However, if you are using the same procedure in the same area each day, if multiple procedures are done, indicate in your operative report that "similar responses were achieved in the previous day's treatment of the same area with the slight difference that I found ___________________." The doctors who have been caught in a "cross-fire" during depositions and court appearances have discovered that, if they used a sample report and did not personalize that report with what we have just presented, it basically put them in the position of trying to explain why each day looked the same.

In addition, the third-party payors are now requesting a brief explanation of what was accomplished and why you feel the need to continue with the next day, especially when your case is a multiple or serial MUA procedure.

In these cases what we are now explaining to the adjustors is that the procedure itself is going to be multiple days. In the authorization phase, you would determine the number of MUA procedures necessary based on National Academy of MUA Physician Standards and Protocols, and would describe this need to the insurance company as a means of clinically justifying the entire procedure.

However, as a precursor to running into this situation with the insurance industry, use a statement such as this:

> "The patient responded as expected on day one of the procedure. We were able to achieve ____ degrees of (flexion, extension, lateral bending, etc.). We are not able to completely mobilize the articulation in the affected area of ________ and will continue with day (2, 3) of the procedure as initially prescribed."

This would alleviate a lot of discrepancies in the reports being sent to the insurance industry.

Finally, remember that when your chart becomes part of the hospital, or ambulatory surgical center, it is open to observation and scrutiny. If you have clinically justified your case, have presented the case in a concise manner, and have described the MUA that follows a specific course, and that representatively is the proper procedure to use to alleviate a particular patient's problem, you have presented all material required for the highest quality standard of care.

## OPERATIVE REPORT (SAMPLE)

This is an operative report for manipulation under anesthesia.

Patient's name: _______________________________________________

Date of the procedure: _________________________________________

Attending physician: ___________________________________________

First assistant: ________________________________________________

Facility: _____________________________________________________

Pre-op diagnosis: _____________________________________________

Post-op diagnosis: ____________________________________________

Anesthesia used (if known): _____________________________________

**Informed Consent**

After adequate explanation of the medical, surgical, and procedural options, this patient has decided to proceed with the recommended spinal manipulation under anesthesia. The patient has been informed that (more than one) (another) procedure may be necessary to achieve satisfactory results.

**Indication**

Upon review of the patient's history and supplied medical records, a plateau has been reached reflecting minimal further improvement with past treatment attempts. Upon examination, less-than-optimum range of motion is present with significant end range pain and myofacial tenderness to palpation and/or including radicular pain or paresthesia. Considering this patient is not a surgical candidate/failed surgery; or has received minimal to no relief from other aggressive treatments/is fearful of other aggressive treatments such as epidural and/or facet and/or trigger point injections and that no other conservative medical intervention other than MUA is available at this point in time, it is deemed appropriate to commence with a series of three MUAs. The standards of protocol being followed are set forth by the National Academy of MUA Physicians.

**Comments**

The patient understands the essence of the diagnosis and the reasons for MUA. The associated risks of the procedure, including anesthesia complications, fracture, vascular accident, disc herniation, and post-procedure discomfort, were thoroughly discussed with the patient. Alternatives to the procedure, including the course of the condition without MUA, were discussed. The patient understands the chances of success from undergoing MUA and that no guarantees are made or implied regarding outcome. The patient has given both verbal and written informed consent for the listed procedure.

**The Procedure in Detail**

The patient was draped in appropriate gowning (and was taken by gurney) (accompanied) to the operative area and asked to lie supine on the operative table. The patient was then placed on the appropriate monitors for this procedure. When the patient and I were ready, the anesthesiologist administered the appropriate medications to assist the patient into twilight sedation using medications that allow the stretching, mobilization, and adjustments necessary for the completion of the outcome I desired.

*The Cervical Spine*

The patient's arms were crossed and the patient was approached from the cephalad end of the table. Long axis traction was applied to the patient's cervical spine and musculature while countertraction was applied by the first assistant. The first assistant was positioned to stabilize the patient's shoulders in order to use this countertraction maneuver. Traction in the same manner was then applied into a controlled lateral coronal plane bilaterally, and then in an oblique manner by rotating the patient's head to 45 degrees and elevating the head toward the patient's chest. This was also accomplished bilaterally. The patient's head was then brought into a neutral posture and cervical flexion was achieved to traction the cervical paravertebral muscles. The cervical spine was then taken into rotatory/lateral traction maneuver to achieve specific closed reduction manipulation of vertebral elements at the level of ______ on the right side and again using the same technique on the left side at the level of ______. During this maneuver, a low-velocity thrust was achieved after taking the vertebrae slightly past the elastic barrier of resistance. Cavitation (was achieved) (was not achieved).

*Shoulder Thoracic Lift*

With the patient in the supine position, the doctor distracted the right/left arm straight cephalad to end range. This was accomplished on both sides to release thoracic elements before the thoracic adjustment.

*Shoulder*

(This technique must not be attempted if the patient has calcific tendonitis or there is a chance for a rotator cuff tear. Both of these conditions must be ruled out before attempting MUA on the shoulder.)

(The cervical and upper thoracic spine MUA procedures are performed prior to the shoulder technique. The adjustment that is part of the shoulder MUA technique needs to be perfected with the patient in the erect position before trying to accomplish the procedure with the patient in the side lying position.)

With the patient in the supine position, the doctor stood on the side of involvement. The doctor took the patient's arm in the bent arm position and tractioned up away from the patient's body and tucked the extremity into the doctor's abdominal area. The doctor had contact at the crook of the patient's bent arm and support contact on the patient's lateral shoulder area over the mid-deltoid area. In this position, the doctor then walked the extremity forward into forward flexion, noting range of motion and patient's resistance. Crepitation would usually occur during the first day of the procedure during this maneuver. Once the doctor had taken the extremity and thus the shoulder into forward flexion, the next move was to leave the contact hand in place and do an adduction traction over the doctor's hand toward the middle of the patient's body. The next move was to relocate the doctor's position so that internal and external ranges of motion were performed (the doctor was standing at the patient's head facing the patient's feet on the side of involvement). The doctor could take the shoulder through simple external and internal ranges of motion on the first day and then become more aggressive on the following days by contacting the upper extremity up near the axial and doing internal and external rotation closer to the body.

The next part of the procedure was the same forward flexion maneuver with the arm straight. Traction was accomplished by contacting the wrist (watch the carpal tunnel), tucking the arm in close to the doctor, and then walking the arm forward into forward flexion. Then the same adduction move was accomplished with the doctor keeping the arm straight and tractioning the arm over his or her hand toward mid-line of the body. Next the doctor stood at the head of the patient and lowered the patient's arm to his side. Forward flexion was then accomplished with a knife edge contact at the acromioclavicular humeral joint area. Traction was made during forward flexion into the knife edge and a slight thrust into the joint was made.

The doctor then assumed the forward position and tractioned the arm up and away and at the same time rotated his or her hip into the axillary area. This opened up the joint space and the doctor contacted the lateral border of the clavicle and administered three short toggle thrusts into the area with a pisiform contact. The thrusts were not directed into the clavicle but the line of drive was more toward the lateral clavicle and the medial border of the humerus.

The patient was then placed in the side lying position and circumduction clockwise and counterclockwise was accomplished by contacting the head of the humerus. This maneuver was accomplished by the doctor cupping the hands with interwoven fingers around the head of the humerus, and the movements were very small and deliberate.

Once all these maneuvers were accomplished, the doctor then completed the A to P adjustive procedure that was originally learned with the patient in the erect position. Contact was at the cephalad border of the pectoralis major with support for the scapula and at the anterior aspect of the humeral glenoid cavity joint. The thrust was a motion that mimics the relocation of the head of the humerus into the glenoid cavity. The movement was up and over the shoulder with respect to line of drive. (This procedure is demonstrated in the class workshops and should not be performed if the doctor has not had manual training in this maneuver.)

*The Thoracic Spine*

With the patient in the supine position on the operative table, the upper extremities were flexed at the elbow and crossed over the patient's chest to achieve maximum traction to the patient's thoracic spine. The first assistant held the patient's arms in the proper position and assisted in rolling the patient for the adjustive procedure. With the help of the first assistant, the patient was rolled to his or her left/right side, selection was made for the contact point, and the patient was rolled back over the doctor's hand. The elastic barrier of the resistance was found, and a low-velocity thrust was achieved using a specific closed reduction anterior to posterior/superior manipulative procedure. (This same procedure was completed at the level of __________.)

*The Lumbar Spine*

With the patient supine on the procedure table, the primary physician addressed the patient's lower extremities which were elevated alternatively in a straight leg raising manner to approximately 90 degrees from the horizontal. Linear force was used to increase the hip flexion gradually during this maneuver. Simultaneously, the first assistant physician applied a myofacial release technique to the calf and posterior thigh musculature. Each lower extremity was independently bent at the knee and tractioned cephalad in a neutral saggital plane, lateral oblique cephalad traction, and medial oblique cephalad traction maneuver. The primary physician then approximated the opposite single knee from his or her position from neutral to medial slightly beyond the elastic barrier of resistance (a piriformis myofascial release was accomplished at this time). This was repeated with the opposite lower extremity. Following this, a Patrick-Fabere maneuver was performed up to and slightly beyond the elastic barrier of resistance.

*Piriformis Bow-String Stretch*

With the patient in the side lying posture and following the adductor stretch, the patient's knee was held slightly past medial and the primary doctor contacted the knee with his or her hand. The force was applied toward the table with the help of the first assistant, and the piriformis muscle was then massaged. The force down the femur into the pelvic basin allowed for relaxation of the piriformis muscle across the obturator foramin.

With the assisting physician stabilizing the pelvis and femoral head (as necessary), the primary physician extended the right lower extremity in the saggital plane, and while applying controlled traction radially stretched the para-articular holding elements of the right hip by means of gradually describing an approximately 30–35 degree horizontal arc. The lower extremity was then tractioned straight caudad and internal rotation was accomplished. Using traction, the lower extremity was gradually stretched into a horizontal arch to approximately 30 degrees. This procedure was then repeated using external rotation to stretch the para-articular holding elements of the hips bilaterally. These procedures were then repeated on the opposite lower extremity.

By approximating the patient's knees to the abdomen in a knee-chest fashion, the lumbo-pelvic musculature was stretched in saggital plane, by both the primary and first assistant, contacting the base of the sacrum and raising the lower torso cephalad, resulting in passive flexion of the entire lumbar spine and its holding elements beyond the elastic barrier of resistance. The knees were kept outside the torso during this stretch to reduce abdominal pressure. With the patient's lower extremities kept in hip/knee flexion, the patient's torso was secured by the first assistant and the lumbar fasciae/musculature elongated obliquely to the right of mid-line, in a controlled manner up to and beyond the elastic barrier of resistance. (Cavitation was noted.) This was repeated on the opposite side.

With the use of undersheets, the patient was carefully placed in the left/right decubitus position and positioned so that the lumbar spine overlay the kidney plate to the point where the lumbar spine attained the horizontal and was derotated to avoid facet imbrication.

*Medial Scapular Border Lift*

With the patient in the side-lying position, the patient's lower arm was moved behind the patient to allow relaxation of the scapular muscles. With the help of the first assistant, the primary doctor reached into the medial scapular area and lifted both vertically and laterally to separate subscapular adhesions. The first assistant applied counter traction from anterior to posterior on the patients shoulder to allow for the continued distraction of the scapular border.

### Iliopsoas Stretch

With the patient in the side-lying position, the upper leg was bent at the knee and distracted in a horizontal manner to stretch the iliopsoas muscle. The leg was then extended more caudally at a 30-degree angle to stretch the TFL (*tensor fasciae latae*).

The patient's body was stabilized by the first assistant. The knee and hip of the upper leg were flexed and the lower leg stabilized in the extended position by the first assistant. Segmental localization of the appropriate lumbar motion-units was made by the primary physician and the elastic barrier of resistance found. A low-velocity impulse thrust was applied achieving cavitation. (The PSIS was then adjusted on the opposite side with the patient in the same position as earlier.)

The patient was then repositioned supine by means of the undersheets. With appropriate assistance, the patient was transferred from the procedure table to the gurney and was returned to the recovery room, where appropriate monitoring equipment was utilized to monitor vital signs. The IV was maintained up to the point where the patient was fully alert and stable. The patient was then transferred to a sitting recovery position and given fluids and a light snack. Following this, the patient was discharged with appropriate home instructions.

### Complications

The patient tolerated the procedure well with no untoward incident or complication. (This would be where any complications would be described.)

### Summary

The patient underwent serial MUA of the cervical spine and/or dorsal spine and/or lumbosacral spine and/or (R), (L) shoulder(s) and/or (R), (L) hip(s). The patient tolerated the procedure well; there were no intra-operative or post-operative complications. The patient was able to achieve increased motion post-MUA with some continued muscle guarding. With the improvement of range of motion, it is medically reasonable to opine that this patient's fibro-adhesive conditions were significantly impacted, increasing the potential for appropriate neuromuscular reeducation of affected myofacial structures and before having reestablishment of collagen deposition during the healing phase.

### PATIENT INSTRUCTIONS (THIS IS PUT IN THE LAST DAY OF A SERIAL PROCEDURE)

The patient will receive post-MUA therapy in the doctor's office or physical therapy suite to include heating the area of involvement; stretching of the involved areas just as they were stretched during the MUA procedure; followed by interferential HVGS and ice. This will be completed each day after the MUA. Following the last MUA, the patient will complete the exact same stretching maneuvers with the addition of the adjustive/manipulative procedure. This will be accomplished for 7–10 days.

This period is then followed by 2 weeks of pre-rehabilitation with emphasis on early strengthening. This is then followed by 4 weeks of formal rehabilitation, which involves strengthening the weakened areas. Adjustive/manipulative therapy should be accomplished 2–3 times per week pre-rehabilitation and for 1–2 times per week during formal rehabilitation.

### Prognosis (This is the continuation of the above report)

Considering the patient's overall improvement in function and diminishing pain, it is opined, absent further injury, that the patient's prognosis is considered to be good. The patient has been instructed that periodic exacerbations/remissions may be experienced. These may be adequately managed by means of palliative care.

### AUTHORIZATION TO ADMIT OBSERVERS

I, __________ authorize Dr. __________ and the __________ Hospital to permit observers in addition to physicians and hospital personnel while I am undergoing the MUA procedure.

Patient: ________________________________________          Date: __________________
(parent or legal guardian)

### FACILITY CHARTING

The properly completed patient's chart is a permanent record of significant current and future value to the patient's well-being. It also can be your best friend if it is evaluated in front of a judge and jury.
   The facility chart generally provides the following information:

1. It is the means of communications between professionals. Any professional involved in the patient care — now or later — needs to be able to understand all of the entries. A remark of a spinal adjustment may mean nothing to your fellow practitioner, let alone a vascular surgeon. The chart must provide communication capabilities, not just a lot of verbiage. Abbreviations may not be used, unless they are on an approved list of same, on file in the medical records department.
2. Plan of individual patient care:
   a. The patient is admitted with a working diagnosis.
   b. The doctor orders special treatment procedures.
   c  The nurse carries out his or her orders.
   d. Consultations are done, including x-rays, lab, etc. to consolidate the diagnosis.
   e. It is hoped that a correction of the condition will result.
3. The patient chart documents evidence of the course of the ailment, the treatment rendered, and results of the treatment.
4. It serves as a basis for the analysis and study of the evaluation of the effectiveness of patient care.
5. It assists in protecting the legal interest of the patient, the doctor and the hospital. It is worth repeating that it can be your best friend when you are confronted by a judge and jury.

The properly completed patient chart tells the story of the patient's stay in the hospital or ambulatory surgical center and protects the patient, doctor, and facility from false, misleading, or derogatory accusations should this occur. The charts are also a track record of the patient care and the provider's quality of treatment.

### PATIENT INFORMATION

Authorization for Release of Patient Information for Insurance Purposes

I authorize _______ (medical practice), their members and employees to furnish
________________________________________________ (insurance company),
a copy of all medical records in their possession regarding __________________
(patient's name).
I further authorize the release of a medical narrative, explanation, or other follow-up information as requested by the above named insurance company, including care rendered up to the time of their request.
I understand that these medical records may contain information from other treating physicians as well as administrative data that is not strictly medical in nature.

I additionally understand that once released as requested, __________ (medical practice), their members and employees, have no responsibility for any further requests of information by the insurance company.

Finally, I release __________ (medical practice), their members and employees, from all responsibility or liability that may arise from their compliance with this authorization.

Signed: __________________________________________

(patient or patient's authorized representative)

Witness: __________________________________________

Date: ___________________________________________

## LEGAL GUIDE FOR PHYSICIANS

Limited Authorization for Release of Patient Information for Insurance Purposes

I authorize __________________ (medical practice), their members and employees, to furnish to __________________ (insurance company), a copy of all medical records in their possession regarding __________________ (patient's name), for the period __________________ to ________________ for the condition of __________________.

I understand that these medical records may contain information from other treating physicians as well as administrative data that is not strictly medical in nature. I additionally understand that once released _____(medical practice), their members and employees, have no responsibility for any further release of the information by the insurance company.

Finally, I release __________________ (medical practice), their members and employees, from all responsibility or liability that may arise from their compliance with this authorization.

Signed __________________________________________

(patient or patient's authorized representative)

Witness: __________________________________________

Date: ___________________________________________

# HOSPITAL/OUTPATIENT MUA PROGRAM

## HOSPITAL ADMISSIONS

A. Inpatient or outpatient services
1. Insurance information
2. Admitting DX
3. Special test/consults/etc.
4. 23-hour admit (short stay)
5. Co-admit doctor
6. Standard orders
B. Co-admit doctors protocols
C. Responsibilities of primary and co-admitting physician
D. Pre-op consultation/education with patient
E. Patient preparation
1. NPO
2. Driver

    3. Jewelry
    4. Makeup
  F.  Anesthesiology
    1. Pre-anesthesia exam
    2. Nursing prep
  G.  Transport to operating room
  H.  Lifting procedure

## Categories:

A.  Same-Day Admit: These are patients who are admitted the day of manipulation under anesthesia and have to remain in the hospital for 24 hours or longer. This is very rare today, but if there were complications that needed to be addressed, the patient might be admitted for observation for a 24-hour period.

B.  Short-Stay Admit: These are patients who are admitted following the spinal manipulation under anesthesia but only stay in the hospital for 23.5 hours or less.

C.  Outpatient Surgery: These are patients who come in for the procedure and leave following recovery. There is no in-house admission or post-op services provided other than standard recovery. This is the standard of care today with the MUA procedure. 99.9% of the MUA procedures completed today have little if any problem that would require further followup in a hospital. Most procedures are now completed in outpatient ambulatory surgical centers with hospitals only as backup should anything occur that would require transport.

D.  Inpatient Admission: These are patients who are admitted to the hospital for other conditions that might also include visits from the chiropractic physician. These cases usually involve patients who have become anatomically immobile due to surgeries, etc., and in need of manipulation to release fixated joints while they are recovering. This is not usually part of the MUA program.

## PROFESSIONAL PROTOCOL FOR THE OPERATIVE AREA AND RECOVERY AREA IN A HOSPITAL OR AMBULATORY SURGICAL CENTER

The chiropractic profession will move into the 21st century with the relationships that will develop by doing the MUA procedure. The medical friendships that have already developed around the country from the knowledge passed on by the chiropractic physicians already doing this procedure are exciting.

"As our profession evolves through change and the growing pains associated with a new environment, it becomes necessary for each of us to observe certain courtesies that are mandated by the seriousness of the responsibility for our patient's safety in and around the hospital operating suite and recovery area."[1]

Protocol in the setting we will find ourselves as we move into outpatient surgical centers and hospitals demands a new sense on common concerns for those around you that the solo practitioner in a chiropractic office does not always encounter. The primary concerns in this setting are patient safety and proper procedural techniques.

Second to this responsibility is the respect and courtesies afforded the primary treating doctor. It is up to the treating doctor to dictate the environment the patient should be in. By this I mean that if the doctor desires to close off the operating room to observation, it should not be a matter for discussion.

The primary treating doctor dictates the procedures to be completed, how they are to be completed, who the first assistant will be, and what kind of help is needed.

Other than the anesthesiologist, the primary treating doctor is the chief during the procedure. The patient and the doctor's wishes are expected to be honored. The primary treating doctor will always honor the wishes of the anesthesiologist and will not question the call to back away from the patient should they be requested to do so during the procedure.

The primary treating doctor should stay in control of the entire procedure until the recovery team takes control of the patient. The recovery team must be respected by the primary treating physician. A visit initially to get the patient psychologically comfortable after the procedure and a return to review progress toward the end of recovery is all that is needed unless the recovery team deems the doctor's presence necessary to make the patient more comfortable. Professional courtesies dictate that the primary treating doctor allow the recovery staff to do their job, and respect them for the job they do.

Many other factors enter into the basic "business" of making the MUA operative area a well-run, efficient arm of the outpatient surgical facility or hospital, but of utmost concern is the behavior of the chiropractic physicians who use the facility.

Every courtesy should be afforded to the patient's admitting/treating chiropractic physician. In our eagerness to observe and assist, we are oftentimes so involved in the excitement of the moment that we may perhaps allow caution and courtesy to slide. It is of utmost importance that we maintain our professionalism at all times. Observing doctors physically present in the operating area should be kept to a minimum to continue the professional atmosphere necessary in the OR to address the patient's problem. The operating area can become very congested at times when professional integrity is forgotten and/or not observed carefully.

When we enter this new environment, especially in a hospital setting, we are going to be highly scrutinized until the mainstay staff and allied physicians become familiar with what we do. That is not to say that we are any different than any other entity that has become part of the hospital setting. As the "new kid on the block," we need to show professional patience and courteous understanding of other disciplines around us. If we do, we will easily be accepted into the natural flow of things.

## CONSIDERATION FOR MUA PATIENT TRANSPORT

The manipulation under anesthesia procedure is completed in an outpatient surgical center or in an outpatient facility of a hospital. The patient will usually walk into the operative area but will be transported out of the operative area on a gurney or rolling bed. The following precautions should be followed when working with an anesthetized patient recovering from the MUA procedure:

1. Make sure you stay with your patient until the patient is transferred to the gurney or rolling bed that will transport the patient to the recovery area.
2. If you are responsible for more than one procedure for the day, make sure the patient in recovery is stabilized before beginning the next procedure. The nursing staff will usually indicate when the next patient is ready and when your previous patient has been stabilized.
3. When having the patient move from the operating table to the gurney (the patient may be responsive to command before moving), make sure the patient's arms and legs are moved together with the torso as the patient slides toward the gurney.
4. If you are responsible for supporting the gurney next to the operative table, make sure that you are leaning on the table to prevent a gap between the operative table and gurney as the patient makes the lateral move to the gurney. This is the responsibility of the OR nursing staff, but assistance is always appreciated.
5. Make sure that the gurney table wheels are locked by pushing on the wheel brake. (Note: Table will move again by putting the brake mechanism in the center position.)
6. The patient will be moved to the center of the gurney, and should be told to do so until the guardrails can be raised. (Guardrails must be up when transporting a patient.)

7. Make sure your patient is comfortable following the MUA procedure (i.e., if the patient is cold, use a blanket to cover him or her). Again, this is the responsibility of the nursing staff, but this is your patient and you can request assistance if you feel there is concern at the time.

8. Be cautious of the patient's extremities when moving the patient from operating area to recovery. The patient's arms or legs can get hit on door jams, etc. while being transported if not careful. Remember, even though you might be having what appears to be a lucid conversation with your patient immediately following the procedure, the patient has not recovered enough from the anesthesia to protect him- or herself in transport.

9. Be aware of the patient's IV while moving the patient to prevent having the IV pulled free from the patient.

10. Be aware of exposed needles in the operative area. This is your responsibility to prevent blood-borne pathogens from being transferred. Precautions are expected by the facility staff and anesthesiologists, but you must remember to protect yourself in this situation as the treating physician and be aware of your surroundings.

11. Give the recovery room staff the courtesy they deserve in transporting your patient to the recovery area.

## DAILY PROGRESS NOTES

The chiropractic/osteopathic physician who controls the progress of a patient under treatment is required to record that progress. In many facilities where MUA is performed today, the only reports that the treating doctor is required to complete is the dictated OP report and discharge summary.

If required by the facility, the progress notes are a daily journal of the way a patient is responding, or not responding, to the care that is being given. Progress notes are necessary as legal documents to protect the physician.

Progress notes must be kept on all patients. They represent the daily worksheet that has occurred in your office, or in the hospital or ambulatory surgical setting, and must be kept concise and accurate.

In the office, the daily journal should contain

- Daily patient comments
- Subjective complaints
- Objective testing (brief)
- Progress from previous visit
- Treatment rendered and area (P.T.)
- Adjustment rendered and level
- Any referral information
- Day and time of treatment
- Record of treating physician (s)

In the hospital setting, the daily journal is in the form of the report that is contained in this section.

## THE DISCHARGE SUMMARY FOR THE MUA PROCEDURE

The discharge summary is a report that is filed following the completion and final observation of the MUA procedures. Since it is being left up to the doctor's discretion as to the number of MUAs required for optimum results from this procedure, this report can be written after 1, 2, 3, or even after 5 procedures have been completed. However, if the MUA procedures are not completed all together on consecutive days, then a discharge summary must be completed after the consecutive

MUAs whatever that might be. (Example: Once MUA is done, the discharge summary would be submitted with the daily operative report and the H&P. If 3 MUAs were completed, the discharge summary would be submitted with the third operative report after the third consecutive manipulation.)

The discharge summary is a summary of findings before and after the completion of the MUA procedure and should also list a follow-up plan of treatment for the patient. It is also wise to indicate the potential for this procedure be repeated at a future time just to leave this option open to you and the patient should you desire to try the procedure again. This would be especially true if the MUA procedure was only done once or twice.

The final segment of the discharge summary is instructions for the patient to follow for that final day and for the next 4–6 weeks following the MUA procedure.

The doctor then signs and dates it.

## SAMPLE DISCHARGE SUMMARY

This is a discharge summary for manipulation under anesthesia.

The patient's name is  _______________________________________________________

The dates of the operation are  _________________________________________________

The physician is  ___________________________________________________________

The first assistant is  _________________________________________________________

The facility is  _____________________________________________________________

The pre-op diagnosis is  ______________________________________________________

The post-op diagnosis is  _____________________________________________________

## Postoperative DX

1. Same
2. Same (These are the pre-op and post-op diagnoses, and they remain the same even after the MUA is completed)

## Indication

Failure of extended conservative care by means of aggressive physical medicine and pharmacological intervention.

## RATIONALE FOR PROCEDURE

Notwithstanding the fact that the patient has improved since the beginning of conservative treatment (physical and manual medicine, trigger point injection, and focused functional restoration exercise), a plateau has been reached that reflects no further improvement. Less-than-optimum ROM is present together with significant end-range pain and myofascial tenderness upon palpation. Considering the fact that the patient was and is not a surgical candidate, and no other conservative medical intervention, other than MUA, was available, it was deemed medically reasonable and appropriate to offer the option to the patient, prior to considering invasive interventional pain medicine procedures (i.e., Epidural Steroid Injection, Selective Nerve Root Blockage, Facet Block, etc.).

The considered opinion of the attending medical team was that MUA was the intervention of choice pertinent to addressing the fibro-adhesive capsulitis/myofascitis and muscle contracture, in an overall effort in restoring normal function and ameliorating the presenting pain syndrome.

## PROCEDURE/POST-PROCEDURE COURSE

Example: The patient underwent serial MUA of the cervical and thoracic spine on ______________. The patient tolerated the procedure well and there were no intraoperative or post-operative complications.

## RESULTS ACCOMPLISHED

The patient was able to achieve near-normal ROM post MUA with a significant reduction of muscle guarding. Immediate post-procedure sequelae were mild/moderate but tolerable and manageable. With the improvement of ROM it is medically reasonable to opine that this patient's fibro-adhesive condition was significantly impacted, increasing the potential for appropriate neuromuscular reeducation of affected myofascial structures and befitting reestablishment of collagen deposition during the healing phase.

## PATIENT INSTRUCTIONS

The patient will receive post-MUA therapy for the next 7–10 days consisting of interferential electrical stimulation, cryotherapy, application of mild myofascial release stretching, with post-therapy discharge to home for rest and additional cryotherapy. Subsequent to this regime, formal functional restoration therapeutics will commence on a frequency basis of 3× weekly for two weeks. This will be followed by 2–3 weeks of formal rehabilitation.

The above protocol is essential in order to maintain the functional gains presently enjoyed by the patient as well as to allow appropriate collagen remodeling of the fibro-adhesive structures and the circumvention of their reformation.

## PROGNOSIS

Considering the patient's overall improvement in function and diminishing in VAS scores, it is opined, absent further injury, that the patient's prognosis is considered to be good. The patient has been instructed that periodic recrudescence and/or exacerbation/remissions may be experienced. These may be adequately managed by means of palliative care, and the patient knows to contact us immediately should these be experienced.

## REFERENCES


1. Capps, S., Texas College of Chiropractic, syllabus: Manipulation under anesthesia, postgraduate course of study, 1992.
2. Gordon, R. with contribution from Furno, P., Cornerstone Professional Education, Inc., MUA syllabus currently sponsored by the National University of Health Sciences, 5th ed., August 1998.
3. Janse, J., in *Principles and Practice of Chiropractic, an Anthology*, R.W. Hildebrandt, DC, Ed., National College of Chiropractic, Kjellberg and Sons Inc., Wheaton, IL, 1976: 47-48, 88–93.
4. Triano, J., Dean of Postgraduate Education, 1992, National College of Chiropractic, Lombard, IL, Correlations.
5. Sandoz, R., "Physical mechanisms of effect of spinal adjustment," *Ann. Swiss Chiro. Assoc.* 6: 91, 1976.

# 15 Risk/Benefit Ratio of Manipulation Under Anesthesia

*Robert C. Gordon*

Since the late 1930s manipulation of the spine requiring anesthesia has been used successfully to treat countless patients who suffer from neuromusculoskeletal discomfort. Most of these patients suffered through years of alternative forms of therapy before reaching the point where they would try anything to overcome the problems that were afflicting them.

When introduced to the MUA procedure, most of the patients who were approached were extremely willing to have an anesthetic incorporated into their treatment because they had tried most forms of therapy and MUA was another alternative prior to surgery, or in some cases following failed surgery.

This book traces the history, scientific basis, protocols, and procedures that have been used for some 70 years in the performance of the MUA procedure. We would not be comprehensive in our presentation of the MUA procedure, however, if we did not present complications that have been noted over the years with the use of this procedure.

Any procedure that uses anesthesia in any form runs the risk of complications. Some patients may be at risk for reactions to anesthesia simply because they have never been placed in the anesthesia environment. The medications used for the MUA procedure have never been introduced into their systems before. Allergic reactions to the medications can occur.

From the standpoint of the manual therapist, the MUA procedure is a procedure that is elective but necessary. The procedure is not an emergency but is required for the patient to fully recover. If the doctor who is performing the MUA does not feel absolutely positive that this is the right treatment for the patient, then the patient should not be considered for the procedure.

The manipulative procedures used in the office are completed with high velocity and low amplitude, and, therefore, if injury were going to occur with manipulative therapy, it would most likely occur in the office. The reason for this is the fact that the patient is placed in a physiological state that allows for relaxation, but there is end-range protection using this type of anesthesia. In other words, as we take the patient through the various movements and adjustive procedures required to accomplish this technique, the patient does not immediately have secondary muscle contraction like they would have in the office setting. Because of this factor, we are able to move the muscles and the articulations around in a protective environment, but in a less restrictive environment than in the office.

By using this form of passive stretch and articular movement, we are able to achieve our objective, but the patient does not immediately resist. This might make the reader who is not familiar with MUA think that this is also a way to tear muscles, and sublux, or dislocate articulations. I would expect this thinking with the untrained person. What must be remembered is that using monitored anesthesia care (MAC) does not take away normal protective processes in the body the way they were once taken away when general anesthesia with intubation techniques were used. Normal end range is maintained, and the certified MUA practitioner is able to feel the end range and move the patient from restricted ranges into fully completed ranges of motion without tearing the muscles or injuring the articular components. The holding elements of the articulation are just mobilized gently to allow for more gentle closed-reduction motion of the articulations with very little resistance or combativeness on the part of the patient. This concept has always been at the core of the debate about the effectiveness of MUA and the risk that using an anesthesia has on the patient. The fact is that the use of MUA is considerably more gentle on the patient than the office manual therapy techniques, and if you add high-velocity forces to the equation as are performed in the office setting, many of the chronic cases that are referred for the MUA technique simply can't tolerate manual therapy of the high-velocity type at all. When manual therapy is the therapy of choice and the patient has tried a conservative course of therapy in the office setting, the most logical choice is to place the patient in an environment where manual therapy can be accomplished in a more gentle form.

## COMPLICATIONS

When addressing the safe and effective nature of the procedure it is necessary to also address complications from the procedure as well as concerns regarding complications. Phil Greenman[1] states that "temporary flare-ups of symptoms after the procedure have been reported by several patients. This flare-up is attributed to stretching of the adhesion and mobilization of inflamed soft tissue joints. It is easily controlled with appropriate post-operative care. Serious complications have been rare." He quotes Poppen[2] who reported in 1945 "two cases of paralysis after manipulation by competent orthopedic surgeons with the patient under anesthesia. This complication occurred in a population of 400 cases of intervertebral disc disease. It appears that serious complications can be avoided by appropriate patient selection, suitable operative technique by a competent practitioner, and consideration for the contraindications and potential complications."

According to Davis,[3] "because of the range of possible adverse reactions, cases must be carefully selected (referring to cervical MUA). Success is directly related to the skill of the anesthesiologist in providing the appropriate sedation and the operator's manipulative skills. Data on complications from cervical MUA are not available. However, the relevant values for severe complications for all cervical manipulations have been estimated at between 1 in 380,000 to over 1 in one million.[4,5] Deaths from chiropractic cervical manipulations are rare.[6] General anesthesia has a higher risk of about 1 death per 200,000 for ambulatory surgery.[7] Though it is possible that the vertebral artery can be compressed or damaged with manipulation throughout the cervical spine, this has generally been reported in the first three segments. Between the C1–C2 transverse process the vertebral arteries are relatively fixed at the C1–C2 transverse foramen; therefore rotation will produce stretching of the vertebral artery. At the C2–C3 level, compression may be due to superior articular facet of C3 on the ipsilateral side of head rotation, and the C1 transverse process can compress the internal carotid artery. An important point to make here is that lateral flexion on the neck apparently has little effect on vertebral artery blood flow in most cases suggesting little stress on the artery."

The procedure of manipulation under anesthesia in the cervical spine is completed with low-velocity, high-amplitude thrusting procedures that put very little torsion into the cervical spine. The primary focus of MUA in the cervical spine is axial and lateral tractioning and oblique tractioning with articular cavitation occurring generally during the stretching maneuvers.[8,9] Also today with the use of conscious sedation (MAC) rather than general anesthesia, the patient is able to discern pain, although neuro-perception is slowed down, and retain end range of muscles and joint during the MUA procedure. This allows for full stretching maneuvers and articular cavitation without the inherent risk of vertebro-vascular accident, tissue rupture, or joint dislocation. The patients have also undergone prerequisite conservative care of at least 4–6 weeks and usually several months prior to having an MUA. Since the office form of manipulation is high velocity, low amplitude, if there were going to be damage to the spinal segments, vertebral arteries, or tissue damage, it certainly would have occurred during the office manipulative therapy program. Again, this is why a regime of conservative manipulative therapy before considering the MUA procedure is recommended and also why there are very few recorded instances of tissue damage, injury, or cerebrovascular accidents (CVAs) from MUA. As with any technique using forms of anesthesia, there are inherent risks that are part of this procedure. Historically there have been very few reports of damage from the MUA procedure, and most of those were either from medication reaction or from the procedure being performed by uncertified, unskilled practitioners.

The safety and effectiveness of manipulation under anesthesia has been widely proven by clinical documentation. The above referenced articles and the information in this book all relate to the educational standards necessary to perform this procedure, proper patient selection for the procedure, and then proper follow-up care once the procedure has been completed. They also relate to the physician being trained to provide proper diagnostic and examination procedures prior to having the patient undergo manipulation under anesthesia. If all of these steps are followed properly, the MUA procedure is safe to perform. It has been performed many thousands of times by using the same or similar techniques, and the effectiveness has greatly outweighed any minimal risks from the types of anesthesia used. All of the malpractice insurance carriers for the chiropractic profession and the osteopathic profession cover these types of physicians for the procedure of manipulation under anesthesia, and I am sure that if there were any questions regarding the safety and effectiveness of this procedure, malpractice insurance carriers would not cover physicians under malpractice parameters. In fact, one of the largest malpractice carriers for the chiropractic profession stopped adding an additional rider to their policies for MUA several years ago due to a low ratio of liability cases involving manipulation under anesthesia.

We must be cognizant of the risks involved in any procedure that is being used to treat our patients. Historically this has always been at the core of health care: "first, do no harm." But if we restrict ourselves to complications that have been shown to be relatively low and the benefits have been shown to greatly outweigh those risks, it is only right that we diligently work to control any risks for this procedure but continue to perform the procedure in the most optimum manner possible. The history of using this procedure tells us that its use has greatly improved the lives of thousands of patients. Since this is the case, then if we were not to use a technique that has a chance to cause the recovery of a select patient population, are we as practitioners not using all of the therapeutic tools at our disposal? Informed consent has a two-sided edge. You must explain to the patient what the treatment technique that you as the practitioner are using, but the other side of that equation is to tell the patient all of the other choices that they have. MUA is a substantially proven treatment to be recommended to the proper patient population, and not to recommend this technique when it is definitely called for in the treatment regime is professionally remiss on the part of the practitioner even if there are some risks, just as there are with many other treatments that are being recommended in today's health-care arena.

## REFERENCES

1. Greenman, P.E., Manipulation with the patient under anesthesia, *J. Am. Osteopath. Assoc.*, 92, 1159, 1992.
2. Poppen, J.L., The herniated intervertebral disk — An analysis of 400 verified cases, *N. Engl. J. Med.*, 232, 211, 1945.
3. Davis, C.G., Chronic cervical spine pain treated with manipulation under anesthesia, *J. Neuromuscu-loskeletal Syst.*, 4, 102, 1996.
4. Eder, M. and Tilscher, H., *Chiropractic Therapy: Diagnosis and Treatment*, Aspen Publishers, Boulder, CO, 1990, 60.
5. Terrett, A.G.J. and Kleynhans, A.M., Cerebrovascular complications of manipulation, in Haldeman, S., Ed., *Modern Development in the Principles and Practice of Chiropractic*, 2nd ed., Appleton-Century-Crofts, New York, 1992, 579.

6.  Terrett, A.G.J., Vascular accidents from cervical spine manipulation: The mechanisms, *ACA J. Chiropractic*, 22, 59, 1988.
7.  Liu, P., *Principles and Procedures in Anesthesiology*, J.B. Lippincott, Philadelphia, 1992, 7.
8.  Gordon, R., Hickman, G., and Gray, J., Proprioception as a pre-requisite to SG cell response in inhibiting musculoskeletal pain using manipulation under anesthesia, *Dynamic Chiropractic*, May, 8, 1999.
9.  Gordon, R., Syllabus on MUA for the course sponsored by The National College of Chiropractic, 4th ed., 1993, 25.

# 16 A Case for MUA

*Robert C. Gordon, David Basch, and Lawrence Petracco*

## CONTENTS

This chapter addresses validating the procedure of manipulation under anesthesia (MUA).

From the early literature written to support clinical outcomes, it is obvious that manual therapy physicians were interested in one primary focus for moving a patient from conservative office care into the MUA arena. That one primary focus was to overcome restrictive barriers in the neuromusculoskeletal system that were creating pain and discomfort in the patients they were treating, and although conservative manual therapy was the therapy of choice, the results were minimal at best.

You've read the chapters in this text that describe the scientific reasons why medication-assisted manipulation with fibrosis-release procedures, also referred to as MUA, works. And you have also read theories and hypotheses as to why we feel this procedure is a significant tool to use in the field of neuromusculoskeletal pain management and, more specifically, spinal pain management.

Our focus in this chapter will be to determine how a case for MUA is decided, how it is organized, what steps need to have taken place prior to becoming an MUA candidate, and then how all of these phases come together to produce great results for the patient undergoing the procedure.

The patients who are selected for MUA are not just taken from the office setting and moved directly into the MUA arena. As you have read in previous chapters, they must follow a prescribed format for selection.

When a patient has undergone a conservative manual therapy program and has not improved as expected, several things need to be on the treating physician's mind:

1. Is this a patient who truly is a manipulation candidate?
2. How much time have I given this patient to respond to conservative manual therapy care?
3. Are there other conservative modalities that I have to offer that the patient has not received?
4. Does this patient have any pathology that I have overlooked that may be causing the slowdown in response to the current therapy program?
5. Does this patient need to have further referral evaluation by a specific specialist to help support my conclusions or suspected pathology?
6. Does this patient fall within the standard types of cases that have responded to MUA historically throughout the U.S. and abroad?
7. Does this patient fit the standard selection criteria of the National and International Academies of MUA Physicians?
8. Has this patient undergone the standard 6–8 weeks of conservative manual therapy care, and if not, what are my reasons for moving the patient into the MUA arena?
9. Have I followed standard office procedures that will support moving the patient from conservative care into advanced manual therapy intervention?
10. What is my rationale for performing MUA?

Once these points have been answered, the choice to place a patient into the MUA procedure program becomes quite obvious. Most health-care practitioners at this point would agree that if all of these points are answered with an affirmative direction for advanced manual therapy intervention, then as long as the candidate is not an outright surgical patient, MUA would be the next logical step to the patient's recovery. My concern here is that in the real world, the insurance industry many times will take steps to prolong conservative care (which continues to help with deterioration), or it will give a blanket approval to questionable surgical intervention. I know surgeons who have worked with me over the years who are sometimes dumbfounded that an insurance carrier will approve surgery that may or may not (10%) improve the patient's condition and deny MUA, which, if properly selected, could have a considerably better outcome (85%–90%) (estimated historically from hundreds of MUAs in the U.S. and abroad).

I believe this becomes an integrity issue that certainly must be addressed in the health-care arena. Do we provide a treatment to the general public that has both a historical and present significant record of improvement when performed by qualified, certified practitioners? Do we rely solely on personal bias and discriminatory practices by questionable carriers who don't have patient improvement and recovery at the forefront of their motivation for reimbursement? And if patient improvement and recovery is at the forefront of their reasoning for debate about this procedure, then why would we be arguing about a procedure that has a track record over the years of returning patients back to work and everyday lifestyles faster than other modalities?

These and other questions are of great concern to practitioners of the MUA procedure because, in the world of reimbursement, many procedures that do not have multiple randomized control studies are being used and approved every day and the results are questionable at best. On the other hand, if the doctor selects the proper case for MUA, not only do the results speak for themselves, but the patients usually do not migrate back into the medical arena for the same condition. Such procedures as intradiscal electro-thermal therapy (IDETT), epidural cortico-steroid injections, neucleoplasty, spinal disc endoscopy, and other more invasive procedures are used and compensated regularly by third-party payers, and, quite frankly, the results are not that great. The reason I know this is that many of the cases we see in this field are cases that have not responded or failed with more invasive types of care, and when MUA is performed on them as described in this text, the patients respond well and move on with their everyday activities.

Somehow this concept makes it hard to comprehend how a third-party payer would want to compensate failure and deny correction and recovery. But this is a fact, and this is happening every day in the field we are presenting in this textbook.

This chapter presents several cases that were compiled from various doctors throughout the U.S. These cases typify the types of patients who are selected for MUA. The histories taken from these cases all indicate the same scenario. They went through standard care to include more invasive procedures before coming to the field of MUA, where they were finally given relief for their problems.

## CASE 1

### CHIEF COMPLAINT

Mr. E presented with persistent headaches, neck pain radiating into both shoulders with pins and needles in both arms, mid-back pain, and lower back pain radiating into both legs with numbness.

### HISTORY OF PRESENT CONDITION

The patient's symptoms are a result of multiple auto accidents, the most recent being on February 27, 2001. He was a passenger in an automobile that was struck in the front. He had chiropractic manipulation, physical therapy, and epidural injections over an 8-year period. He stated that treatment helped only for short periods of time. He would get recurring pain when he sat, stood, or lifted for any length of time. His injuries had really interfered with his work, causing him to miss multiple days.

### PAST MEDICAL HISTORY

The patient's past medical history was unremarkable.

## Past Treatment History

The patient has had chiropractic treatment, physical therapy, massage, acupuncture, and epidural injections. He had some relief with treatment, but the pain would always return in a short period of time.

## Family, Social, Occupational History

The patient stated that his father had prostate cancer and kidney problems. He stated that he has only an occasional drink and does not smoke. He is currently working as a laborer.

## Physical Examination (Pre-MUA)

### Physical Examination

Height:   5'11"
Weight:   210 lbs.

The patient appeared to have a mesomorph body type.

### Deep Tendon Reflex Testing

Left biceps — hypomobile (1+); Left patellar — hypomobile (1+).

### Sensory Perception

Areas of hypoesthesia were noted within the dermatome areas corresponding to the nerve root levels of C6 and L5 on the left.

### Orthopedic Evaluation

Fabere Patrick test for hip muscle spasm/low back strain, positive bilateral producing tension.
Gaenslens test for sacroiliac lesion reproduced mild pain bilaterally.
Kemp's test for intervertebral disk rupture reproduced moderate pain bilaterally.
Lasegue's test for sciatic nerve irritation was positive bilaterally, reproducing mild pain.
Goldthwait's (L/S Les.) for lumbar differentiation was positive bilaterally, producing mild pain.
Milgram's test was positive bilaterally, producing moderate pain.
Jackson's comp. for nerve root compression was positive, reproducing mild pain.
Shoulder depression for radicular pain was positive bilaterally, producing moderate pain.
Soto Hall for vertebral trauma was positive, producing mild pain.

### Palpation

*Tenderness*: The paravertebral muscles in the cervical, thoracic, and lumbar spinal areas reproduced moderate pain upon palpation. Subluxations were found at the cervical region, the thoracic region, and the lumbar region. Osseous palpation over the spinous processes was mildly tender; the posterior cervical spine area revealed moderate tenderness, with concomitant moderate spasm; the trapezius muscles bilaterally revealed moderate tenderness, with accompanying moderate spasm.

Cervical ROM testing

| | |
|---|---|
| Flexion: (Normal = 50°) | 50 due to mild pain |
| Extension: (Normal = 60°) | 40 due to moderate pain |
| Left lat. flex: (Normal = 45°) | 40 due to moderate pain |
| Right lat. flex: (Normal = 45°) | 40 due to moderate pain |
| Left rotation: (Normal = 80°) | 50 due to moderate pain |
| Right rotation: (Normal = 80°) | 50 due to moderate pain |

Lumbosacral ROM testing

| | |
|---|---|
| Flexion: (Normal = 60°) | 50 due to severe pain |
| Extension: (Normal = 25°) | 15 due to severe pain |
| Left lat. flex: (Normal = 25°) | 20 due to mild pain |
| Right lat. flex: (Normal = 25°) | 20 due to mild pain |
| Left rotation: (Normal = 30°) | 20 due to mild pain |
| Right rotation: (Normal = 30°) | 20 due to mild pain |

## DIAGNOSIS

Disc herniation at C4–5
Posterior herniation of the disc at L4–5 and L5–S1
    Posttraumatic cephalgia
    Cervical/brachial syndrome
    Compression of lumbo/sacral plexus
    Thoracic spine pain
    Subluxation complex (cervical)
    Subluxation complex (lumbar)

## TREATMENT PLAN

Due to the patient's recurrent cervical, thoracic, and lumbar pain over the past 8 years and the continual need for therapy, the patient was advised that manipulation under anesthesia may be beneficial for his condition. The patient agreed to having the procedure done and was scheduled.

## DISCUSSION

Mr. E had been under conservative care for an 8-year period. He would feel better immediately following treatment, but the pain would return several hours later. This had a tremendous impact on his life. It interfered with his finances, his marriage, and his overall personality. His pain would cause him to be angry all the time and cause him to lash out at others.

Mr. E underwent three days of MUA as indicated by his condition and protocols. He stated that he felt 40% better after the first day, 70% better the second day, and was almost 100% better the third day. He then followed up with the recommended post-therapy.

## PHYSICAL EXAMINATION (POST-MUA)

### Deep Tendon Reflex Testing

WNL (within normal limits)

**Sensory Perception**

WNL

**Orthopedic Evaluation**

Milgram's Test was positive bilaterally, producing mild pain.
Shoulder depression for radicular pain was positive bilaterally, producing mild pain.

**Palpation**

*Tenderness*: The cervical region mild; the lumbar region mild. Subluxations were found at the cervical region, the thoracic region, and the lumbar region. Nonspinal tend.: Posterior cervical revealed mild tenderness, without spasm; trapezius revealed mild tenderness, without spasm; paraspinal revealed no tenderness, no spasm.

Cervical ROM testing

| | |
|---|---|
| Flexion: (Normal = 50°) | 50 without pain |
| Extension: (Normal = 60°) | 60 without pain |
| Left lat. flex: (Normal = 45°) | 45 without pain |
| Right lat. flex: (Normal = 45°) | 50 without pain |
| Left rotation: (Normal = 80°) | 80 without pain |
| Right rotation: (Normal = 80°) | 80 without pain |

Lumbosacral ROM testing

| | |
|---|---|
| Flexion: (Normal = 60°) | 80 without pain |
| Extension: (Normal = 25°) | 30 without pain |
| Left lat. flex: (Normal = 25°) | 25 without pain |
| Right lat. flex: (Normal = 25°) | 25 without pain |
| Left rotation: (Normal = 30°) | 30 without pain |
| Right rotation: (Normal = 30°) | 30 without pain |

Mr. E stated that the procedure changed his life. He is now able to hold a job and not miss days of work. He has a better relationship with his wife and friends. He claims this is the procedure that gave him his life back.

Mr. E is still on a once a month care plan, as are many patients, to help maintain good health, but the main symptoms that he originally came in for have abated. It has been approximately 9 months and he is still feeling great.

## CASE 2

### CHIEF COMPLAINT

Miss D was referred to the office by her parents after receiving notification from her middle school that she had scoliosis. Miss D's primary complaint was lower back pain localized to the left side and radiating into the upper hip.

## History of Present Condition

The patient has had low back and left hip pain for approximately 6 weeks prior to her initial visit in this office. The ideology, from what the patient related, was a jump from a small trampoline during cheerleading practice. Following the practice, Miss D. noticed a moderate strain in her low back that radiated into the iliac crest on the left. She related to jumping from the trampoline into the air for a specific type of maneuver related to her cheerleading and landing awkwardly. The pain was immediate and sharp with intermittent burning, and was relieved with sitting and ice. Walking short distances did not inflame the condition, but walking longer distances, such as to class, did irritate the condition. The patient has been seeing her general practitioner for anti-inflammatory medication and has been told to stop cheerleading, rest, and use heat. The patient was referred to our clinic because of the report sent home from the scoliosis screeners at her middle school and because of our background in sports medicine and scoliosis. Her mother and father are patients in our clinic and felt their daughter should have our biomechanical evaluation completed.

## Past Medical History

The patient's past medical history was unremarkable

## Past Medical Treatment

The patient has been seen twice in 6 weeks by her family practitioner and was prescribed NSAID's. She was told to stop cheerleading, rest at home after school, and use heat on the left hip area as needed. She had not been evaluated prior to this time for scoliosis. The patient has had viruses and flu-like symptoms from time to time in the past, but has not been hospitalized and is generally in good health. She did not relate to any other accidents other than this present complaint.

## Family, Social, Occupational History

The patient is an eighth grader at a local middle school. She is actively involved in a cheerleading organization with the Optimist program and participates in cheerleading competitions regularly. The patient's mother does not have scoliosis, nor does her grandmother on either her mother's side or her father's side. There is no family history of scoliosis in any siblings or in any of the parents' siblings. Her grandmother on her mother's side has rheumatoid arthritis and is 68. Her grandfather on her mother's side has cardiac dysfunction and is 72. Her father's mother has some osteoarthritis but is in general good health at 70, and her father's father is deceased. Her mother and father are in relatively good health but both suffer from periodic low back pain and dysfunction.

## Physical Examination (Pre-MUA)

The patient is a healthy 14-year-old female. She weighs 120 lbs and is 5'3" tall. Her vital signs are all within normal limits. Her heart rate and respirations are normal and unremarkable. The patient favors her left hip when ambulating but does not have a decidedly uneven gate.

### Observations

The patient has a noticeably high right hip compared to the left, and there is mild compensation with a right shoulder drop when observing the patient from the posterior. When gowned, the patient has the appearance of a spinal curvature in the lumbar spinal segments, with a drop on the left side of the pelvis. There is not much compensation noted in the thoracic spine when observing the spine from the posterior. There are no obvious birth defects or markings on the patient's skin. The patient appears quite relaxed and has a very good outlook on her lifestyle. She does not feel that this problem should slow down her goals in the cheerleading program, nor does she let it. She has not followed the recommendations of her general practitioner with regard to discontinuing cheerleading; however, she has discontinued jumping from the trampoline and no longer participates in the gymnastics portion of the cheering. The patient appears in general good health.

### Neurological Evaluation

Deep tendon reflexes were 2+ and brisk in both upper and lower extremities. Sensory and motor functions were unremarkable and within normal limits. The patient had no nystagmus, tremors, pallor, or decreased sensations to palpations, and her pupils were equal and reactive. She did have pain upon palpation over the paravertebral muscles in the mid- to lower lumbar spinal area. On a visual analogue scale (VAS), the patient related the pain on palpation to 6/10.

### Orthopedic Evaluation

Laseque's test reproduced the patient's discomfort in the low back when completed on the left side when lowering the leg from vertical and reproduced the low back pain on the left when completed on the right at 40 degrees. Anatomical leg length was equal bilaterally, but there was mild hamstring spasm and shortening on the left side. Gaenslen's test for sacroiliac dysfunction reproduced the patient's discomfort bilaterally but was more prominent on the left. Kemp's test was completed but did not cause the patient discomfort. Goldthwait's test reproduced the patient's discomfort in the lumbar spine but was limited to paraspinal muscle spasm bilaterally. Palpation over the sacral base was tender, and localized pinpoint pressure over the sacroiliac joints bilaterally reproduced the patient's discomfort. The patient had an anterior/inferior drop in pelvis on the left and a concomitant posterior rotation of the pelvis on the right.

### Radiological Evaluation

The patient was x-rayed in the anterior/posterior plane in the standing position. Full spine x-rays were taken to evaluate posture, and anterior/posterior, lateral, and bilateral side bending plane films in the lumbar and lumbosacral area were taken to evaluate for pathology. Of note was a left lateral scoliosis in the lumbar spine measured at 28 degrees using Cobb's angle measurements. The apex of the lumbar curvature was at L-3–4. There was only slight compensatory thoracic curvature starting in the thoracic spine at T12, but the apex of the curvature could not be clearly delineated and Cobb's angle was essentially negative. The right ilium was measured and found to be rotated posterior as compared to the left. The left ilium was decreased in size and dropped on the left, indicating concomitant left side anterior pelvic rotation. Sacral base measurement indicated a 20-mm drop on the left. There were no fractures, dislocations, or osseous abnormalities noted in the films. Since it was obvious to this examiner that this was a postural abnormality, potentially brought on by trauma during cheerleading practice, further diagnostic radiological evaluation in the form of MRI or CT was not indicated at the time of the initial exam.

Essentially the patient had maintained normal ranges of motion in the lumbar spine and was only limited by spasm in the paravertebral muscles during right lateral bending. Rotation to the right was slightly reduced, but again this was more related to paravertebral muscle spasm.

### DIAGNOSIS

Thoracic spine segmental dysfunction at T7–10
Post-traumatic lumbago
Segmental dysfunction of L3–4–5

Secondary compensatory scoliosis of the lumbar spine
Pelvic distortion syndrome
Paravertebral muscle spasm with secondary myofascitis

## TREATMENT PLAN

The patient will undergo an initial 4 weeks of Leander traction, stretching exercises both in-office and at home, postural correction adjustive therapy in the lumbar spine and pelvis, and mild rehabilitation in the form of treadmill and cycling with mild to moderate resistance.

## DISCUSSION

The patient underwent the prescribed 4 weeks of in-office therapy. The patient experienced only minimal improvement but received relief when adjustive therapy was completed. Cavitation was noted, but the joint never really fully completed articular motion. It was decided that manipulation under anesthesia was warranted because of the minimal response to office therapy. (To clarify this, it is this author's experience with a patient of this age,, and with the active/athletic nature of this patient's lifestyle, that response to in-office therapy would be excellent.) When the 4 weeks had passed and the patient was only minimally improved, but had responded favorably to manipulation, I determined that getting the patient to relax would help achieve the needed corrective pelvic rotation to also correct the secondary lumbar scoliosis.

At the time this patient underwent MUA there were no protocols for the numbers of MUAs that should be completed. Based on this patient's age and her athletic background, I determined that two MUAs were needed to correct her problem.

The patient underwent the first MUA, and after stretching the area in specific manners relative to her scoliosis and pelvic drop, and completing the desired adjustive procedure, the patient responded with a very loud cavitation. Following the procedure the patient was almost immediately out of discomfort. Her range of motion had decidedly increased in the recovery area, as well as in the post-MUA therapy program in the office.

Following this patient's first MUA it was determined that she had reached the desired level of improvement that was expected from the MUA procedure. On average, it has been this author's experience that most patients undergoing MUA need the usual serial MUA and most often have the prescribed three procedures to complete the desired results. This case is an example of why standards of care have been established by the National Academy of MUA Physicians. One procedure was necessary in this case because the patient was not responding to conservative care in the office setting, as was expected given her age, and the fact that she had not injured this area previously. In completing this procedure it was evident by the response that she only needed one MUA, and now, with the standards that are available, we reason that in this particular type of case, this was the proper course of treatment. The patient recovered completely from this procedure, and her lumbar curvature changed from the 28 degrees to 3 degrees using Cobb's angle measurement within a month of the procedure when new x-rays were taken.

This was a case that was completed early in this author's introduction to the MUA procedure. However, the results were so dramatic that the course of treatment has helped to add to the current standards that are part of the National Academy of MUA Physicians protocols for patient selection criteria. It is evident that there was a real need for the MUA technique in this case by the very noticeable cavitation that occurred when the pelvis was corrected and a unilateral lumbar adjustment took place in a relaxed physiologic environment. It is because of this case and many more that have been completed by many physicians with similar case histories that MUA is worthy of continued use.

## MUA HAS BOTH A DIAGNOSTIC AND THERAPEUTIC USE

The following case illustrates the diversity of the MUA procedure. For many years, MUA has been used as a therapeutic modality, and a diagnostic tool to help patients recover from neuro-musculoskeletal dysfunction, and to help physicians determine a more definitive approach to continued treatment.

This case below illustrates this concept by having the patient seen on a multidisciplinary basis by both an orthopedic surgeon and a chiropractic physician. The basis of the care rendered was to help the patient achieve successful recovery with options including surgical intervention and MUA. Although these cases are not as successful as some other MUA cases, the results are significant in helping to continue the diverse patient selection criteria and promote better patient outcome assessment guidelines.

## CASE 3

### CHIEF COMPLAINT

Mrs. L is a 60-year-old female who comes to this office after having back pain of insidious onset. The latest bout of severe low back pain has been for approximately 6 weeks. She is experiencing pain in her lower back with numbness into the right thigh. She is unable to sleep at night, and she is slow in standing from a seated position. Sitting as she has to do at work aggravates the low back pain and appears to increase the right thigh numbness. She has been absent on numerous occasions from the work site. Her pain at present is rated at constant and a VAS of 9/10, but she also has intermittent bouts of pain that are rated at 8/10. The numbness in her right thigh is relieved slightly by rest and increased during movement, and is of an achy quality with periodic sharp burning sensations.

### HISTORY OF PRESENT CONDITION

The pain that the patient is experiencing has been coming on progressively over several years and has an unknown etiology with onset insidious. At present she is having one of her "severe bouts," which has lasted the longest at 6 weeks. She does not relate to any bowel or bladder dysfunction. The patient has been seen by her general practitioner, who gave her Demerol, and she has also undergone periodic sessions of chiropractic manual therapy. The patient has had only minimal relief from both manual therapy and pharmocologic intervention. The relief from treatment she has received lasts for a few hours but then returns. This last bout of pain has lasted the longest, and the numbness has been more prominent than she has ever experienced. The patient related to having gone to the emergency room on occasion to get relief from her pain. At that time she received Demerol and was prescribed heat and rest. She is currently disabled from her job. The patient presently takes Demerol, Nexium, and cyclobenzaprine.

### PAST MEDICAL HISTORY

She denies any major illnesses.

### ALLERGIES

Penicillin

### PHYSICAL EXAMINATION

On physical examination the patient is a pleasant female appearing her stated age. She is ambulating with a mild antalgic gait secondary to right thigh pain. There is mild tenderness over the lower lumbar spine as well as the right sciatic notch. There is mild stiffness of the lumbar spine in flexion and extension with concomitant pain throughout the ranges. Straight leg raising is positive on the right at 90 degrees for reproduction of right leg pain. She has pain and numbness in the distribution of L3 in the right thigh. There is no obvious atrophy, and on neurological testing there is good strength in both lower extremities. Sensation is slightly diminished over the right thigh to light touch and reflexes are 2+ brisk and symmetric bilaterally. There is good range of motion of both hips and knees without pain.

## RADIOLOGICAL EVALUATION

An MRI of the lumbar spine brought in by the patient is reviewed. This MRI shows a large herniated disc at the level of L2–3 on the right side. By report this is causing nerve root impingement. Also noted is some mild neural foraminal narrowing at the L4–5 and L5–S1 levels bilaterally.

## DISCUSSION

Approximately 2 months after her initial visit in this office, the patient underwent a laminectomy and excision of the far lateral disc herniation at L2–3 on the right side. Her progress immediately following surgery was very good. She noticed good relief of her preoperative right thigh pain and numbness. She had some mild incisional pain in her back and stated that she experienced a short bout of nausea and vomiting from some of the pain medication that she was given. She was given home exercises to perform and was still disabled from the work site.

Approximately 2 months after surgery she was recommended to start physical therapy three to four times per week, including lumbar flexibility, McKensie, and trunk stabilization exercises. The patient is still noticing some low back pain similar to surgery without the numbness; however, she also has some arthritis and degenerative disc disease of the lower spine, specifically at L4–5 and L5–S1. Pain medication in the form of Ultracet has been renewed.

## HISTORY LEADING TO MUA

The patient underwent laminectomy with discectomy of the far lateral disc herniation at L2–3 in September. The patient felt relief from the numbness she was experiencing in her right thigh. Her lumbar pain, however, has not resolved. It is felt that this patient could benefit from undergoing manipulation under anesthesia.

At this time I have discussed other treatment options with her. I do feel we should obtain an EMG for further evaluation of her radiculopathy to see if it is coming from the area of her surgery or from the lower lumbar spine. I have given her a prescription for this. In addition, I have discussed other treatment options with her, including continued further treatment with epidural steroid injections, which she is currently undergoing, and possible further surgical intervention. At this time, the patient states that she would like to proceed with manipulations under anesthesia. I do feel that she is a candidate for this and that this is medically necessary. I have discussed this with her in detail and we will go ahead and set this up on an elective basis. She wants to return to work as soon as possible and this makes her an excellent MUA candidate psychologically. MUA will be performed and we will see how she does in follow-up.

## STATUS POST-MUA

The patient returns after having both epidural steroid injections (3) and manipulation under anesthesia. The patient also had an EMG, which was positive for radiculopathy in the L4–5 and S1 area bilaterally. The MUA did give this patient considerable relief; however, she still remains symptomatic. Her VAS is now rated at 4/10 constantly and 8/10 periodically. The patient is returning to the work site but will modify her workstation and will move about at frequent intervals to help with her motion and flexibility. She continues to take Valium at night to sleep. I have discussed further surgical options with the patient, and she states that she will continue with conservative care for now. Overall she has responded favorably to the MUA procedure and is now able to return to the work site. Her lifestyle has been improved by this procedure, but she must maintain modified activity and exercises in order to potentially avoid undergoing future surgery.

## A CASE FOR MUA

MUA is not the only modality that works, but it deserves its fair assessment and evaluation as a real alternative to prolonged conservative care, injection therapy, IDETT, endoscopy, neuroplasty, or full surgical intervention.

In recent months MUA has begun to move into mainstream medicine as another modality to use when other more recognized forms of therapy have been tried with little or no success. I am hoping that by presenting the material in this textbook we can ensure that the scientific community will start to open dialogue with those of us who have been involved in MUA for these many years so that as more is learned about this procedure, more practitioners will understand its place in mainstream pain management.

If our goal as health-care practitioners is to offer treatment methods that express our true empathy for creating an environment for patient recovery, then we must not turn away from treatment modalities that are benefiting certain patient populations greatly, just because further research is continuing. If we were to do that, most if not all of the various methods that are now being brought to the forefront of expanded medical care would not be used. I would hate to see medicinal assistance in all of its many forms be based on biased, opinionated outcomes because when that happens, years of intellectual invention will be lost to outdated, monopolizing thought. Today we are too talented in our understanding of the human body to let small thinkers dictate how patients will be treated, and have patient recovery based on how much an insurance policy will reimburse.

# 17 Sample Forms and Reports

## SAMPLE 1

### SAMPLE GUIDELINE FOR CREATING AN H&P (TO BE WRITTEN IN NARRATIVE FORM)*

Patient's full name
Date of examination
Attending physician
Patient vitals
History
Chief complaint
    Present complaint
    Location (use P2 QRST format for each area)
        P — Palliative (what makes discomfort better)
        P — Provocative (what makes discomfort worse)
        Q — Quality (aching, sharp, burning, numbness)
        R — Radiation (location - P2 QST)
        S — Severity Scale 1–4 (mild, moderate, severe)
    Temporal — (rare 10%, occasional 25%, intermittent 50%, frequent 75%, constant 100%)
History of present illness — Concise, with all treatment the patient has received, including the duration, type, and P: response.
Past medical history — All past accidents, falls, other injuries; surgeries; illnesses; past history of present chief complaint.
Social history — Work type and duties, smoking habits, drinking habits, recreational drugs, etc.
Allergies
Medications — All prescription and OTC presently taking including any vitamins, herbs, or other natural remedies.
Review of systems — All current medical conditions. Include names of doctors being seen presently. Include a current pre-anesthesia consult if under care for cardiac, respiratory, kidney, or other condition that may be adverse for anesthesia use.
Physical examination
    General — Well developed, well nourished, alert, acute, distress, gait, posture, antalgic, etc.
    Cervical — Spinal tenderness, paraspinal muscle tenderness spasm, trigger points, ROM, ortho tests, etc.
    Thoracic — Spinal tenderness, paraspinal muscle tenderness spasm, trigger points, notable articular dysfunction (rib head subluxation)
    Lumbar — Spinal tenderness, paraspinal muscle tenderness spasm, trigger points, ROM, ortho tests, etc.

---

* B.H. Rubin contributed to this section.

Extra spinal — Based on allowable procedures in each state.

Neurological — DTRs, sensory, motor testing, EMGs, etc.

Radiographic imaging — Reports attached, or interpretation of all films, MRIs, CTs, etc.

Clinical impression — Record your diagnosis verbally, which will coincide with your OP report. Do not use insurance dx code numbers. Recommendations: state your rationale for MUA and whether single or multiple procedures will be rendered and why.

Rationale Example: The patient has chronic recurrent headaches, which manifest in the occipital area with radiation to the forehead. Review of systems is unremarkable for systemic pathology. Imaging studies in the form of plain film x-rays reveal hypomobility of the C4–5 motion units and static movement at C5–6. The patient continues to suffer from chronic paravertebral muscle contracture in the cervical and mid- to upper thoracic spinal areas from C2 to T9. A working diagnosis of torticollis with secondary cervico-thoracic myofascial radiculitis has been used and the patient has undergone three months of noninvasive conservative care to include physical therapy and specific chiropractic manipulation with minimal articular motion. The patient is also under a regime of medical care to include both pain management and muscle relaxants with little improvement. To date this patient has responded only minimally to his therapy program. This patient falls within the standard acceptable forms of conditions that have responded favorably to MUA as documented in other cases and referenced case studies throughout the country. I am recommending MUA as an alternative to chronic prolonged conservative care or possible future surgical intervention. The patient will receive a series of two MUAs in accordance with chronicity and patient response to previous therapy. This follows protocols as established by the National Academy of MUA Physicians (NAMUAP).

## SAMPLES OF HISTORY AND PHYSICAL

### Case 1

*Chief Complaint — Neck Pain, Headache, and Low Back Pain*

Mrs. S. is a 36-year-old woman of Caucasian descent. She stated that she exercises occasionally. She drinks alcohol occasionally and also smokes tobacco (1 pack per day.) She is currently employed as a nurse. She is 5 foot 1 and weighs 190 pounds. Her resting pulse was 72 bpm. The left brachial blood pressure was 136/92. Today, Mrs. S. described having frequent moderate right upper neck symptoms that were dull in character. She states that her "neck catches" when she turns to the right. She further reported having right occipital pain. She describes that it feels like a stick in her right upper neck. She was also experiencing intermittent moderate diffuse right upper back symptoms of an achy and dull nature. She further reported having mid-line lower back pain that seems to come and go since the auto accident. She also states that she has some intermittent right ear pain that she has noticed since the accident. The symptoms were first noticed after this automobile accident. She was the driver of her vehicle and was wearing her seatbelt. She stated that the other vehicle failed to stop and struck the right front quarter panel of her vehicle. She reports that this caused her to be thrown into the driver's side door. She does have a past history of neck and lower back pain but not to this extent. She states that in the past usually a couple of adjustments would fix the problem. She states that since the accident after she is treated she will feel better for a while but that her symptoms gradually return. She also related that a couple of weeks ago she thought for a few days that she was over it but that her symptoms have returned. Her diagnostic workup for this condition has included plain lumbar and cervical x-rays. Treatment has consisted of physiotherapy (interferential electrical muscle stimulation), progressive resistance exercises of the cervical spine, ice/heat, traction, and spinal manipulation. She is using a cervical pillow and lordotic cervical traction at home. She denies having any known drug allergies. She is currently taking Prozac. She states that her family physician prescribed this to her about one month ago and she states it is helping her get through some mild depression. I asked if she feels her symptoms and/or the accident are related to the depression and she said she did not think so. She said that she was on Prozac a few years ago for a while when she was going through a divorce. She also takes ibuprofen occasionally for the pain. Neck Disability Index (NDI) is graded at 22%, which is considered by the questionnaire to be a mild disability. The review of systems was unremarkable.

On palpitation, moderate spasm and tenderness were noticed in the superior trapezius on the right and to a lesser degree on the left; moderate tenderness was found in the levator scapulae and superior trapezius bilaterally. On further digital palpitation, mild tenderness was found in the sacroiliac region bilaterally and tenderness was found in the lumbo-sacral region. Active trigger points were found in the superior trapezius on the right. On active testing in the cervical region, extension was painful, right lateral flexion was mildly restricted by pain, and right rotation was mildly restricted by pain. All other active cervical ranges of motion were unrestricted. All active thoraco-lumbar ranges of motion were mildly restricted. The head was positioned slightly anterior when viewed from the side. There was no antalgia present. All heart sounds were normal to auscultation. The lungs were normal to auscultation and percussion. Routine examination of the eyes, ears, nose, and oral cavity was unremarkable. She is somewhat obese. All of the standard upper extremity muscle strengths were graded 5/5. All of the standard lower muscle strengths were grade 2/2. Dermatomes were found to be unremarkable with the use of pinwheel. Cervical compression was found to be negative. Cervical distraction decreased the neck pain. Shoulder depression was found to be positive bilaterally for the neck pain. George's test was found to be negative during the standard procedure. Seated straight leg raise was negative bilaterally to 90 degrees. Kemp's test was found to be negative bilaterally. Routine x-rays of the cervical and lumbar spinal areas were taken. On spinal evaluation, moderate joint dysfunctions were noted at the right occiput, C1, C5, T2, T3, L5, and the right sacroiliac joint.

The primary diagnosis is cervicocranial syndrome with associated myofascitis. The secondary diagnosis is lumbar somatic dysfunction, which is complicated by L5 grade 1 spondylolisthesis.

I have spoken with the patient and her husband in detail with regard to other options of treatment for her condition. We spoke in depth about manipulation under anesthesia (MUA). I have given her written research information and a video to watch about the MUA procedure. I feel that due to her plateaued response to her recent care she would be an excellent candidate for the procedure. She has failed to gain prolonged relief of her symptoms with the recent care given.

I feel that MUA is a viable alternative to continued prolonged conservative care. Given the chronicity of her condition, I believe that a series of three MUA procedures will be needed to achieve the expected gain. This follows protocols as established by the National Academy of MUA Physicians.

Sincerely,


## Case 2

*History*

*Chief Complaint*

Ms. Y described her neck pain as follows. She stated that it felt like she had to hold her head up with her hands. She described a deep soreness to the neck and upper trapezius area, which got to be a throbbing type of pain occasionally. She stated that it occurs almost daily. She further stated that her neck pain worsened as the day progressed and that this was consistent 7 days a week. Her neck pain was aggravated by prolonged sitting, which was required in her duties as an administrative secretary. At the time of presentation she reported no numbness or tingling into the upper extremities, but she did report some immediately following the motor vehicle accident.

The pain was mostly on the left side of her neck and into her shoulders; however, there was also persistent pain on the right side of her neck. Ms. Y described her headaches initially as starting at the base of her skull and in the neck, and the pain then radiates forward to behind the eyes in a C type pattern on each side of her head. These were very severe at least a few times per month and lasted from three to four days. She had severe nausea accompanying these headaches and also vomiting on a regular basis. On her initial presentation the headaches had returned full blown and were worsening once again, and even waking her through the night occasionally. Her low back pain was initially described as an irritating kind of pain where she could not sit down. It had eased up a little bit over the few days prior to her initial visit, but it had overall been a very persistent problem. She also noticed some constipation relative to increases in back pain. There was a sharp component to the low back pain with certain movements, but by and large this was a dull achy soreness.

*History of Present Illness*

Following a traffic accident, the patient did not go to the hospital. On her way home the patient started feeling neck pain and started feeling a severe headache coming on. The pain got worse through the night and her low back started hurting quite badly. She did not go to work the next day and she thought "she was going to die because of the low back and neck pain." At that time she called her family physician, Dr. R, who scheduled her in right away. Upon examination, he diagnosed her condition as a cervical strain. He prescribed for her exercises, stretching, ibuprofen, and Norflex. These treatments did not seem to help Ms. Y very much, although Dr. R did monitor her weekly for 3 to 4 weeks, at which time due to lack of progress, he referred her to Dr. H. Dr. H performed x-rays that revealed no broken bones, and he diagnosed her as having a soft tissue injury. Ms. Y reports that Dr. H gave her a book of stretches and exercises and referred her to a physical therapy program. Ms. Y was given physical therapy for 3 to 4 months. Her physical therapy treatments involved heat, muscle stimulation, ultrasound, home ice, in-office exercises, and some home exercises. She was released after this period of time.

*Past Medical History*

Prior medical history involved a motor vehicle accident in which she was rear-ended. She was a passenger in that vehicle. She did sustain some facial cuts and stitches due to the fact that she was not wearing a seatbelt and struck an object in the vehicle. She also reported previous accidents where her car was barely hit in the front end. No injuries were sustained in that accident. All of these injuries had resolved and she had no similar complaints prior to this most recent motor vehicle accident. All other past medical history was unremarkable.

*Social History*

Patient is a nonsmoker and a light drinker. Patient reports no use of recreational drugs. Patient is an administrative secretary, which requires prolonged periods of sitting and typing, which aggravate her neck pain. Social activities of daily living include Nordictrack, line dancing, some light weight lifting at the YMCA, and playing tennis.

*Allergies*

Patient states no known allergies.

*Medications*

Ibuprofen.

*Review of Symptoms*

Patient was referred by Dr. H for present condition. Patient reports no other current medical conditions.

## Physical Exam

*General* — On initial physical exam, Ms. Y presented as a well-developed, well-nourished alert 38-year-old Caucasian female with good blood pressure of 102/62. She weighed 125 lbs. and is 5'6" tall.

*Cervical* — Numerous myofascial trigger points were found in the paravertebral musculature. Specific areas of tenderness and dysfunction were noted as well. There was an exquisite amount of tenderness found over the greater and lesser occipital nerves bilaterally. Ranges in motion were markedly diminished due to pain and muscle spasms. Foraminal compression tests were found to be positive bilaterally as well as a positive left Spurling's test.

*Thoracic* — Digital palpation revealed myofascial trigger points and multiple vertebral misalignments.

*Lumbar* — Noted decrease in all ranges of motion with paraspinal muscular spasms. A positive right Yeoman's test with localized pain to the sacroiliac joint and slightly positive left Yeoman's also localizing to the left sacroiliac region indicating bilateral SI lesions. Lumbar joint dysfunction was identified.

*Neurological* — Examination at this time was essentially unremarkable and this included scans of cranial nerve function, posterior column function, cerebellar function, deep tendon reflexes in the upper and lower extremities, and sensitivity to the pin wheel and dermatomal ranges in the upper and lower extremities.

*Radiographic imaging* — A-P and lateral full spine radiographs were taken. X-ray revealed decreased cervical curve with vertebral rotational disc relationships in cervical, thoracic, and lumbar spine. Pelvic distortion was noted. Neither osseous interruptions nor gross pathologies were identified as visualized.

*Clinical impressions* — My impression is that the patient was suffering from occipital neuralgia secondary to the most recent motor vehicle accident; chronic myofascitis secondary to cervical sprain/strain, which occurred as a result of the most recent motor vehicle accident; chronic lumbar myofascitis and dysfunction as a sequel to her lumbar sprain/strain, which was resultant from the accident; sacroilititis and fibromyositis both secondary to the motor vehicle accident.

*Recommendations* — My initial recommendations were that the patient undergo spinal manipulative therapy with passive modalities with the possibility of needing to progress treatment to manipulation under anesthesia due to the chronicity of her condition at the time of initial presentation. Patient is recommended at this time for three MUA procedures.

## Rationale Example

The patient has chronic recurrent headaches that manifest in the occipital area with radiation behind the eyes. Review of systems is unremarkable for systemic pathology. Imaging studies in the form of plain film x-rays reveal decreased cervical curve with multiple rotational disrelationships of the cervical thoracic and lumbar spines. The working diagnosis at this time is chronic myofascitis secondary to cervical sprain/strain, chronic lumbar myofascitis and dysfunction, sacroilitis, and fibromyositis bilaterally. After undergoing 18 months of conservative chiropractic care, including electro-muscle stimulation and specific adjusting with minimal articular motion, pharmacological intervention, and pain management, the patient's treatment has plateaued and she has slowed her recovery, making minimal progress toward returning to normal activities. Therefore I am recommending MUA as an alternative to chronic prolonged conservative care or possible future surgical intervention. The patient will receive a series of three MUAs. This follows protocols as established by the National Academy of MUA Physicians.

*History (Sample Form)*

Patient's name _______________________________________________

Date _______________________________________________

Chief Complaint _______________________________________________

_______________________________________________

Allergies (leave room for responses) _________________ Meds. _________________

Social History _________________ Referred by _________________

Could you be pregnant? Yes _________ No _________

## Patient Review of Systems

☐ Ulcer, hiatal hernia　　　　　　☐ Palpitations
☐ Pneumonia, lung problems　　　☐ Pacemakers
☐ Asthma, wheezing　　　　　　　☐ Chest pain
☐ Heart condition　　　　　　　　☐ Diabetes
☐ High blood pressure　　　　　　☐ Heart failure
☐ Heart attack date　　　　　　　☐ Kidney failure
☐ Thyroid disease　　　　　　　　☐ Hepatitis, liver problem
☐ Stroke　　　　　　　　　　　　☐ Rheumatic fever
☐ Back problems　　　　　　　　　☐ Steroid Rx
☐ Blindness, deafness　　　　　　 ☐ Heart murmur
☐ Nervous disorder　　　　　　　 ☐ Dizziness, epilepsy
☐ Polio

## X-ray

## EKG

## Medical History

## Surgical History

## Physical Examination

Height　　Wt.　　　Age　　B/P　　P
General
Head
Neck
Eyes
Heart
Lungs
Back
Extremities

## Assessment/Disposition

## SAMPLE 2

### SAMPLE OPERATIVE REPORT

This is an operative report for manipulation under anesthesia.

Patient's name: ______________________________________________________________

Date of the procedure: ________________________________________________________

Attending physician: __________________________________________________________

First assistant: _______________________________________________________________

Facility: ____________________________________________________________________

Pre-op diagnosis: _____________________________________________________________

Post-op diagnosis: ____________________________________________________________

Anesthesia used (if known): ____________________________________________________

## Informed Consent

After adequate explanation of the medical, surgical, and procedural options, this patient has decided to proceed with the recommended spinal manipulation under anesthesia. The patient has been informed that (more than one) (another) procedure may be necessary to achieve satisfactory results.

## Indication

Upon review of the patient's history and supplied medical records, a plateau has been reached reflecting minimal further improvement with past treatment attempts. Upon examination, less-than-optimum range of motion is present with significant end-range pain and myofacial tenderness to palpation and/or including radicular pain and/or paresthesias. Considering this patient is not a surgical candidate/failed surgery; or has received minimal to no relief from other aggressive treatments/is fearful of other aggressive treatments such as epidural and/or facet and/or trigger point injections and that no other conservative medical intervention other than MUA is available at this point in time, it is deemed appropriate to commence with a series of three MUAs. The standards of protocol being followed are set forth by the National Academy of MUA Physicians.

## Comments

The patient understands the essence of the diagnosis and the reasons for MUA. The associated risks of the procedure, including anesthesia complications, fracture, vascular accident, disc herniation, and post-procedure discomfort, were thoroughly discussed with the patient. Alternatives to the procedure, including the course of the condition without MUA, were discussed. The patient understands the chances of success from undergoing MUA and that no guarantees are made or implied regarding outcome. The patient has given both verbal and written informed consent for the listed procedure.

## The Procedure in Detail

The patient is draped in appropriate gowning and (is taken by gurney) (accompanied) to the operative area and asked to lie supine on the operative table. The patient is then placed on the appropriate monitors for this procedure. When the patient and I are ready, the anesthesiologist administers the appropriate medications to assist the patient into twilight sedation using medications that allow the stretching, mobilization, and adjustments necessary for the completion of the outcome I desire.

*The Cervical Spine*

The patient's arms are crossed and the patient is approached from the cephalad end of the table. Long axis traction is applied to the patient's cervical spine and musculature while countertraction is applied by the first assistant. The first assistant is positioned to stabilize the patient's shoulders in order to use this countertraction maneuver. Traction in the same manner is then applied into a controlled lateral coronal plane bilaterally, and then in an oblique manner by rotating the patient's head to 45 degrees and elevating the head toward the patient's chest. This is also accomplished bilaterally. The patient's head is then brought into a neutral posture and cervical flexion is achieved to traction the cervical paravertebral muscles. The cervical spine is then taken into rotatory/lateral traction maneuver to achieve specific closed reduction manipulation of vertebral elements at the level of ______ on the right side and again using the same technique on the left side at the level of ______. During this maneuver, a low-velocity thrust is achieved after taking the vertebrae slightly past the elastic barrier of resistance. Cavitation (is achieved) (is not achieved).

*Shoulder Thoracic Lift*

With the patient in the supine position, the doctor distracts the right/left arm straight cephalad to end range. This is accomplished on both sides to release thoracic elements before the thoracic adjustment.

*Shoulder*

(This technique must not be attempted if the patient has calcific tendonitis or there is a chance for a rotator cuff tear. Both of these conditions must be ruled out before attempting MUA on the shoulder.)

(The cervical and upper thoracic spine MUA procedures are performed prior to the shoulder technique. The adjustment that is part of the shoulder MUA technique needs to be perfected with the patient in the erect position before trying to accomplish the procedure with the patient in the side lying position.)

With the patient in the supine position the doctor stands on the side of involvement. The doctor takes the patient's arm in the bent arm position and tractions up away from the patient's body and tucks the extremity into the doctor's abdominal area. The doctor has contact at the crook of the patient's bent arm and support contact on the patient's lateral shoulder area over the mid deltoid area. In this position, the doctor then walks the extremity forward into forward flexion, noting range of motion and patient's resistance. Crepitation will usually occur during the first day of the procedure during this maneuver. Once the doctor has taken the extremity and thus the shoulder into forward flexion, the next move is to leave the contact hand in place and do an adduction traction over the doctor's hand toward the middle of the patient's body. The next move is to relocate the doctor's position so that internal and external ranges of motion are performed (the doctor is standing at the patient's head facing the patient's feet on the side of involvement). The doctor can take the shoulder through simple external and internal ranges of motion on the first day and then become more aggressive on the following days by contacting the upper extremity up near the axial and doing internal and external rotation closer to the body.

The next part of the procedure is the same forward flexion maneuver with the arm straight. Traction is accomplished by contacting the wrist (watch the carpal tunnel), tucking the arm in close to the doctor, and then walking the arm forward into forward flexion. Then the same adduction move is accomplished with the doctor keeping the arm straight and tractioning the arm over his or her hand toward mid line of the body. Next the doctor stands at the head of the patient and lowers the patient's arm to his side. Forward flexion in then accomplished with a knife edge contact at the acromioclavicular humeral joint area. Traction is made during forward flexion into the knife edge and a slight thrust into the joint is made.

The doctor then assumes the forward position and tractions the arm up and away and at the same time rotates his hip into the axillary area. This opens up the joint space, and the doctor contacts the lateral border of the clavicle and administers three short toggle thrusts into the area with a pisiform contact. The thrusts are not directed into the clavicle, but the line of drive is more toward the lateral clavicle and the medial border of the humerus.

The patient is then placed in the side lying position, and circumduction clockwise and counterclockwise is accomplished by contacting the head of the humerus. This maneuver is accomplished by the doctor cupping the hands with interwoven fingers around the head of the humerus, and the movements are very small and deliberate.

Once all these maneuvers are accomplished, the doctor then completes the A to P adjustive procedure that was originally learned with the patient in the erect position. Contact is at the cephalad border of the pectoralis major with support for the scapula and at the anterior aspect of the humeral glenoid cavity joint. The thrust is a motion that mimics the relocation of the head of the humerus into the glenoid cavity. The movement is up and over the shoulder with respect to line of drive.

## The Thoracic Spine

With the patient in the supine position on the operative table, the upper extremities are flexed at the elbow and crossed over the patient's chest to achieve maximum traction to the patient's thoracic spine. The first assistant holds the patient's arms in the proper position and assists in rolling the patient for the adjustive procedure. With the help of the first assistant, the patient is rolled to his/her left/right side, selection is made for the contact point, and the patient is rolled back over the doctor's hand. The elastic barrier of the resistance is found, and a low-velocity thrust is achieved using a specific closed reduction anterior to posterior/superior manipulative procedure. (This same procedure is completed at the level of _________.)

## The Lumbar Spine

With the patient supine on the procedure table, the primary physician addresses the patient's lower extremities, which are elevated alternately in a straight leg–raising manner to approximately 90 degrees from the horizontal. Linear force is used to increase the hip flexion gradually during this maneuver. Simultaneously, the first assistant physician applies a myofacial release technique to the calf and posterior thigh musculature. Each lower extremity is independently bent at the knee and tractioned cephalad in a neutral saggital plane, lateral oblique cephalad traction, and medial oblique cephalad traction maneuver. The primary physician then approximates the opposite single knee from his/her position from neutral to medial slightly beyond the elastic barrier of resistance (a piriformis myofascial release is accomplished at this time). This is repeated with the opposite lower extremity. Following this, a Patrick-Fabere maneuver is performed up to and slightly beyond the elastic barrier of resistance.

## Piriformis Bow-String Stretch

With the patient in the side lying posture and following the adductor stretch, the patient's knee is held slightly past medial and the primary doctor contacts the knee with his/her hand. The force is applied toward the table with the help of the firstt assistant and the piriformis muscle is then massaged. The force down the femur into the pelvic basin allows for relaxation of the piriformis muscle across the obturator foramin.

With the assisting physician stabilizing the pelvis and femoral head (as necessary), the primary physician extends the right lower extremity in the saggital plane, and while applying controlled traction radially, stretched the para-articular holding elements of the right hip by means of gradually describing an approximately 30–-35 degree horizontal arc. The lower extremity is then tractioned straight caudad and internal rotation is accomplished. Using traction, the lower extremity is gradually stretched into a horizontal arch to approximately 30 degrees. This procedure is then repeated using external rotation to stretch the para-articular holding elements of the hips bilaterally. These procedures are then repeated on the opposite lower extremity.

By approximating the patient's knees to the abdomen in a knee-chest fashion, the lumbo-pelvic musculature is stretched in saggital plane, by both the primary and first assistant, contacting the base of the sacrum and raising the lower torso cephalad, resulting in passive flexion of the entire lumbar spine and its holding elements beyond the elastic barrier of resistance. With the patient's lower extremities kept in hip/knee flexion, the patient's torso is secured by the first assistant and the lumbar fasciae/musculature is elongated obliquely to the right of mid-line, in a controlled manner up to and beyond the elastic barrier of resistance. (Cavitation is noted.) This is repeated on the opposite side.

With the use of undersheets, the patient is carefully placed in the left/right decubitus position and positioned so that the lumbar spine overlays the kidney plate to the point where the lumbar spine attains the horizontal and is derotated to avoid facet imbrication.

### Medial Scapular Border Lift

With the patient in the side lying position, the lower portion of the patient's arm is moved behind the patient to allow relaxation of the scapular muscles. With the assistance of the first assistant, the primary doctor reaches into the medial scapular area and lifts both vertically and laterally to separate subscapular adhesions.

### Iliopsoas Stretch

With the patient in the side lying position, the upper leg is bent at the knee and distracted in a horizontal manner to stretch the iliopsoas muscle. The leg is then extended more caudad at a 30 degree angle to stretch the TFL.

### Lumbar Segmental Manipulation (Adjustment)

The patient's body is stabilized by the first assistant. The knee and hip of the upper leg are flexed and the lower leg stabilized in the extended position by the first assistant. Segmental localization of the appropriate lumbar motion-units is made by the primary physician and the elastic barrier of resistance found. A low-velocity impulse thrust is applied, achieving cavitation. (The PSIS is then adjusted on the opposite side with the patient in the same position as above.)

The patient is then repositioned supine by means of the undersheets. With appropriate assistance, the patient is transferred from the procedure table to the gurney and is returned to the recovery room, where appropriate monitoring equipment is utilized to monitor vital signs. The IV is maintained up to the point where the patient is fully alert and stable. The patient is then transferred to a sitting recovery position and given fluids and a light snack. Following this, the patient is discharged with appropriate home instructions.


## Complications

### Summary

The patient underwent serial MUA of the cervical spine and/or dorsal spine and/or lumbosacral spine and/or (R), (L) shoulder(s) and/or (R), (L) hip(s). The patient tolerated the procedure well; there were no intra-operative or post-operative complications. The patient was able to achieve increased motion post-MUA with significant muscle guarding. With the improvement of range of motion, it is medically reasonable to opine that this patient's fibro-adhesive conditions were significantly affected, increasing the potential for appropriate neuromuscular reeducation of affected myofacial structures and before having reestablishment of collagen deposition during the healing phase.

## Patient Instructions:

The patient will receive post-MUA therapy in the doctor's office or physical therapy suite to include heating the area of involvement and stretching of the involved areas just as they were stretched during the MUA procedure, followed by interferential HVGS and ice.

# SAMPLE 3

### SAMPLE DISCHARGE SUMMARY

This is a discharge summary for manipulation under anesthesia.

The patient's name is __________________________________________________

The dates of the operation are _______________________________________

The physician is _________________________________________________

The first assistant is ____________________________________________

The facility is ___________________________________________________

The pre-op diagnosis is __________________________________________

The post-op diagnosis is _________________________________________

## Postoperative DX

1. Same
2. Same

## Indication

Failure of extended conservative care by means of aggressive physical medicine, and pharmacological intervention.

## Rationale for Procedure

Notwithstanding the fact that the patient has improved since the instigation of conservative treatment (physical and manual medicine, trigger point injection, and focused functional restoration exercise), a plateau has been reached that reflects no further improvement. Less-than-optimum ROM is present together with significant end-range pain and myofascial tenderness upon palpation. Considering the fact that the patient is not a surgical candidate, and no other conservative medical intervention other than MUA was available, it was deemed medically reasonable and appropriate to offer the option to the patient, prior to considering invasive interventional pain medicine procedures (i.e., Epidural Steroid Injection, Selective Nerve Root Blockage, Facet Block, etc.).

The considered opinion of the attending medical team was that MUA was the intervention of choice pertinent to addressing the fibro-adhesive capsulitis/myofascitis and muscle contracture, in an overall effort in restoring normal function and ameliorating the presenting pain syndrome.

The rationale from the H&P should be included here, or incorporated into this section of the discharge summary.

**Procedure/Postprocedure Course**

Ex: The patient underwent serial MUA of the _______________ and ______________ ______________ on _______________ and___________. The patient tolerated the procedure well, and there were no intraoperative or postoperative complications.

**Results Accomplished**

The patient was able to achieve near-normal ROM post-MUA with a significant reduction of muscle guarding. Immediate post-procedure sequelae were mild/moderate but tolerable and manageable. With the improvement of ROM it is medically reasonable to opine that this patient's fibro-adhesive condition was significantly affected, increasing the potential for appropriate neuromuscular reeducation of affected myofascial structures and befitting reestablishment of collagen deposition during the healing phase of post-MUA therapy.

**Patient Instructions**

The patient will receive post-MUA therapy for the next 7–10 d consisting of interferential electrical stimulation, cryotherapy, applicaton of mild myofascial release stretching, with post-therapy discharge to home for rest and additional cryotherapy. Subsequent to this regime, formal functional restoration therapeutics will commence on a frequency basis of 3× weekly for 2 weeks. This will be followed by 2–3 weeks of formal rehabilitation.

The above protocol is essential in order to maintain the functional gains presently enjoyed by the patient as well as to allow appropriate collagen remodeling of the fibro-adhesive structures and the circumvention of their reformation.

**Prognosis**

Considering the patient's overall improvement in function and diminishing in VAS scores, it is opined, absent further injury, that the patient's prognosis is considered to be good. The patient has been instructed that periodic recrudescence and/or exacerbation/remissions may be experienced. These may be adequately managed by means of palliative care, and the patient knows to contact us immediately should these be experienced.

# MUA Pathway

Patient has responded to some degree but not fully (see guidelines)
No positive response to D.C. manipulation treatment
Appropriate consultation referral
Patient continues to improve
Patient becomes refractory to standard office-based TX
Continues standard office-based manipulation/TX
Referral (ortho/neuro) consultation for MUA or alternate TX or combination
Full Resolution
NO
Additional DX studies
Yes
MUA indicated
MRI, CT, discogram, mylogram, VideoFloro motion study, EMG/NCV/SSEP blood lab studies
Seriel MUA 1st MUA 80% Improvement
Therapeutic Injection
<50%–70% improved
2nd MUA 80% improved
Surgery
<50%–70% improved
Post-MUA care 7-10 days, heat, ice, Inf/EMS, Stretching (Same as MUA)
Post-surgical rehab
3rd MUA 80% improved
4th or 5th MUA if indicated in extremely difficult cases
Post-MUA rehab exercises

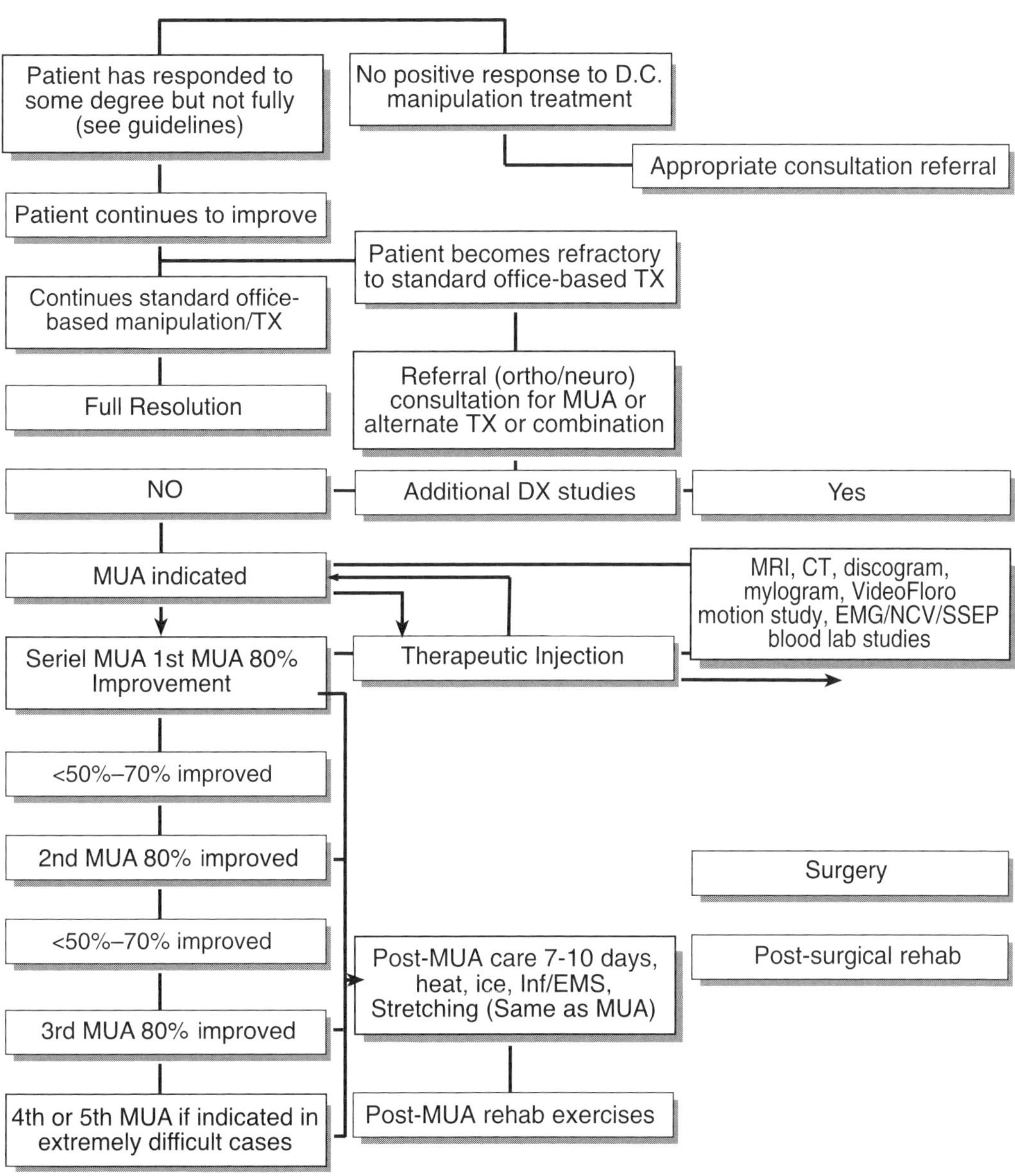

**Gordon Pain Assessment Form**

**Name:** _______________________________________**Date:** _________________

Please indicate the type and area of your pain on the drawings below, by using the abbreviations provided:

**D = Dull Pain**        **T = Tingling**        **B = Burning**
**N = Numbness**      **P = Sharp Pain**     **S = Stiffness**

**RIGHT**            **LEFT**          **LEFT**            **RIGHT**

**FRONT**                              **BACK**

**Please Check The Face That Most Accurately Depicts Your Pain.**

Please Give A Numeric Value To Your Pain On The Pain Scale Below.

**1** _______________________________**5**_______________________________**10**
**No Pain**                                                                **As Bad As**
                                                                           **It Can Be**

# Index

## C



## D